FORWARD

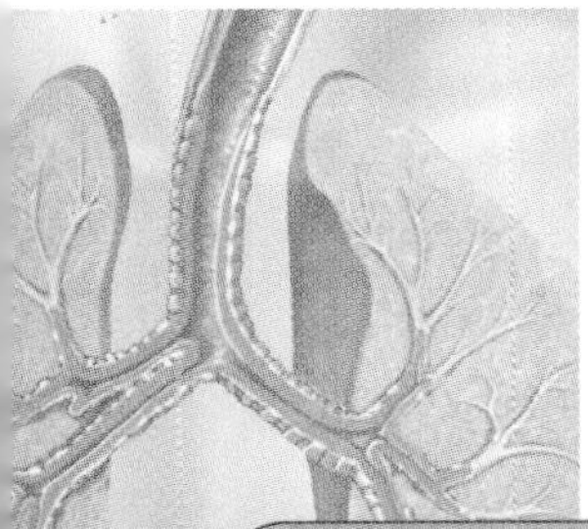
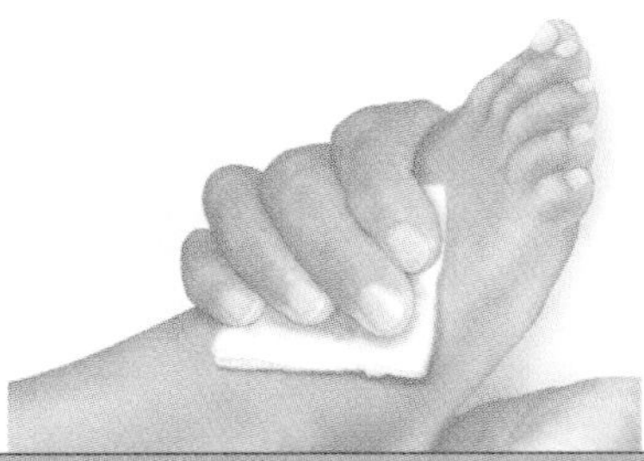
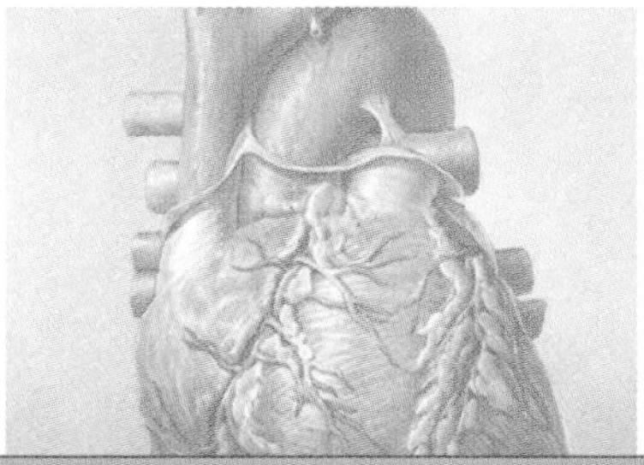
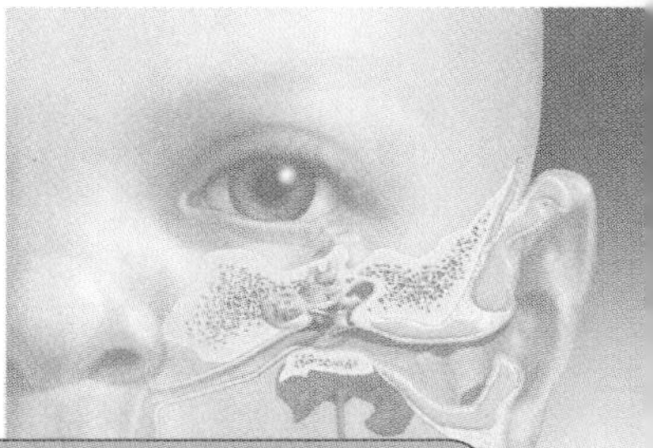

Today more than ever, people need to be actively involved in their own health care. Numerous studies have shown that patients who understand their condition and **actively participate in their care** are more likely to follow through and have positive results. In addition, increasing evidence in the medical literature demonstrates that there are wide variations in the care delivered, based on region of the country, race, gender, language spoken, and other factors.

Studies also show that while the American healthcare system can produce miracle cures, it does not deliver care without errors. In fact, for some conditions, patients who passively move through the process are only receiving recommended treatment about half of the time.

Faced with these facts, patients must become an active participant in the process. The *A.D.A.M. Illustrated Family Health Guide* is an excellent tool to assist us all in this effort. By using this book, you will be better able to understand your health issues, know recommended treatments, provide first aid, recognize symptoms of concern, take better care of yourself, and work in better concert with your doctor and other health professionals. This should lead to improved follow through with treatment, reduced variations in care, fewer errors, greater use of recommended guidelines of care, and, as a consequence, better outcomes of care.

Keep this book close at hand. Your family will benefit from its use.

~ Ray Fabius, M.D.
GE Global Medical Leader

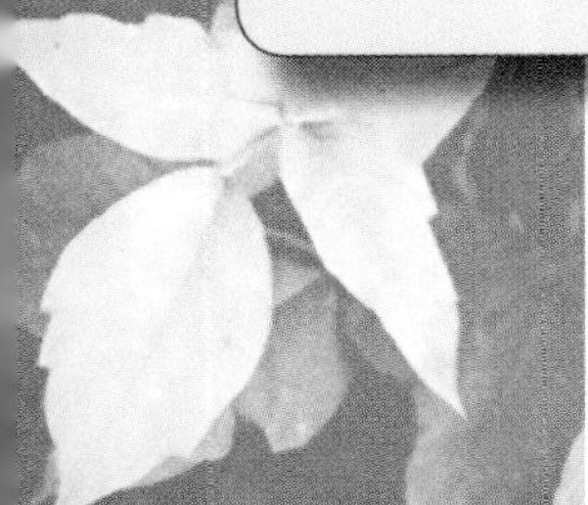
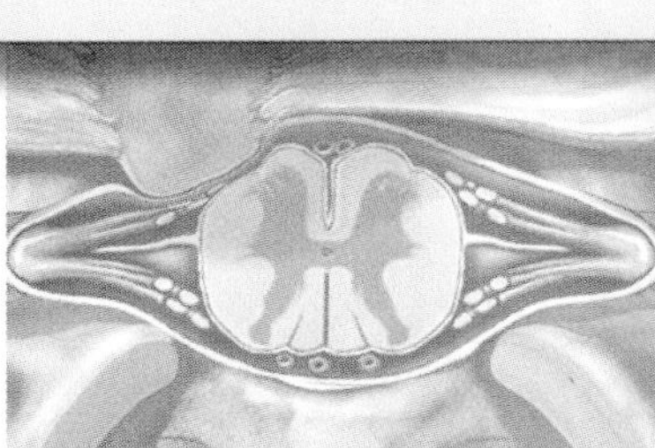
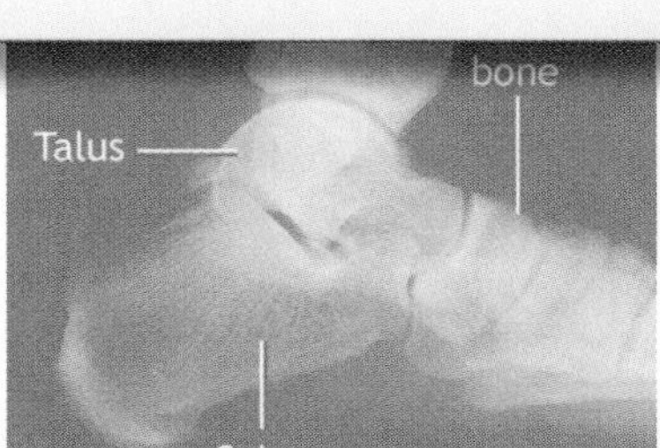

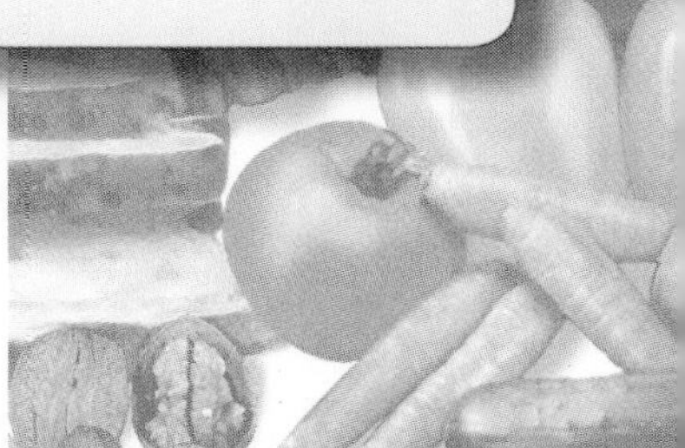

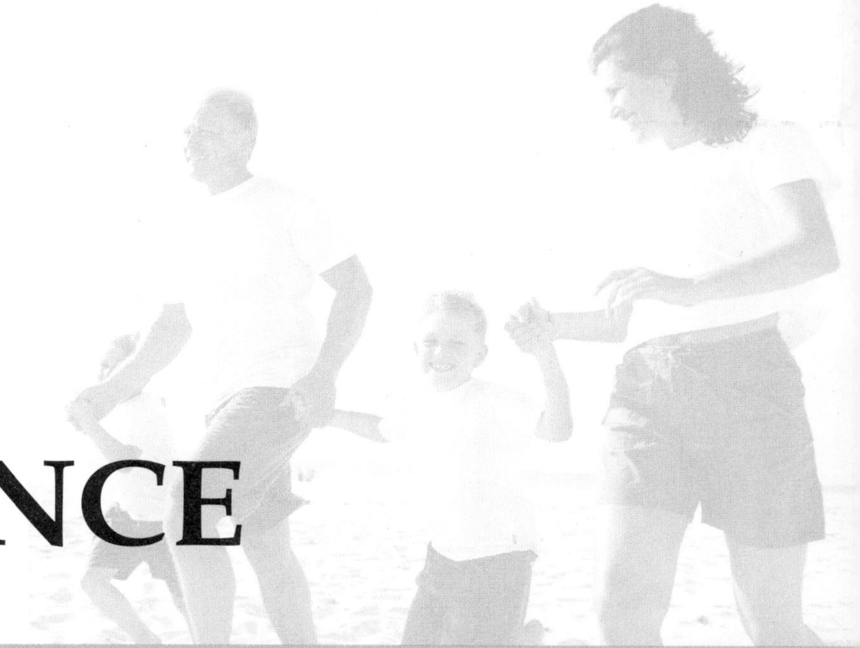

QUICK PHONE REFERENCE

Keep track of your important numbers on this page.

Ambulance		Fire	
Poison Control	1-800-222-1222	Police	
Provider Name		Phone Number	
Specialty		Best Time to Call	
Office Staff		Address	
Provider Name		Phone Number	
Specialty		Best Time to Call	
Office Staff		Address	
Provider Name		Phone Number	
Specialty		Best Time to Call	
Office Staff		Address	
Pharmacist		Phone Number	

A.D.A.M., Incorporated
1600 Riveredge Parkway
Suite 100
Atlanta, GA 30328
Nasdaq: ADAM

Find us online at www.adam.com

Bring the power of health information to your organization! For information on discount orders and customization opportunities, please contact sales@adamcorp.com.

A.D.A.M. ILLUSTRATED FAMILY HEALTH GUIDE, FIRST EDITION

This book is intended to help consumers work with their health care providers in the management of their health. It is not a substitute for diagnosis and treatment by a licensed medical professional.

ISBN: 1-57245-300-1

A.D.A.M.

TABLE OF CONTENTS

Body atlas

Healthy living

THE NEW DOCTOR - PATIENT RELATIONSHIP

In August 2003, a Reuters News report had the astounding headline:

Man With Ear Ache Gets Vasectomy

How could such a thing happen? It turns out that the gentleman was sitting in a clinic waiting room and misheard whose name was called as the next to be seen. The Reuters story reports that "the strangest thing is that he asked no questions when the doctor started preparations in the area which had so little to do with his ear."

This is an extreme example of the old style doctor-patient relationship. The now-snipped man let others take complete responsibility for his health. He didn't ask adequate questions. He didn't enjoy productive communication with his doctor. He didn't expect his doctor to explain how the treatment would help his problem. He was an un-informed, passive patient.

Hippocrates set the pattern for the passive patient with his famous oath, which asks doctors to swear to keep the knowledge of the medical arts a well-guarded secret. When our parents were growing up, this passive approach to our health was considered the norm.

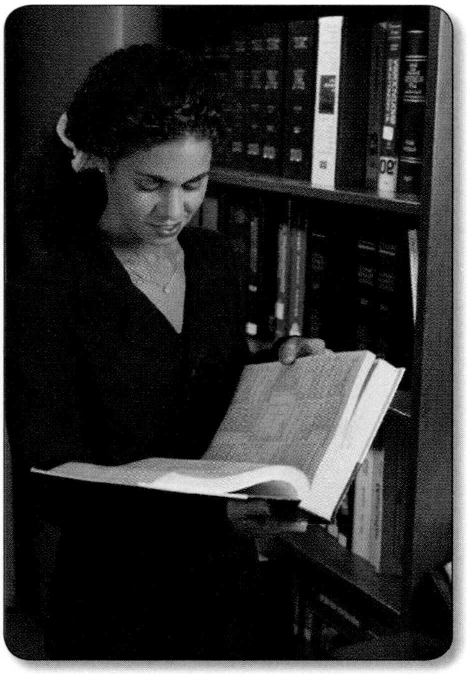

But we are living in one of the most exciting times in the history of healthcare. Our understanding of health and disease is unprecedented. Technical advances continue at a staggering pace. But perhaps most importantly, people in the 21st century can expect a new kind of doctor-patient relationship.

PATIENT, HEAL THYSELF

Ultimately, we are each responsible for our own health. The new doctor-patient relationship turns the Hippocratic Oath upside down, urging physicians to commit themselves to teaching their patients to understand illness and health.

A generation ago, access to medical libraries was restricted to healthcare professionals. Today, the world's medical knowledge is readily available in books and online. Most of our important healthcare choices take place between, not during, doctor visits. Physicians are becoming expert consultants to help you manage your own health.

Here are some ways you can benefit from the new doctor-patient relationship:

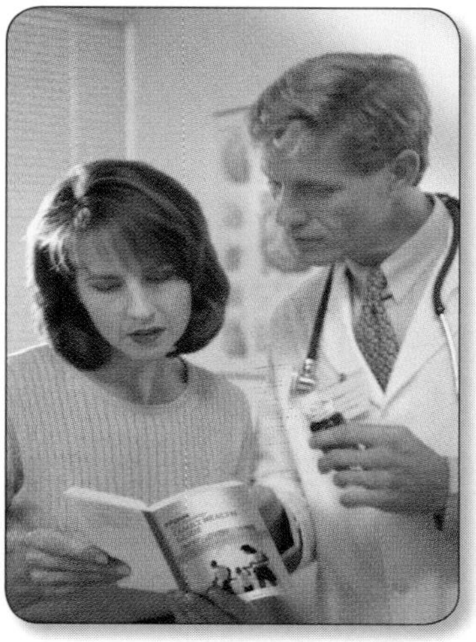

1. **Take responsibility.**

2. **Learn about your health and illness. This book is a great resource for that.**

3. **Ask your doctor to explain what you need to know.**

4. **Ask focused questions until you understand.**

5. **Choose together from among your treatment options.**

Make your choices based on solid science

"Evidence-based medicine" is an important part of the new doctor-patient relationship. With the support of your doctor, choose what to do based on *solid evidence of what really works*. Learn to weigh the benefits of treatment against the costs. This is the opposite of the vasectomy-for-earache approach.

One thing that evidence has taught us is that **prevention** is more powerful than treatment. We will spend time, attention, and money on our heath, *one way or another.* How much better to spend your time enjoying a brisk walk, than sitting in a waiting room for a sick visit… or eating a delicious, healthy meal, than swallowing a handful of prescriptions!

Evidence has shown that some gentle home treatments are as powerful as prescription drugs, and without all the unwanted side effects. Other home remedies are ineffective or even harmful. Learn which are which. Sometimes lifestyle choices fit together hand-in-hand with prescription medicines. For example, the evidence has been clear for years that broccoli can help prevent some cancers. Newer research suggests that it might work alongside chemotherapy to help destroy cancer cells.

A friend indeed

We designed this book to teach you about your own family's health and many common illnesses. We introduce you to treatment options and help you start weighing the pros and cons. We also include the latest recommendations of practical steps you can take to prevent illness, and why you'll want to take them.

This book is intended to spark questions. It's not an attempt to replace your doctor. On the contrary, we are working to make your relationship with your doctor richer and more productive than ever before.

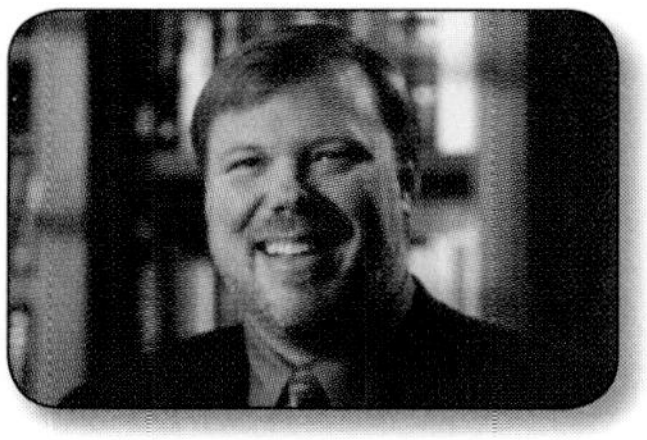

We'll also explain when you might and might not want a vasectomy. And we're pretty sure you'll prefer our suggestions for treating earaches – though they might surprise you!

~ Alan Greene, M.D.

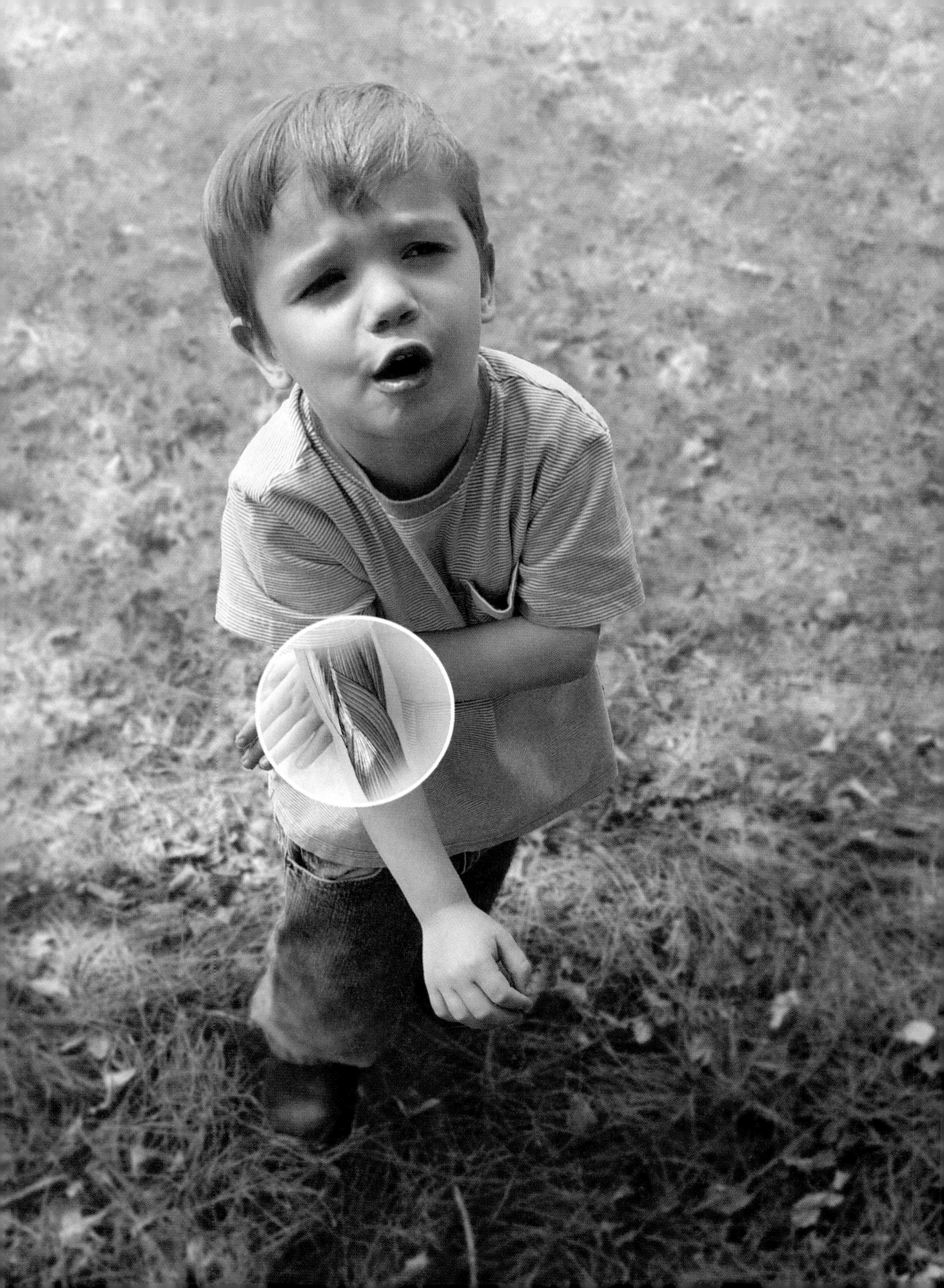

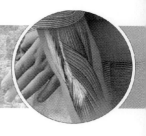

FIRST AID AND EMERGENCIES

Bites - Animal

An animal bite can result in a break in the skin, a bruise, or a puncture wound.

If the bite is a puncture wound, it has a greater chance of becoming infected.

Rabies is a rare, but potentially fatal, disease transmitted by the saliva of a rabid animal.

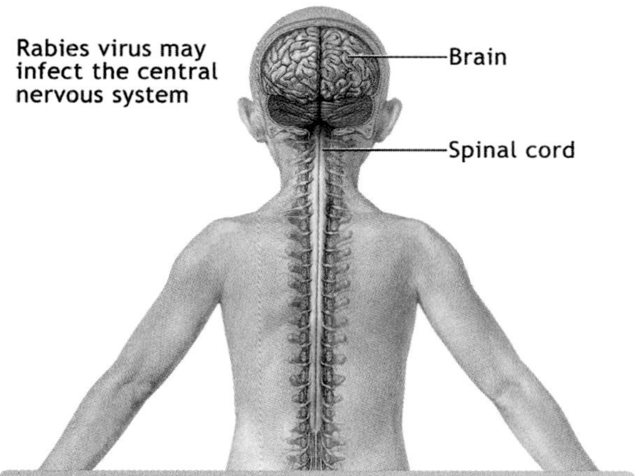

If left untreated, rabies may cause significant damage to the central nervous system.

If you believe an animal may be rabid, notify the proper authorities. DON'T go near an animal that may be rabid. Examples include a raccoon who is active during the day, a stray pet, an animal that is acting strangely, or one for whom the biting was unprovoked.

If you believe you may have been exposed to rabies, you must get vaccinated immediately.

While transmission of rabies to a human is extremely rare, be particularly cautious with bats. Some doctors believe that any potential contact with a bat, even simply seeing a bat in your house, requires a rabies vaccination.

If you are bitten by a wild animal or an unknown pet, try to keep it in view while you notify animal control authorities for help in capturing it. They will determine if the animal needs to be impounded and checked for rabies. Any animal whose rabies vaccination status is unknown should be captured and quarantined.

First Aid

1. Calm and reassure the person. Wear latex gloves or wash hands thoroughly before attending to the wound. Wash hands afterwards as well.

2. If the bite is not bleeding severely, wash the wound thoroughly with mild soap and running water for 3 to 5 minutes. Then, cover the bite with antibiotic ointment and a clean dressing.

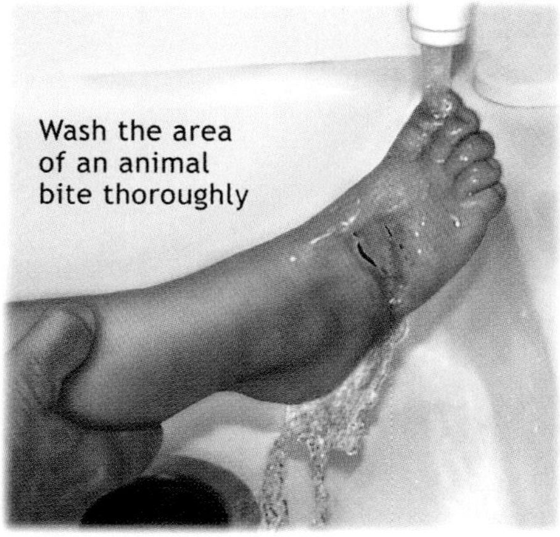

Wash the area of an animal bite thoroughly

3. If the bite is actively bleeding, apply direct pressure with a clean, dry cloth until the bleeding subsides. Elevate the area of the bite.

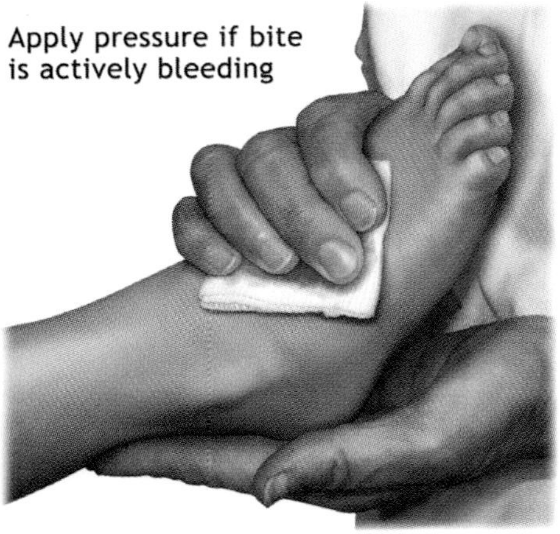
Apply pressure if bite
is actively bleeding

4. If the bite is on the hand or fingers, call the doctor right away.

5. Over the next 24 to 48 hours, observe the bite for signs of infection (increasing skin redness, swelling, and pain).

6. If the bite becomes infected, call the doctor or take the person to an emergency facility.

When to contact a medical professional

Call 911 if the person has been seriously wounded – for example, if the person is bleeding significantly and it will not stop with simple first aid measures.

Call your doctor or go to a hospital emergency room if:

- The person was bitten by an unknown or wild animal.
- The person has not had a tetanus shot within the past 10 years. (If a person has not had a tetanus shot in 10 years, a tetanus shot is recommended within 24 hours of any skin break.)
- There is swelling, redness, pus draining from the wound, or pain.
- The bite is on the face, neck, or hands.
- The bite is deep or large.
- You aren't sure if the wound needs stitches.

Bites - human

Human bites that break the skin, like all puncture wounds, have a high risk of infection. They also pose a risk of injury to tendons and joints.

Bites are very common among young children. Children often bite to express anger or other negative feelings.

First aid

1. Calm and reassure the person. Wash your hands thoroughly with soap.

2. If the bite is NOT bleeding severely, wash the wound with mild soap and running water for 3 to 5 minutes and then cover the bite with a clean dressing.

3. If the bite is actively bleeding, apply direct pressure with a clean, dry cloth until the bleeding subsides. Elevate the area.

4. Get medical attention.

When to contact a medical professional

All human bites that break the skin should be promptly evaluated by a doctor. Bites may be especially serious when:

- There is swelling, redness, pus draining from the wound, or pain.
- The bite occurred near the eyes or involved the face, hands, wrists, or feet.
- The person who was bitten has a weakened immune system (for example, from HIV or receiving chemotherapy for cancer). The person is at a higher risk for the wound to become infected.

Bites - tick

Ticks are small, insect-like creatures that live in woods and fields. They attach to you as you brush past bushes, plants, and grass.

Once on you, ticks often move to a warm, moist location, like the armpits, groin, and hair. At that point they typically attach firmly to your skin and begin to draw blood.

Ticks can be fairly large – about the size of a pencil eraser – or so small that they are almost impossible to see. Ticks can cause a variety of health conditions ranging from harmless to serious.

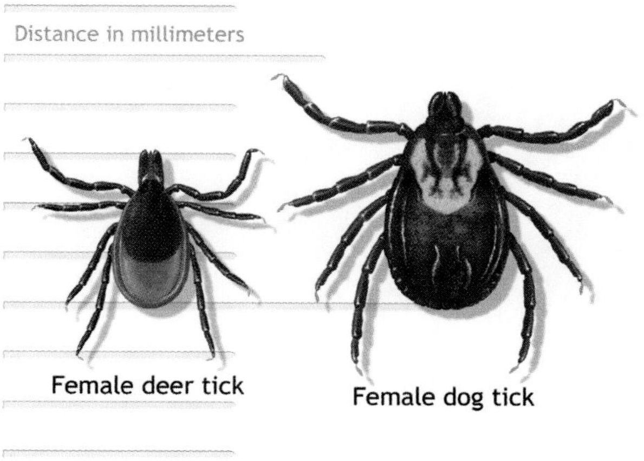

Symptoms

While most ticks do not carry diseases, some ticks can cause Lyme disease, Rocky Mountain spotted fever, Colorado tick fever, and tularemia. Watch for the symptoms of these diseases in the weeks following a tick bite – muscle or joint aches, stiff neck, headache, weakness, fever, swollen lymph nodes, and other flu-like symptoms. Watch for a red spot or rash starting at the location of the bite.

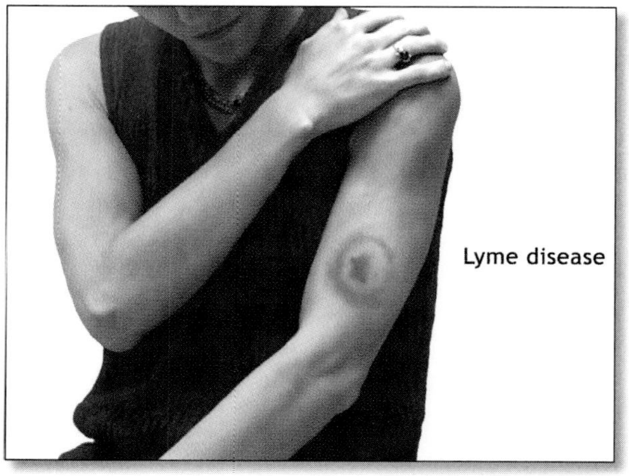

The tick itself can cause tick paralysis. Symptoms include numbness, tingling, weakness, incoordination, and spreading paralysis.

First aid

If a tick is attached to you, follow these steps to remove it.

1. Grasp the tick close to its head or mouth with tweezers or your fingernails. Pull it straight out with a slow and steady motion. Be careful not to leave the head embedded in the skin.

2. Clean the area thoroughly with soap and water.

3. Save the tick in a jar and watch carefully for the next week or two for signs of Lyme disease.

4. If all the parts of the tick cannot be removed, get medical help.

Do not

- DO NOT try to burn the tick with a match or other hot object.
- DO NOT twist the tick when pulling it out.
- DO NOT try to kill, smother, or lubricate the tick with oil, alcohol, Vaseline, or similar material.

When to contact a medical professional

Call your doctor if you have not been able to remove the entire tick. Also call if you develop a rash, joint pain or redness, flu-like symptoms, or swollen lymph nodes following a tick bite.

Call 911 if you have any signs of severe headache, paralysis, trouble breathing, chest pain, heart palpitations, or other serious symptoms.

Prevention

Wear long pants and long sleeves when walking through heavy brush, tall grass, and densely wooded areas. Pull your socks over the outside of your pants to prevent ticks from crawling up inside. Keep your shirt tucked into your pants. Wear light-colored clothes so that ticks can be spotted easily. Spray your clothes with insect repellent. Check your clothes and skin frequently while in the woods.

After returning home, remove your clothes and thoroughly inspect all skin surface areas, including your scalp. Ticks can quickly climb up the length of your body. Some ticks are large and easy to locate. Other ticks can be quite small, so carefully evaluate all black or brown spots on the skin.

Bites and stings - insect and spider

The bite from fire ants and the sting from bees, wasps, and hornets usually cause an immediate painful skin reaction. Mosquitoes, fleas, mites, and spiders have bites that are more likely to cause itching than pain.

In most cases, bites and stings can be easily treated at home. However, some people have a severe allergic reaction to insect bites and stings. This is a life-threatening allergic reaction known as anaphylaxis, and it requires urgent emergency care. Severe reactions can affect the whole body and may occur very quickly, often within minutes. These severe reactions can be rapidly fatal if untreated. Call 911 if you are with someone who has trouble breathing or goes into shock.

Some spider bites, like those of the black widow or brown recluse, are also serious and can be life-threatening. Most spider bites, however, are harmless. If bitten by an insect or spider, bring it for identification if this can be done quickly and safely.

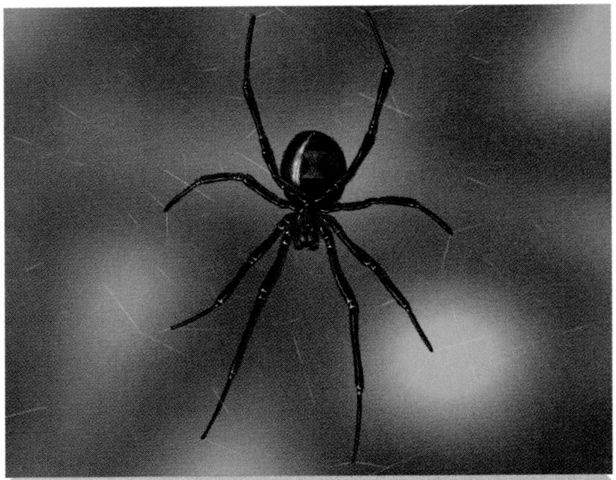

A black widow spider can be identified by the bright red hour glass marking on the back of its body.

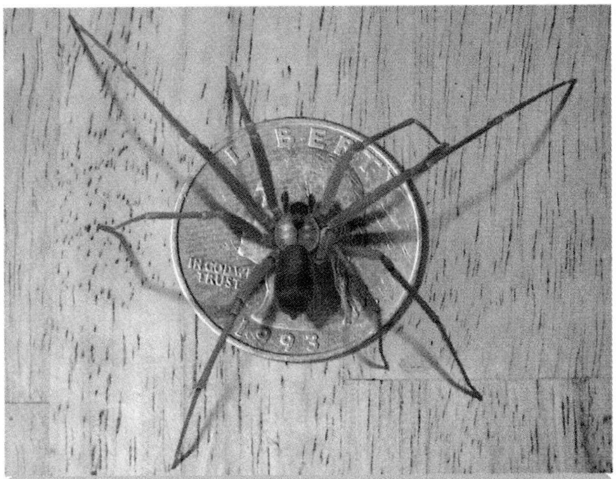

Most species of the brown recluse spider have a dark brown violin-shaped mark on their back. The neck of the "violin" points away from the spider's head.

Symptoms

The non-emergency symptoms vary according to the type of insect and the individual. Most people have localized pain, redness, swelling, or itching. You may also feel burning, numbness, or tingling.

First aid

For emergencies (severe reactions):

1. Check the person's airway and breathing. If necessary, call 911 and begin rescue breathing and CPR.

2. Reassure the person. Try to keep him or her calm.

3. Remove nearby rings and constricting items because the affected area may swell.

4. Use the person's Epi-pen or other emergency kit, if they have one. (Some people who have serious insect reactions carry it with them.)

5. If appropriate, treat the person for signs of shock. Remain with the person until medical help arrives.

General steps for most bites and stings:

1. Remove the stinger if still present by scraping the back of a credit card or other straight-edged object across the stinger. Do not use tweezers – these may squeeze the venom sac and increase the amount of venom released.

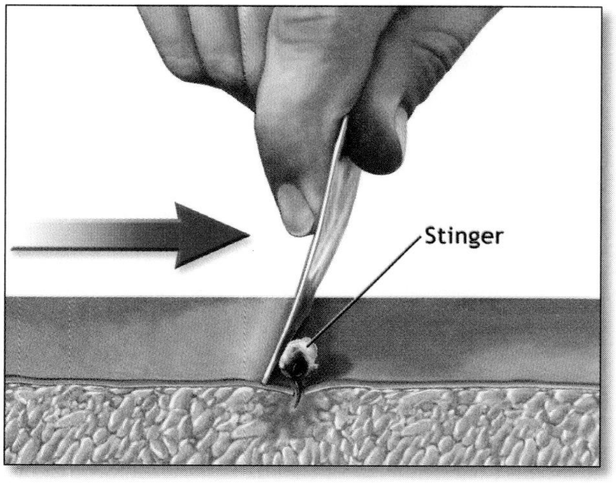

2. Wash the site thoroughly with soap and water.

3. Place ice (wrapped in a washcloth) on the site of the sting for 10 minutes and then off for 10 minutes. Repeat this process.

4. If necessary, take an antihistamine or apply creams that reduce itching.

5. Over the next several days, watch for signs of infection (such as increasing redness, swelling, or pain).

Do not

- DO NOT apply a tourniquet.
- DO NOT give the person stimulants, aspirin, or other pain medication unless prescribed by the doctor.

When to contact a medical professional

Call 911 if the person is having a severe reaction:

- Trouble breathing, wheezing, shortness of breath
- Swelling anywhere on the face
- Throat feels tight
- Feeling weak
- Turning blue

Prevention

- Avoid provoking insects whenever possible.
- Avoid rapid, jerky movements around insect hives or nests.
- Avoid perfumes and floral-patterned or dark clothing.
- Use appropriate insect repellents and protective clothing.
- Use caution when eating outdoors, especially with sweetened beverages or in areas around garbage cans, which often attract bees.
- For those who have a serious allergy to insect bites or stings, carry an emergency epinephrine kit (which requires a prescription). Friends and family should be taught how to use it if you have a reaction. Wear a medical ID bracelet.

Breathing problems

Breathing difficulties can be described in several different ways. You may feel "winded," short of breath, unable to take a deep breath, "air hunger," not getting enough air, or like you are gasping for air.

If you are having difficulty breathing, it is almost always a medical emergency (other than feeling slightly winded from normal activity like exercise or climbing a hill).

Symptoms

The following symptoms are often associated with difficulty breathing:

- Gurgling, wheezing, or whistling sounds
- Using chest and neck muscles to breathe
- Bluish lips, fingers, and fingernails
- Cough (if the person also has phlegm/sputum, this may be pneumonia; a barking cough in a child is croup)
- Chest pain (could be a heart attack or injury; sharp chest pain could be pulmonary embolism or collapsed lung)
- Chest moving in an unusual way as the person breathes (may indicate an airway or chest injury)
- Confusion, light-headedness, weakness, or sleepiness
- Fever

First aid

1. Call 911 immediately.

2. Check the person's airway, breathing, and circulation. If necessary, begin rescue breathing, CPR, and first aid for bleeding.

3. Loosen any tight clothing.

4. Help the person use any prescribed medication (such as an asthma inhaler or home oxygen).

Common causes of breathing difficulty

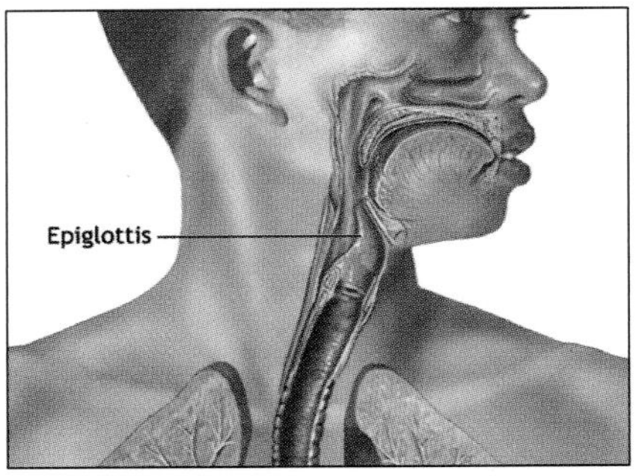

Inflammation of the epiglottis

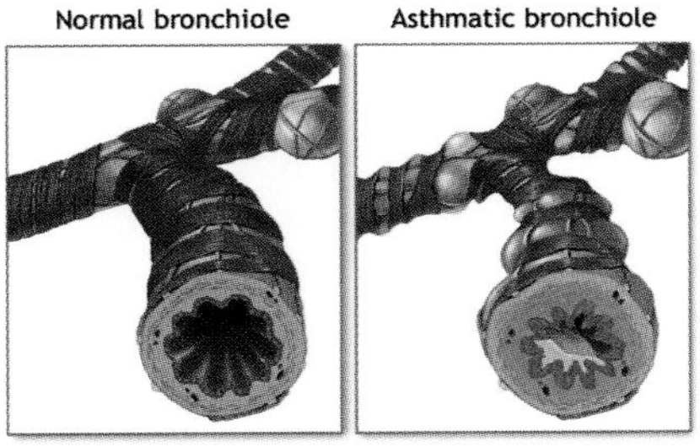

Medical problems like asthma

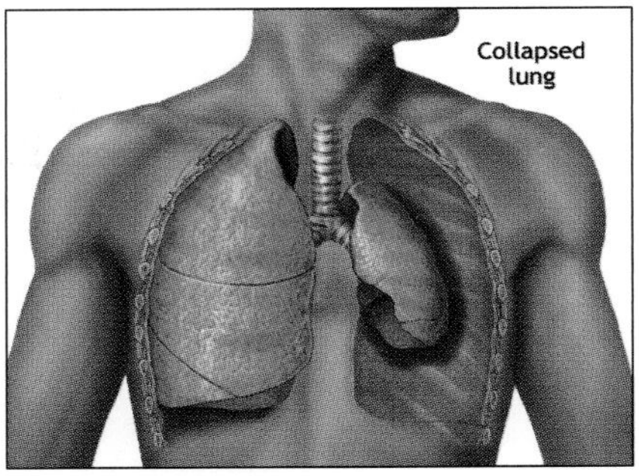

Collapsed lung caused by disease or trauma

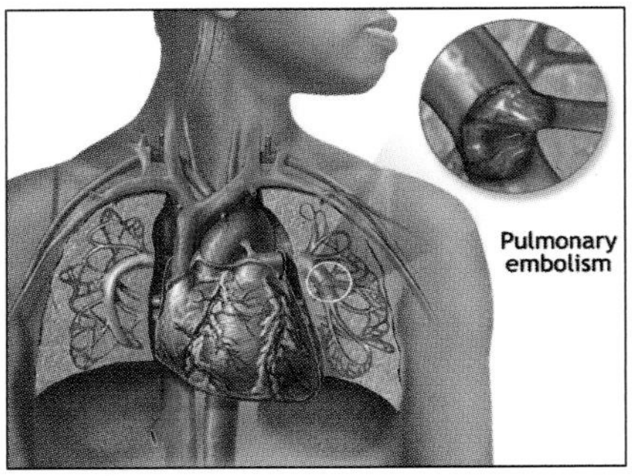

Pulmonary embolism (blood clot in the lung)

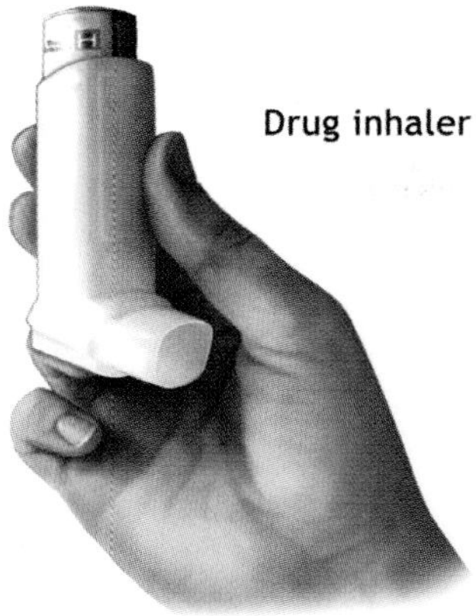

Inhalers come in different shapes and sizes.

5. Continue to monitor the person's breathing and circulation until medical help arrives. DO NOT assume that the person's condition is improving if you can no longer hear wheezing.

6. If there are open wounds in the neck or chest, they must be closed immediately, especially if air bubbles appear in the wound. Bandage such wounds at once.

7. A "sucking" chest wound allows air to enter the person's chest cavity with each breath. This can cause a collapsed lung. Bandage the wound with plastic wrap, a plastic bag, or gauze pads covered with petroleum jelly, sealing it except for one corner. This allows trapped air to escape from the chest, but prevents air from entering the chest through the wound.

Do not

- DO NOT give the person any foods or drinks.
- DO NOT move the person if there has been a chest or airway injury, unless it is absolutely necessary.
- DO NOT place a pillow under the person's head if he or she is lying down. This can close the airway.
- DO NOT wait to see if the person's condition improves before getting medical help. Get help immediately.

When to contact a medical professional

Call 911 if you or someone else has labored breathing, especially if accompanied by:

- Chest pain
- Sweating
- Nausea or vomiting
- Dizziness or lightheadedness
- Blue lips, fingers, or fingernails
- Inability to speak
- High pitched or wheezing sounds
- Facial, tongue, or throat swelling
- Hives
- Rapid or irregular heart beat
- Coughing up large amounts of blood
- Excessive drooling

Call your doctor right away if:

- Your shortness of breath is brought on by coughing, especially productive coughing.
- Your child's cough has a barking sound.
- You have a fever, green or yellow phlegm, night sweats, weight loss, loss of appetite, or swelling in your legs.
- You are coughing up small amounts of blood.

For those with congestive heart failure

If you have been diagnosed with heart failure, see *Taking Charge of Congestive Heart Failure*. Ask your doctor or local hospital about programs to help you manage this condition.

Prevention

- Wear a medical alert tag if you have a pre-existing breathing condition, such as asthma.

- If you have a history of severe allergic reactions, carry an epinephrine pen and wear a medical alert tag. Your doctor will teach you how to use the Epi-pen.
- If you have asthma or allergies, eliminate household allergy triggers like dust mites and mold.
- Don't smoke and keep away from second-hand smoke. Don't allow smoking in your home.
- If you have asthma, see the article on asthma to learn ways to manage it.
- Make sure your child obtains the pertussis (whooping cough) vaccine.
- When traveling by airplane, get up and walk around once in awhile to avoid forming blood clots in your legs. Clots can break off and lodge in your lungs. If traveling by car, stop and walk around regularly.
- Lose weight. You are more likely to feel winded if you are overweight. You are also at greater risk for heart disease and heart attack.

Broken bones

If more pressure is put on a bone than it can stand, it will split or break. A break of any size is called a fracture. If the broken bone punctures the skin, it is called an open fracture (compound fracture).

It is hard to tell a dislocated bone from a broken bone. However, both are emergency situations, and the basic first aid steps are the same.

Symptoms

- A visibly out-of-place or misshapen limb or joint
- Swelling, bruising, or bleeding
- Intense pain
- Numbness and tingling
- Broken skin with bone protruding
- Limited mobility or inability to move a limb

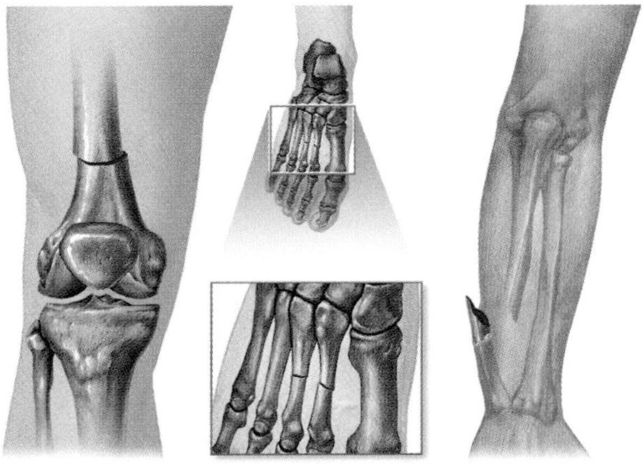

Types of fractures

First aid

1. Check the person's airway and breathing. If necessary, call 911 and begin rescue breathing, CPR, or bleeding control.
2. Keep the person still and calm.
3. Examine the person closely for other injuries.
4. In most cases, if medical help responds quickly, allow the medical personnel to take further action.
5. If the skin is broken, it should be treated immediately to prevent infection. Don't breathe on the wound or probe it. If possible, lightly rinse the wound to remove visible dirt or other contamination, but do not vigorously scrub or flush the wound. Cover with sterile dressings.
6. If needed, immobilize the broken bone with a splint or sling. Possible splints include a rolled up newspaper or strips of wood. Immobilize the area both above and below the injured bone.
7. Apply ice packs to reduce pain and swelling.

8. Take steps to prevent shock. Lay the person flat, elevate the feet about 12 inches above the head, and cover the person with a coat or blanket. However, DO NOT move the person if a head, neck, or back injury is suspected.

TREAT BLEEDING

1. Place a dry, clean cloth over the wound to dress it.

2. If the bleeding continues, apply direct pressure to the site of bleeding. DO NOT apply a tourniquet to the extremity to stop the bleeding unless it is life-threatening.

Do not

- DO NOT move the person unless the broken bone is stable.
- DO NOT move a person with an injured hip, pelvis, or upper leg unless it is absolutely necessary. If you must move the person, pull the person to safety by his clothes (such as by the shoulders of a shirt, a belt, or pant-legs).
- DO NOT move a person who has a possible spine injury.
- DO NOT attempt to straighten a bone or change its position unless blood circulation appears hampered.
- DO NOT try to reposition a suspected spine injury.
- DO NOT test a bone's ability to move.

When to contact a medical professional

Call 911 if:

- There is a suspected broken bone in the head, neck, or back.
- There is a suspected broken bone in the hip, pelvis, or upper leg.
- You cannot completely immobilize the injury at the scene by yourself.
- There is severe bleeding.
- An area below the injured joint is pale, cold, clammy, or blue.
- There is a bone projecting through the skin.

Even though other broken bones may not be medical emergencies, they still deserve medical attention. Call your health care provider to find out where and when to be seen.

If a young child refuses to put weight on an arm or leg after an accident, won't move the arm or leg, or you can clearly see a deformity, assume the child has a broken bone and get medical help.

The danger of falls

Did you know that more than a third of adults over age 65 fall each year, and that falls are a leading cause of death in the elderly? For more information on how to address this serious problem, see *Preventing Falls* in the Healthy Living chapter.

Bruises

A bruise is an area of skin discoloration. A bruise occurs when small blood vessels break and leak their contents into the soft tissue beneath the skin.

The main symptoms are pain, swelling, and skin discoloration. The bruise begins as a pinkish red color that can be very tender to touch. It is often difficult to use the muscle that has been bruised. For example, a deep thigh bruise is painful when you walk or run.

Eventually, the bruise changes to a bluish color, then greenish-yellow, and finally returns to the normal skin color as it heals.

Do not

- DO NOT attempt to drain the bruise with a needle.
- DO NOT continue running, playing, or otherwise using the painful, bruised part of your body.
- DO NOT ignore the pain or swelling.

> **Key point**
>
> Children often have bruises on their shins. This is usually no cause for concern. However, if a child has multiple bruises on other parts of his or her body, you should bring the child in for evaluation.

First aid

1. Place ice on the bruise to help it heal faster and to reduce swelling. Place the ice in a cloth – DO NOT place ice directly on the skin. Apply the ice for up to 15 minutes per hour.

2. Keep the bruised area raised above the heart, if practical. This helps keep blood from pooling in the bruised tissue.

3. Try to rest the bruised body part by not overworking your muscles in that area.

4. If needed, take acetaminophen (Tylenol) to help reduce pain.

When to contact a medical professional

Call your doctor immediately if you feel extreme pressure in a bruised part or your body, especially if the area is large or very painful. This may be due to a condition known as "compartment syndrome." Increased pressure on the soft tissues and structures beneath the skin can decrease the supply of vital blood and oxygen to the tissues. This is potentially life-threatening and you should receive emergency care promptly.

Also call your doctor if:

- You are bruising spontaneously without any injury, fall, or other reason.
- There are signs of infection around the bruised area including streaks of redness, pus or other drainage, or fever.

Healing process – visible changes to a subcutaneous (skin) bruise

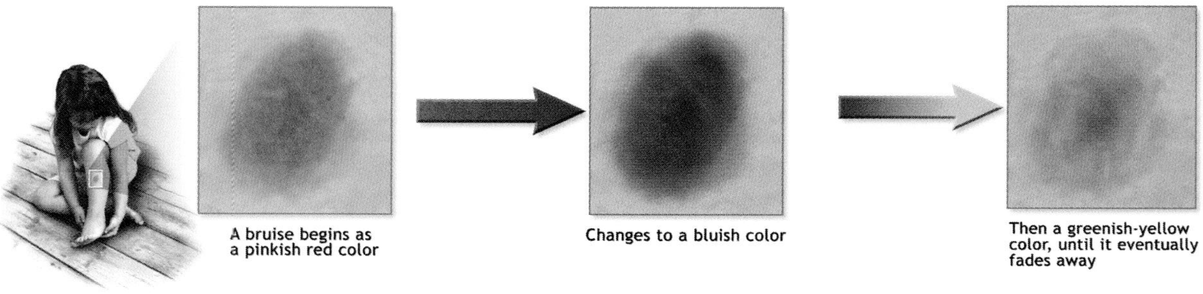

A bruise begins as a pinkish red color
Changes to a bluish color
Then a greenish-yellow color, until it eventually fades away

Bruises occur when a force causes blood vessels to break. Blood leaks into areas under the skin, resulting in pain, swelling, and discoloration.

The bruise will darken. The color change occurs from a biochemical breakdown of a blood component called hemoglobin.

The bruise then fades, turns a pale yellow, and disappears. The healing process usually takes a couple of weeks.

Burns

There are three levels of burns:

- **First-degree** burns affect only the outer layer of the skin. They cause pain, redness, and swelling.
- **Second-degree** (partial thickness) burns affect both the outer and underlying layer of skin. They cause pain, redness, swelling, and blistering.
- **Third-degree** (full thickness) burns extend into deeper tissues. They cause white or blackened, charred skin that may be numb.

Before giving first aid, evaluate how extensively burned the person is and try to determine the depth of the most serious part of the burn. Then treat the entire burn accordingly. If in doubt, treat it as a severe burn.

By giving immediate first aid before professional medical help arrives, you can help lessen the severity of the burn. Prompt medical attention to serious burns can help prevent scarring, disability, and deformity. Burns on the face, hands, feet, and genitals can be particularly serious.

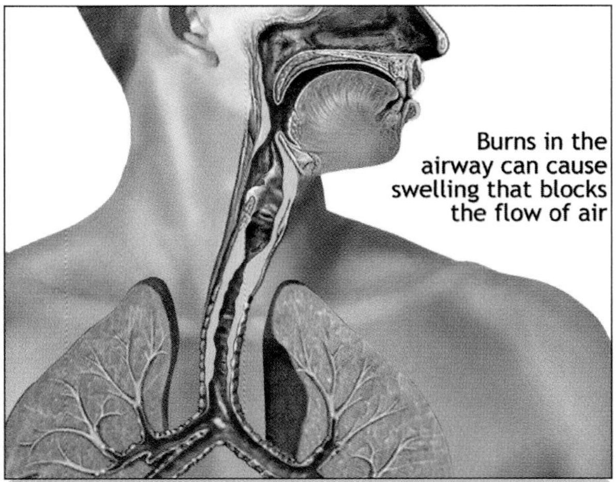

Burns in the airway can cause swelling that blocks the flow of air

Burns can be caused by inhaling smoke, steam, superheated air, or toxic fumes, especially in a poorly ventilated space.

Children under age 4 and adults over age 60 have a higher chance of complications and death from severe burns.

Degrees of a Burn

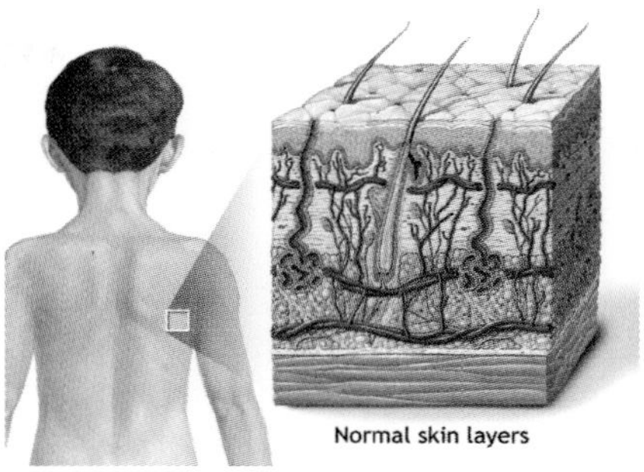

Skin is composed of 3 main layers: epidermis, dermis, and hypodermis

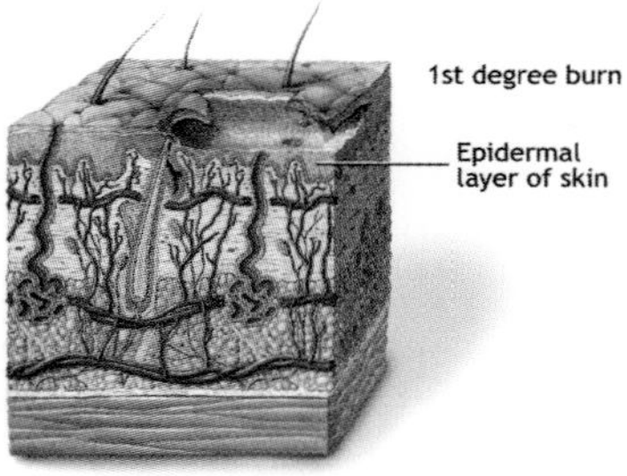

1st degree burn penetrates the top layer of skin (epidermis).

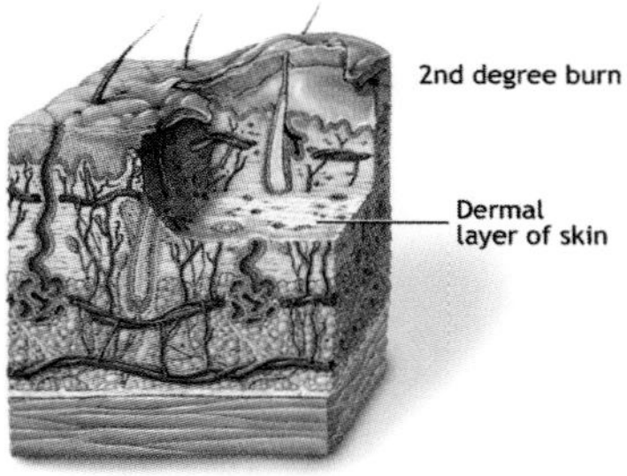

2nd degree burn penetrates the middle layer of skin (dermis).

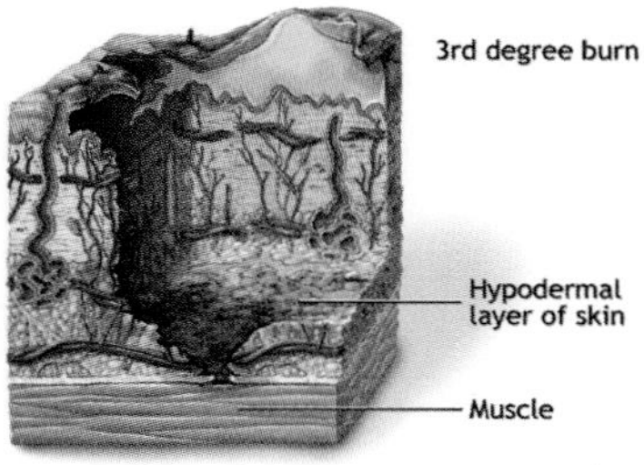

3rd degree burn penetrates down to the bottom layer of skin (hypodermis) or underlying layer of muscle.

In case of a fire, you and the others there are at risk for carbon monoxide poisoning. Anyone with symptoms of headache, numbness, weakness, or chest pain should be tested.

First aid for minor burns

1. If the skin is unbroken, run cool water over the area of the burn or soak it in a cool water bath (not ice water). Keep the area submerged for at least 5 minutes. A clean, cold, wet towel will also help reduce pain.

Run cool water over area of burn

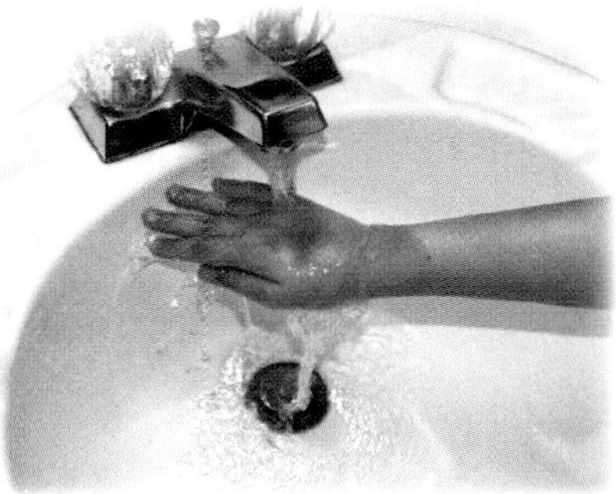

2. Calm and reassure the person.
3. After flushing or soaking, cover the burn with a dry, sterile bandage or clean dressing.

Cover the burn with a sterile bandage

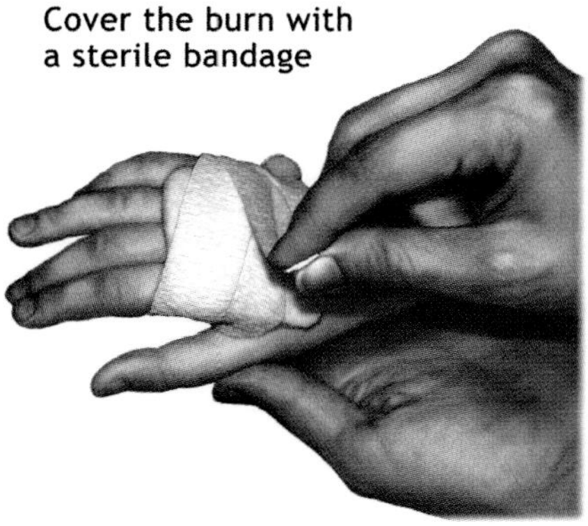

4. Protect the burn from pressure and friction.
5. Over-the-counter ibuprofen or acetaminophen can help relieve pain and swelling. DO NOT give children under 12 aspirin. Once the skin has cooled, moisturizing lotion also can help.
6. Minor burns will usually heal without further treatment. However, if a second-degree burn covers an area more than 2 to 3 inches in diameter, or if it is located on the hands, feet, face, groin, buttocks, or a major joint, treat the burn as a major burn.
7. Make sure the person is up-to-date on tetanus immunization.

First aid for major burns

1. If someone is on fire, tell the person to STOP, DROP, and ROLL. Wrap the person in thick material to smother the flames (a wool or cotton coat, rug, or blanket). Douse the person with water.
2. Call 911.
3. Make sure that the person is no longer in contact with smoldering materials. However, DO NOT remove burnt clothing that is stuck to the skin.
4. Make sure the person is breathing. If breathing has stopped, or if the person's airway is blocked, open the airway. If necessary, begin rescue breathing and CPR.
5. Cover the burn area with a dry sterile bandage (if available) or clean cloth. A sheet will do if the burned area is large. DO NOT apply any ointments. Avoid breaking burn blisters.
6. If fingers or toes have been burned, separate them with dry, sterile, non-adhesive dressings.
7. Elevate the body part that is burned above the level of the heart. Protect the burnt area from pressure and friction.

8. Take steps to prevent shock. Lay the person flat, elevate the feet about 12 inches, and cover him or her with a coat or blanket. However, DO NOT place the person in this shock position if a head, neck, back, or leg injury is suspected or if it makes the person uncomfortable.

9. Continue to monitor the person's vital signs until medical help arrives. This means pulse, rate of breathing, and blood pressure.

Do not

- DO NOT apply ointment, butter, ice, medications, cream, oil spray, or any household remedy to a severe burn.
- DO NOT breathe, blow, or cough on the burn.
- DO NOT disturb blistered or dead skin.
- DO NOT remove clothing that is stuck to the skin.
- DO NOT give the person anything by mouth, if there is a severe burn.
- DO NOT immerse a severe burn in cold water. This can cause shock.
- DO NOT place a pillow under the person's head if there is an airway burn. This can close the airway.

When to contact a medical professional

Call 911 if:

- The burn is extensive (the size of your palm or larger).
- The burn is severe (third degree).
- You aren't sure how serious it is.
- The burn is caused by chemicals or electricity.
- The person shows signs of shock.
- The person inhaled smoke.
- Physical abuse is the known or suspected cause of the burn.

Call a doctor if your pain is still present after 48 hours.

Call immediately if signs of infection develop. These signs include increased pain, redness, swelling, drainage or pus from the burn, swollen lymph nodes, red streaks spreading from the burn, or fever.

Also call immediately if there are signs of dehydration: thirst, dry skin, dizziness, lightheadedness, or decreased urination. Children, elderly, and anyone with a weakened immune system (e.g., HIV) should be seen right away.

Prevention

To help prevent burns:

- Install smoke alarms in your home. Check and change batteries regularly.
- Teach children about fire safety and the hazards of matches and fireworks.
- Keep children from climbing on top of a stove or grabbing hot items like irons and oven doors.
- Turn pot handles toward the back of the stove so that children can't grab them and they can't be accidentally knocked over.
- Place fire extinguishers in key locations at home, work, and school.
- Remove electrical cords from floors and keep them out of reach.
- Know about and practice fire escape routes at home, work, and school.
- Set temperature of water heater at 120 degrees or less.

Choking - Adult or Child

A choking person's airway may be completely or partially blocked. A complete blockage is an urgent medical emergency. A partial obstruction can quickly become life threatening if the person loses the ability to breathe in and out sufficiently.

Without oxygen, permanent brain damage can occur in as little as 4 minutes. Rapid first aid for choking can save a life.

Symptoms

The universal distress signal for choking is grabbing the throat with one or both hands.

Other danger signs include:

- Inability to speak
- Weak, ineffective coughing
- Noisy breathing or high-pitched sounds while inhaling
- Difficulty breathing
- Bluish skin color
- Loss of consciousness if blockage is not cleared

First aid

1. Ask, "Are you choking? Can you speak?"

   DO NOT perform first aid if the person is coughing forcefully and able to speak – a strong cough can dislodge the object.

2. Stand behind the person and wrap your arms around the person's waist.
3. Make a fist with one hand. Place the thumb side of your fist just above the person's navel, well below the breastbone.
4. Grasp the fist with your other hand.
5. Make quick, upward and inward thrusts with your fist.
6. Continue these thrusts until the object is dislodged or the person loses consciousness.

IF THE PERSON LOSES CONSCIOUSNESS

- Lower the person to the floor.
- Call 911 – or tell someone to call 911.
- Begin CPR.
- If you see something blocking the airway, try to remove it.

FOR PREGNANT OR OBESE PEOPLE

1. Wrap your arms around the person's CHEST.
2. Place your fist on the MIDDLE of the breastbone between the nipples.
3. Make firm, backward thrusts.

Do not

- DO NOT interfere if the person is coughing forcefully, able to speak, or is able to breathe in and out adequately. However, be ready to act immediately if the person's symptoms worsen.
- DO NOT try to grasp and pull out the object if the person is conscious or if you CANNOT see the object.

When to contact a medical professional

When the person is choking:

- Tell someone to call 911 while you begin first aid.
- If you are alone, shout for help and begin first aid.

Prevention

- Eat slowly and chew food thoroughly.
- Make sure dentures fit properly.
- Don't drink too much alcohol before or during eating.
- Keep small objects away from young children.

Choking – First Aid

1. Ask the person:

   "Are you choking?"

   "Can you speak?"

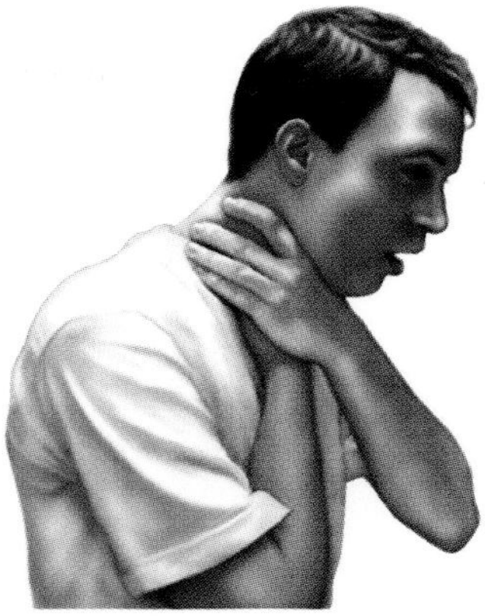

Universal sign of choking

DO NOT perform first aid if the person is coughing forcefully and able to speak – a strong cough can dislodge the object on its own.

Adult

Child

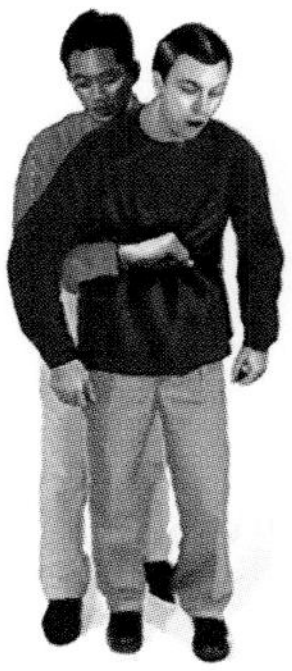

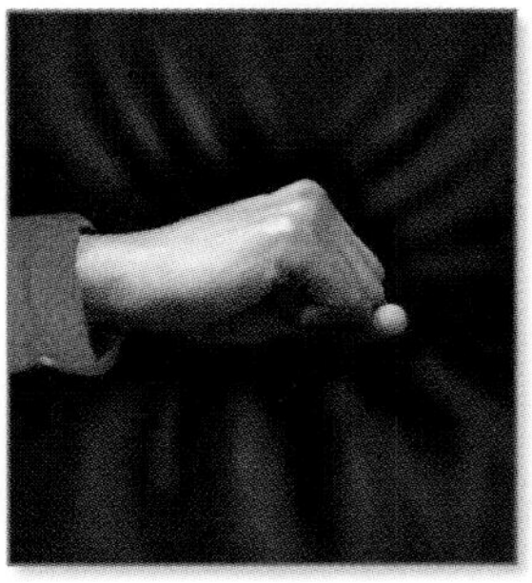

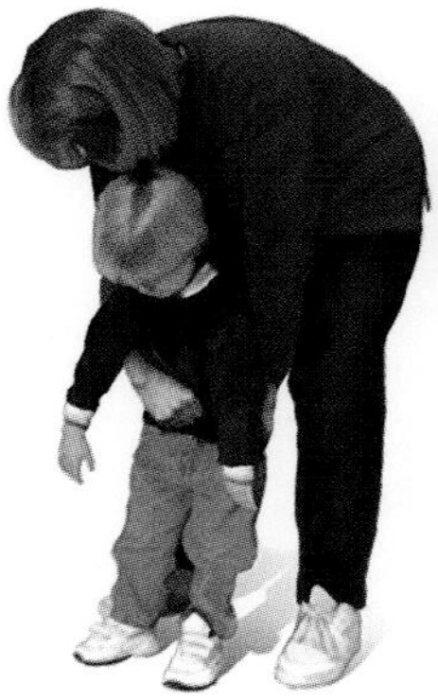

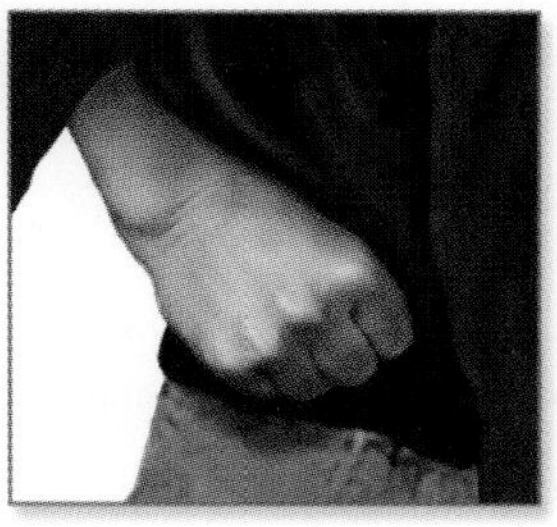

2. Stand behind the person and wrap your arms around the person's waist.

3. Make a fist with one hand. Place the thumb side of your fist just above the person's navel, well below the breastbone.

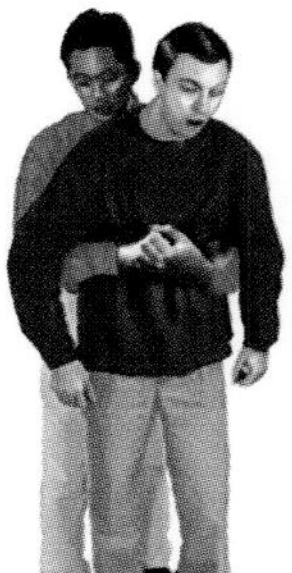

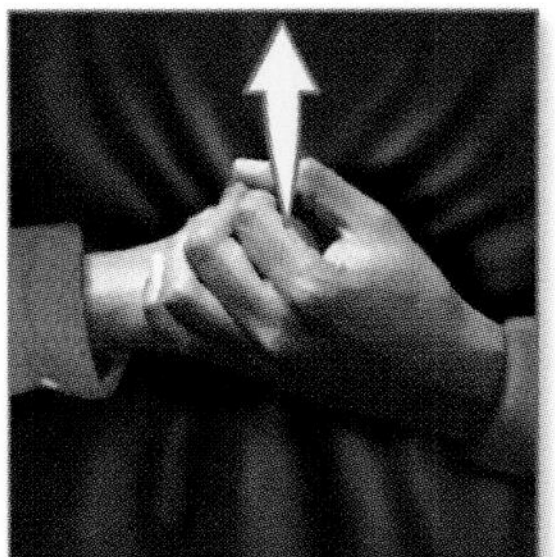

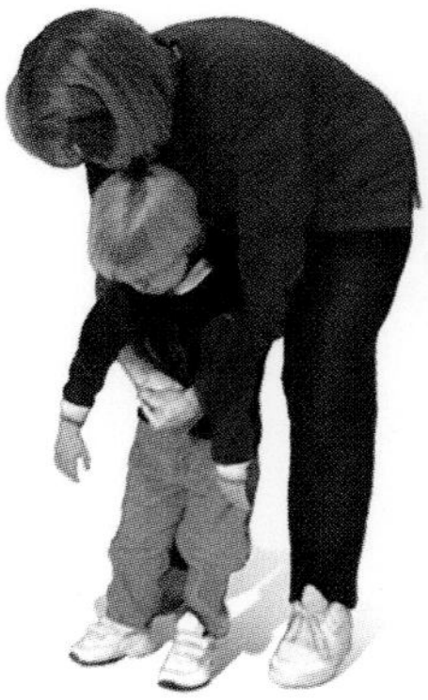

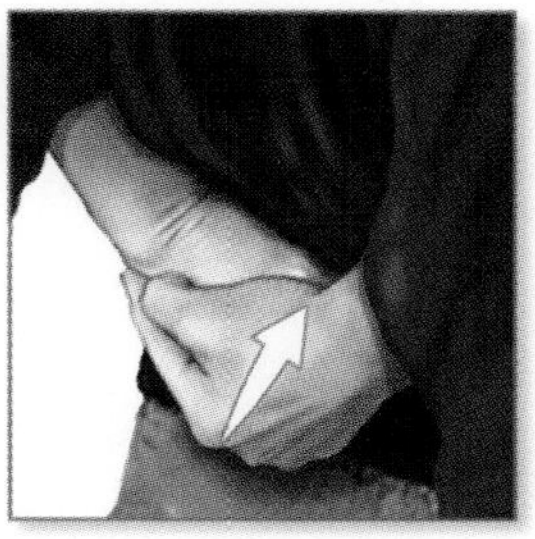

4. Grasp the fist with your hand.

5. Make quick, upward and inward thrusts with your fists.

6. Continue thrusts until the object is dislodged or the person loses consciousness. If the person becomes unconscious, lower person to the floor, call 911, and begin CPR. If you see the object blocking the airway, try to remove it.

Choking - infant

The danger signs of true choking are:

- Inability to cry or make much sound
- Weak, ineffective coughing
- Soft or high-pitched sounds while inhaling
- Difficulty breathing - ribs and chest retract
- Bluish skin color
- Loss of consciousness if blockage is not cleared

First aid

1. DO NOT perform these steps if the infant is coughing forcefully or has a strong cry – either of which can dislodge the object on its own.

2. Lay the infant face down, along your forearm. Use your thigh or lap for support. Hold the infant's chest in your hand and jaw with your fingers. Point the infant's head downward, lower than the body.

3. Give up to 5 quick, forceful blows between the infant's shoulder blades. Use the heel of your free hand.

Place the infant stomach-down across your forearm and give five quick, forceful blows on the infant's back with heel of your hand

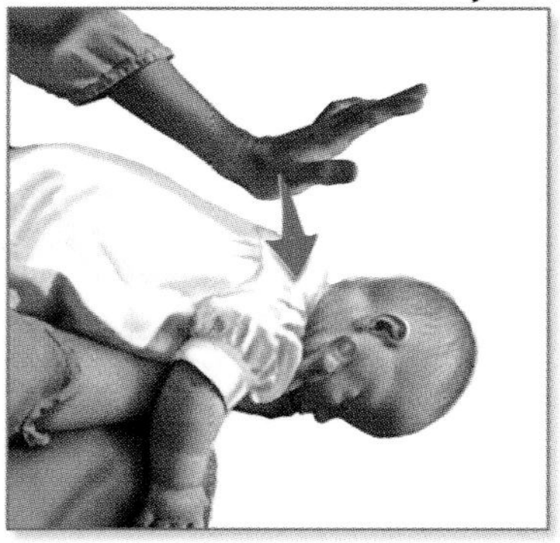

IF OBJECT ISN'T FREE AFTER 5 BLOWS

1. Turn the infant face up. Use your thigh or lap for support. Support the head.

2. Place 2 fingers on the middle of his breastbone just below the nipples.

3. Give up to 5 quick thrusts down, compressing the chest 1/3 to 1/2 the depth of the chest.

4. Continue this series of 5 back blows and 5 chest thrusts until the object is dislodged or the infant loses consciousness.

Place two fingers in the middle of the infant's breastbone and give five quick downward thrusts

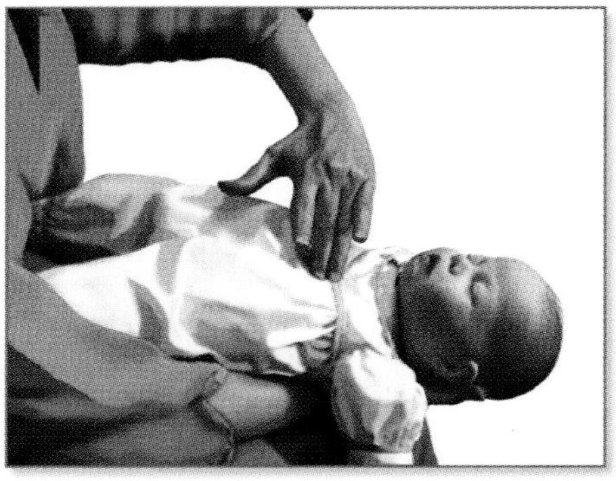

IF THE INFANT LOSES CONSCIOUSNESS

If the child becomes unresponsive, stops breathing, or turns blue:

- Shout for help.
- Give infant CPR. Call 911 after one minute of CPR.
- Try to remove an object blocking the airway ONLY if you can see it.

Remove the object with your finger ONLY if you can see it

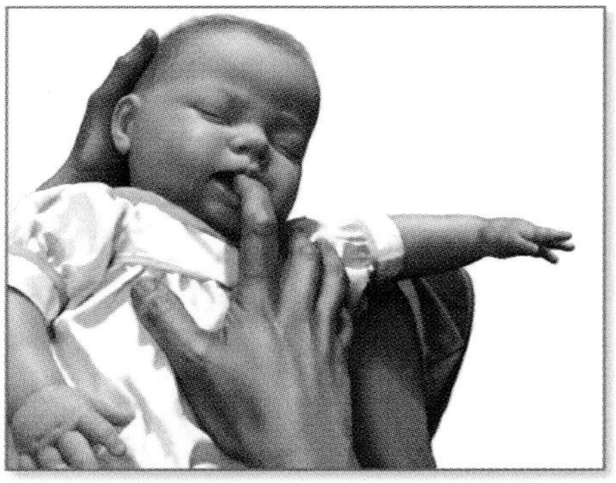

Do not

- DO NOT interfere if the infant is coughing forcefully, has a strong cry, or is breathing adequately. However, be ready to act if the symptoms worsen.
- DO NOT try to grasp and pull out the object if the infant is conscious.
- DO NOT perform these steps if the infant stops breathing for other reasons, such as asthma, infection, swelling, or a blow to the head.

When to contact a medical professional

If an infant is choking:

- Tell someone to call 911 while you begin first aid.
- If you are alone, shout for help and begin first aid.

Even if you successfully dislodge the object and the infant seems fine, call a doctor for further instructions.

Prevention

- Don't give children under 3 years old balloons or toys with fragile or small parts.
- Keep infants away from buttons, popcorn, coins, grapes, nuts, or similar items.
- Watch infants and toddlers while they are eating. Do not allow a child to crawl around while eating. Childproof your home.
- The earliest safety lesson is "No!"

Confusion

Confusion is the inability to think with your usual speed or clarity. When confused, you have difficulty focusing your attention and may feel disoriented. Confusion interferes with your ability to make decisions.

Confusion may come on suddenly or gradually over time, depending on the cause. Some confused people may behave aggressively.

Many times, confusion is temporary. Other times it is permanent and not curable. Confusion is more common in the elderly, and often occurs during hospitalization.

Confusion may be caused by:

- Alcohol intoxication
- Low blood sugar
- Head trauma or head injury

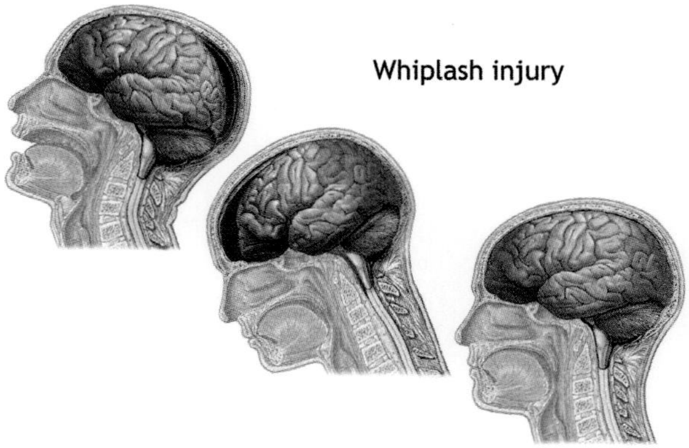

Whiplash injury may cause head and brain trauma.

- Concussion
- Fluid and electrolyte imbalance
- Nutritional deficiencies, particularly niacin , thiamine, vitamin C, or vitamin B-12
- Fever
- Sudden drop in body temperature (hypothermia)
- Low levels of oxygen (for example, from chronic lung disorders)
- Medications
- Infections
- Brain tumor
- Illness in an elderly person
- Sleep deprivation
- Seizures

Home care

A good way to test to see if a person is confused is to ask the person his or her name, age, and the date. If they are unsure or answer incorrectly, they are confused.

A confused person should not be left alone. To ensure a confused person's safety, physical restraints may be required in some situations. Try to keep the surroundings calm, quiet, and peaceful.

For sudden confusion due to low blood sugar (for example, from diabetes medication), the person should drink a sweet drink or eat a sweet snack. If the confusion lasts longer than 10 minutes, call the doctor.

When to contact a medical professional

Call 911 if:

- Confusion has come on suddenly or is accompanied by other symptoms like headache, feeling dizzy or faint, rapid pulse, slow or rapid breathing, cold or clammy skin, uncontrolled shivering, or fever.
- Confusion has come on suddenly in someone with diabetes.
- Confusion came on following a head injury.
- The person becomes unconscious at any time.

If you have had ongoing confusion that came on gradually, call for an appointment with your doctor if you have never been evaluated for this problem.

Convulsions

Convulsions are when a person's body shakes rapidly and uncontrollably. During convulsions, the person's muscles contract and relax repeatedly.

The term "convulsion" is often used interchangeably with "seizure," although there are many types of seizure, some of which have subtle or mild symptoms instead of convulsions. Seizures of all types are caused by disorganized and sudden electrical activity in the brain.

Convulsions can be unsettling to watch. Despite their appearance, most seizures are relatively harmless. They usually last from 30 seconds to 2 minutes. However, if a seizure is prolonged, or if multiple seizures happen and the person doesn't awaken in between, this is a medical emergency.

If a person has recurring seizures, and there are no underlying causes that can be identified, that person is said to have epilepsy. Epilepsy can usually be controlled well with medication.

Symptoms

- Brief blackout followed by period of confusion
- Sudden falling
- Drooling or frothing at the mouth
- Grunting and snorting
- Breathing stops temporarily
- Uncontrollable muscle spasms with twitching and jerking limbs
- Loss of bladder or bowel control
- Eye movements
- Teeth clenching
- Unusual behavior like sudden anger, sudden laughter, or picking at one's clothing

The person may have warning symptoms prior to the attack, which may consist of fear or anxiety, nausea, visual symptoms, or vertigo.

First aid

1. When a seizure occurs, the main goal is to protect the person from injury. Try to prevent a fall. Lay the person on the ground in a safe area. Clear the area of furniture or other sharp objects.

2. Cushion the person's head.

3. Loosen tight clothing, especially around the person's neck.

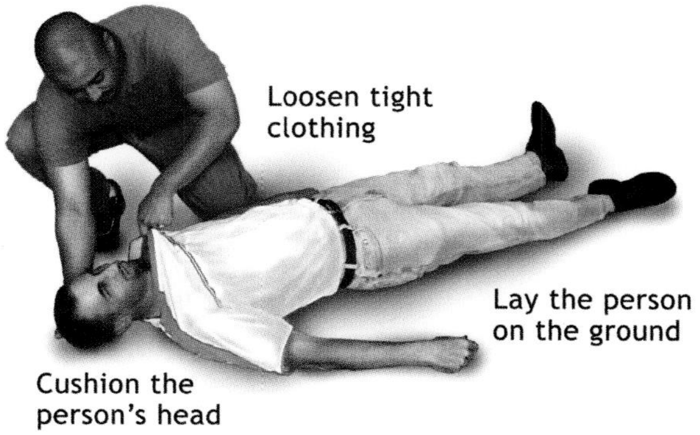
Loosen tight clothing
Lay the person on the ground
Cushion the person's head

4. Turn the person on his or her side. If vomiting occurs, this helps make sure that the vomit is not inhaled into the lungs.

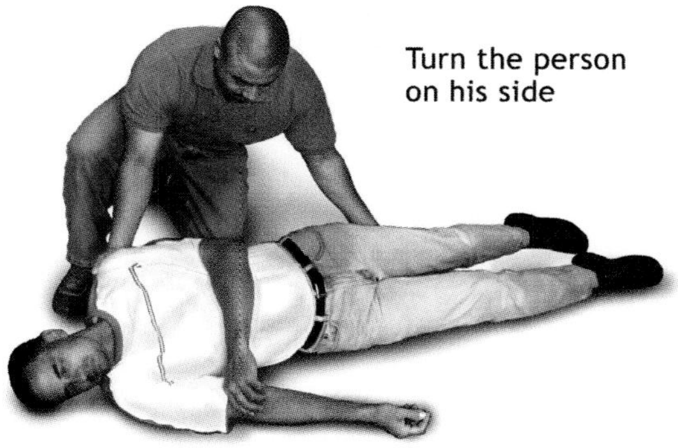
Turn the person on his side

5. Look for a medical I.D. bracelet with seizure instructions.

6. Stay with the person until recovery or until you have professional medical help. Meanwhile, monitor the person's vital signs (pulse, rate of breathing).

7. In an infant or child, if the seizure occurs with a high fever, cool the child gradually with tepid water. You can give the child acetaminophen (Tylenol), especially if the child has had fever convulsions before. DO NOT immerse the child in a cold bath. See *Fever Convulsions*.

When to contact a medical professional

Call 911 if:

- This is the first time the person has had a seizure.
- A seizure lasts more than 2 to 5 minutes.
- The person does not awaken or have normal behavior after a seizure.
- Another seizure starts soon after a seizure ends.
- The person had a seizure in water.
- The person is pregnant, injured, or has diabetes.
- The person does not have a medical ID bracelet (instructions explaining what to do).
- There is anything different about this seizure compared to the person's usual seizures.

CPR - for Adults

CPR is a lifesaving procedure that is performed when someone's breathing or heartbeat has stopped, as in cases of electric shock, drowning, or heart attack. CPR is a combination of:

- Rescue breathing, which provides oxygen to a person's lungs
- Chest compressions, which keep the person's blood circulating.

Permanent brain damage or death can occur within minutes if a person's blood flow stops. Therefore, you must continue these procedures until the person's heartbeat and breathing return, or trained medical help arrives.

CPR can be lifesaving, but it is best performed by those who have been trained in an accredited CPR course. The procedures described here are not a substitute for CPR training. (See www.americanheart.org for classes near you.)

When a bystander – whether friend, family, or stranger – starts CPR before emergency support arrives, the chance of surviving is tripled! Nevertheless, when most emergency workers arrive at a cardiac arrest, they usually find *no one giving CPR*. This would be a good time to find a convenient CPR class and learn how to save lives.

First Aid

The following steps are based on instructions from the American Heart Association.

1. **Check for responsiveness.** Shake or tap the person gently. See if the person moves or makes a noise. Shout, "Are you OK?"

2. **Call 911 if there is no response.** Shout for help and send someone to call 911. If you are alone, call 911 even if you have to leave the person.

3. Carefully place the person on his or her back. If there is a chance the person has a spinal injury, two people are needed to move the person without twisting the head and neck.

4. **Open the airway.** Lift up the chin with 2 fingers. At the same time, push down on the forehead with the other hand.

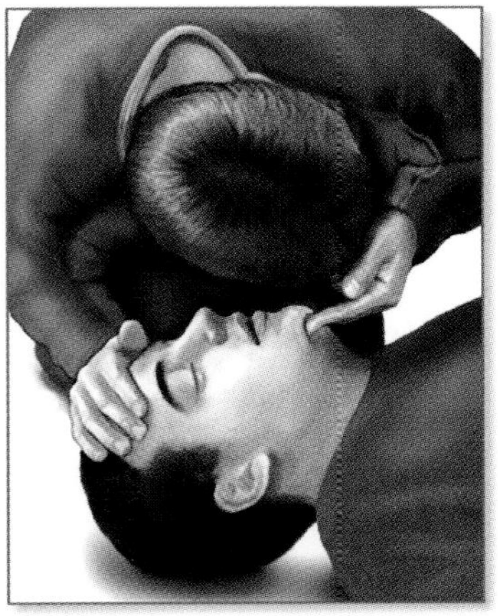

Look, listen, and feel for breathing and pulse

5. **Look, listen, and feel for breathing.** Place your ear close to the person's mouth and nose. Watch for chest movement. Feel for breath on your cheek.

6. **If the person is not breathing:**

- Cover the person's mouth tightly with your mouth
- Pinch the nose closed
- Keep the chin lifted and head tilted
- Give 2 slow, full breaths

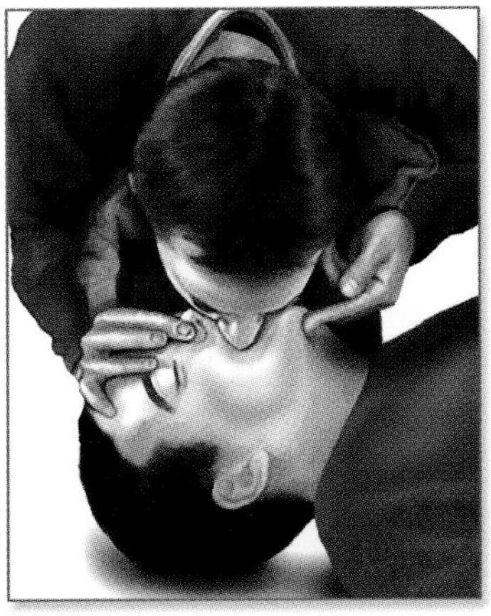

Place your mouth over the person's mouth and exhale

7. If the chest does NOT rise, try the chin lift-head tilt again, and give 2 more breaths. If the chest still doesn't rise, check to see if something is blocking the airway and try to remove it.

8. **Look for signs of circulation** – normal breathing, coughing, or movement. If these signs are absent, begin chest compressions.

9. **Perform chest compressions:**

- Place the heel of one hand on the breastbone – right between the nipples.
- Place the heel of your other hand on top of the first hand.
- Position your body directly over your hands. Your shoulders should be in line with your hands. DO NOT lean back or forward. As you gaze down, you should be looking directly down on your hands.
- Give 15 chest compressions. Each time, press down about 2 inches into the chest. These compressions should be FAST with no pausing. Count the 15 compressions quickly: "a, b, c, d, e, f, g, h, i, j, k, l, m, n, off."

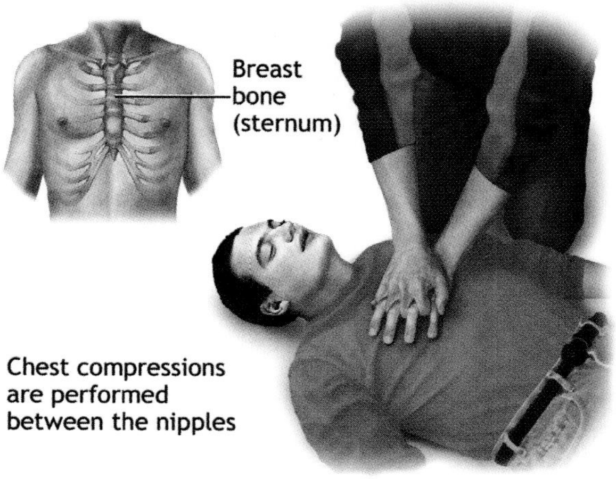
Breast
bone
(sternum)
Chest compressions
are performed
between the nipples

10. **Give the person 2 slow, full breaths.** The chest should rise.

11. Continue cycles of 15 chest compressions followed by 2 slow, full breaths.

12. After about 1 minute (four cycles of 15 compressions and 2 breaths), re-check for signs of circulation.

13. Repeat steps 11 and 12 until the person recovers or help arrives.

If the person starts breathing again, place him or her in the recovery position. Periodically re-check for breathing and signs of circulation until help arrives.

CPR - FOR CHILDREN (1-8 YEARS OLD)

All parents and those who take care of children should learn *infant and child* CPR if they haven't already. This jewel of knowledge is something no parent should be without. (See www.americanheart.org for classes near you.)

FIRST AID

The following steps are based on instructions from the American Heart Association.

1. **Check for responsiveness.** Shake or tap the child gently. See if the child moves or makes a noise. Shout, "Are you OK?"

2. **If there is no response, shout for help.** Send someone to call 911. Do not leave the child yourself to call 911 until you have performed CPR for about one minute.

3. **Carefully place the child on his or her back.** If there is a chance the child has a spinal injury, two people are needed to move the child without twisting the head and neck.

4. **Open the airway.** Lift up the chin with one hand. At the same time, push down on the forehead with the other hand.

5. **Look, listen, and feel for breathing.** Place your ear close to the child's mouth and nose. Watch for chest movement. Feel for breath on your cheek.

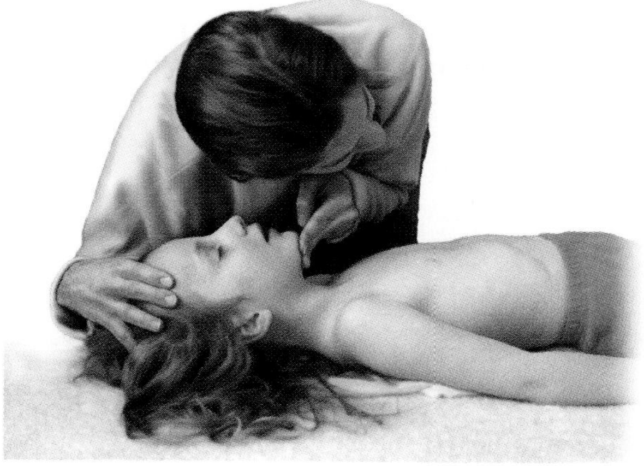

6. **If the child is not breathing:**

- Cover the child's mouth tightly with your mouth
- Pinch the nose closed
- Keep the chin lifted and head tilted
- Give 2 slow breaths. DO NOT give large, full, forceful breaths.

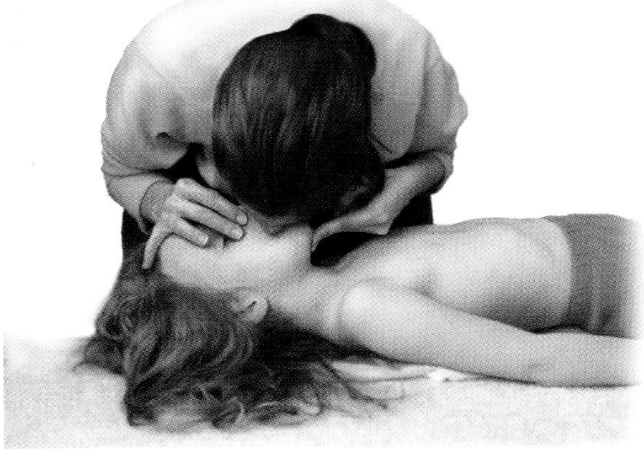

7. If the chest does NOT rise, try the chin lift-head tilt again, and give 2 more breaths. If the chest still doesn't rise, check to see if something is blocking the airway and try to remove it.

8. **Look for signs of circulation** – normal breathing, coughing, or movement. If these signs are absent, begin chest compressions.

9. **Perform chest compressions:**

- Place the heel of one hand on the breastbone – just below the nipples. Make sure your heel is not at the very end of the breastbone.
- Keep your other hand on the child's forehead, keeping the head tilted back.
- Press down on the child's chest so that it compresses about 1/3 to 1/2 the depth of the chest.

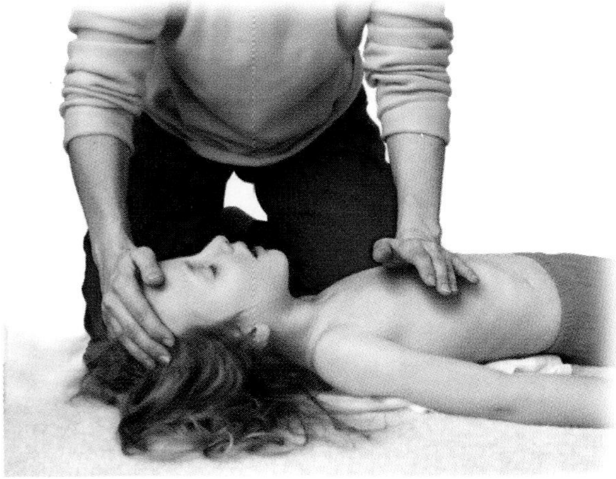

- Give 5 chest compressions. Each time, let the chest rise completely. These compressions should be FAST with no pausing. Count the 5 compressions quickly: "a, b, c, d, off."

10. **Give the child 1 slow, full breath.** The chest should rise.

11. Continue cycles of 5 chest compressions followed by 1 slow, full breath.

12. After about 1 minute, check again for signs of circulation.

13. At this time, if the child still does not have normal breathing, coughing, or any movement, leave the child to **call 911**.

14. Repeat steps 11 and 12 until the child recovers or help arrives.

If the child starts breathing again, place him or her in the recovery position. Periodically re-check for breathing and signs of circulation until help arrives.

Learn about the AED!

Machines called automated external defibrillators (AEDs) are now available in many public locations and are very easy to use. They have pads or paddles to place on the chest during a life-threatening emergency, and automatically administer a sudden shock if needed to get the heart back into the right rhythm. Look for AEDs in malls, airports, and other public places. *Find out if your workplace has one.* Also, if you are at risk for a heart attack, they can be purchased for your home.

CPR - FOR INFANTS

All parents and those who take care of children should learn *infant and child* CPR if they haven't already. This jewel of knowledge is something no parent should be without. (See www.americanheart.org for classes near you.)

First aid

The following steps are based on instructions from the American Heart Association.

1. **Check for responsiveness.** Shake or tap the infant gently. See if the infant moves or makes a noise. Shout, "Are you OK?"

2. **If there is no response, shout for help.** Send someone to call 911. Do not leave the infant yourself to call 911 until you have given about one minute of CPR.

3. **Carefully place the infant on his or her back.** If there is a chance the infant has a spinal injury, two people are needed to move the infant without twisting the head and neck.

4. **Open the airway.** Lift up the chin with one hand. At the same time, push down on the forehead with the other hand.

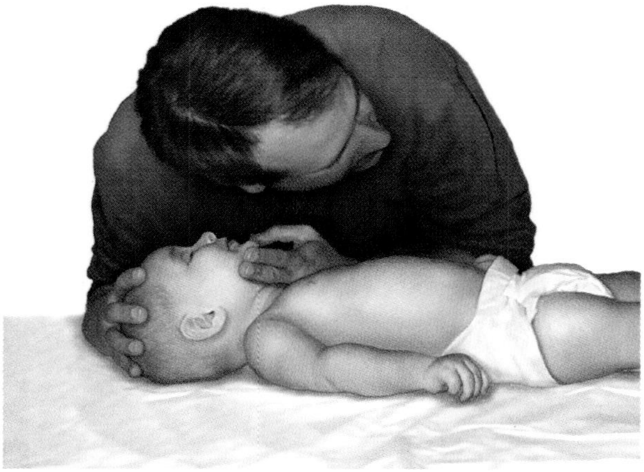

5. **Look, listen, and feel for breathing.** Place your ear close to the infant's mouth and nose. Watch for chest movement. Feel for breath on your cheek.

6. **If the infant is not breathing:**

- Cover the infant's mouth and nose tightly with your mouth
- Alternatively, cover just the nose. Hold the mouth shut.
- Keep the chin lifted and head tilted
- Give 2 slow breaths. Do NOT give large, full, forceful breaths.

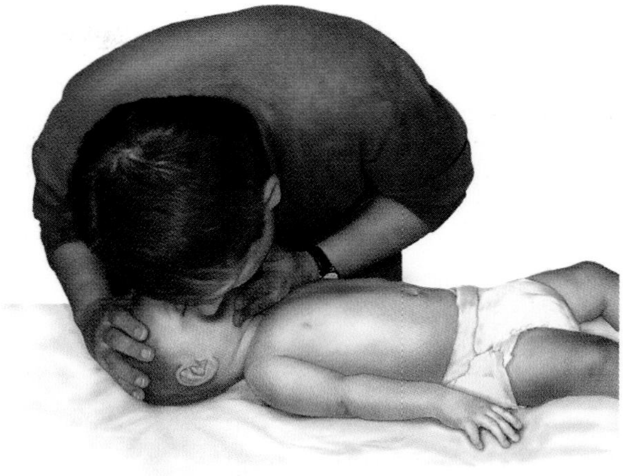

7. If the chest does NOT rise, try the chin lift-head tilt again, and give 2 more breaths. If the chest still doesn't rise, check to see if something is blocking the airway and try to remove it.

8. **Look for signs of circulation** – normal breathing, coughing, or movement. If these signs are still absent, begin chest compressions.

9. **Perform chest compressions:**

- Place 2-3 fingers on the breastbone – just below the nipples. Make sure not to press at the very end of the breastbone.
- Keep your other hand on the infant's forehead, keeping the head tilted back.
- Press down on the infant's chest so that it compresses about 1/3 to 1/2 the depth of the chest.

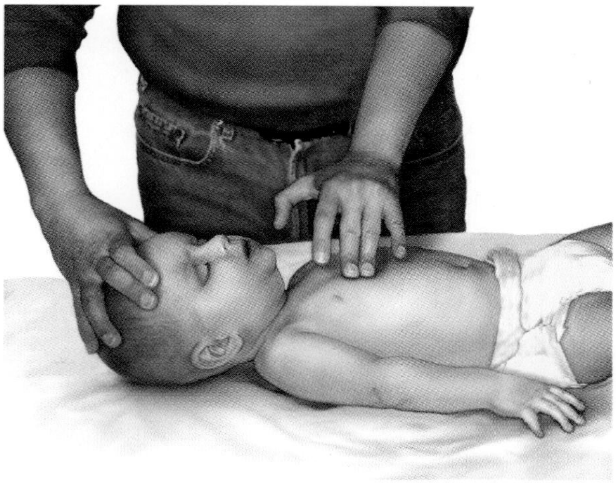

- Give 5 chest compressions. Each time, let the chest rise completely. These compressions should be FAST with no pausing. Count the 5 compressions quickly: "a, b, c, d, off."

10. **Give the infant 1 slow, full breath.** The chest should rise.

11. Continue cycles of 5 chest compressions followed by 1 slow, full breath.

12. After about 1 minute, check again for signs of circulation.

13. At this time, if the infant still does not have normal breathing, coughing, or any movement, leave the infant to **call 911**.

14. Repeat steps 11 and 12 until the infant recovers or help arrives.

If the infant starts breathing again, place him or her in the recovery position. Periodically re-check for breathing and signs of circulation until help arrives.

Cuts and puncture wounds

A cut is an injury that results in a break or opening in the skin. A laceration is a jagged, irregular cut. A puncture is a wound made by a pointed object (like a nail, knife, or sharp tooth).

Laceration

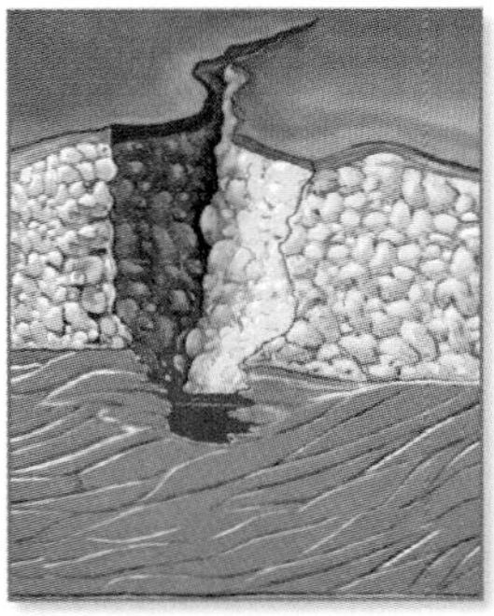

Puncture wound

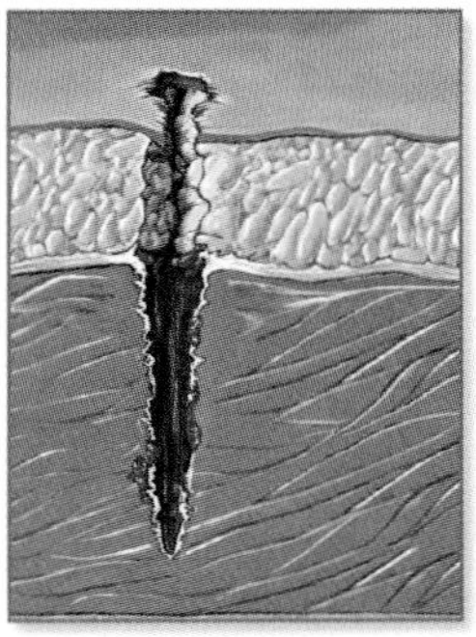

First aid

If the wound is bleeding severely, call 911.

Minor cuts and puncture wounds can be treated at home. Take the following steps.

FOR MINOR CUTS

1. Wash your hands with soap to avoid infection.
2. Wash the cut thoroughly with mild soap and water.
3. Use direct pressure to stop the bleeding.
4. Apply an antibacterial ointment.
5. If the cut is likely to get dirty or be reopened by friction, cover it (once the bleeding has stopped) with a bandage that will not stick to the injury.

FOR MINOR PUNCTURES

1. Wash your hands.
2. Use a stream of water for at least five minutes to rinse the puncture wound. Wash with soap.
3. Look (but DO NOT probe) for objects inside the wound. If found, DO NOT remove – go to the emergency room. If you cannot see anything inside the wound, but a piece of the object that caused the injury is missing, also seek medical attention.
4. Apply antibacterial ointment and a clean bandage.

Do not

- DO NOT assume that a minor wound is clean because you can't see dirt or debris inside. Wash it.
- DO NOT breathe on an open wound.
- DO NOT try to clean a major wound, especially after the bleeding is under control.

How to treat a minor cut

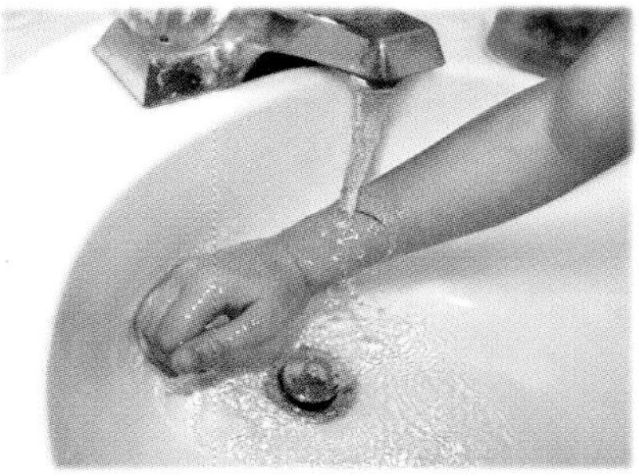

Wash the cut with mild soap and water.

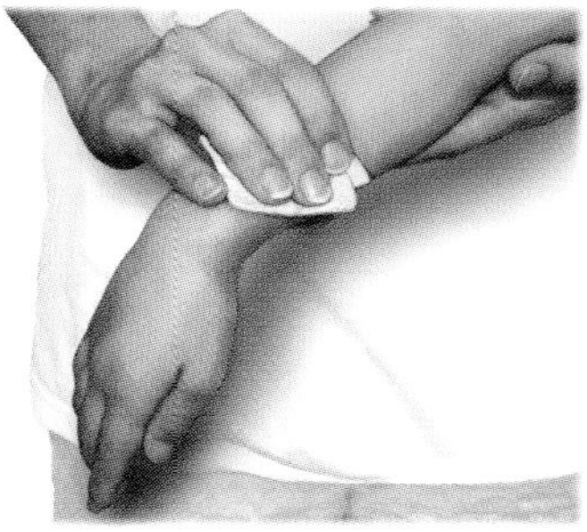

Apply direct pressure to stop bleeding.

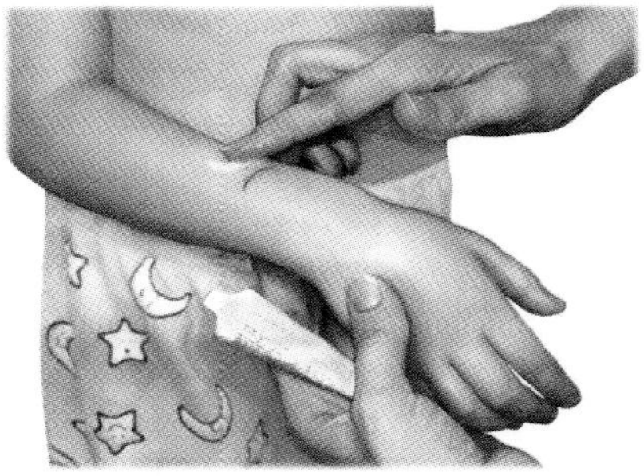

Apply an antibacterial ointment.

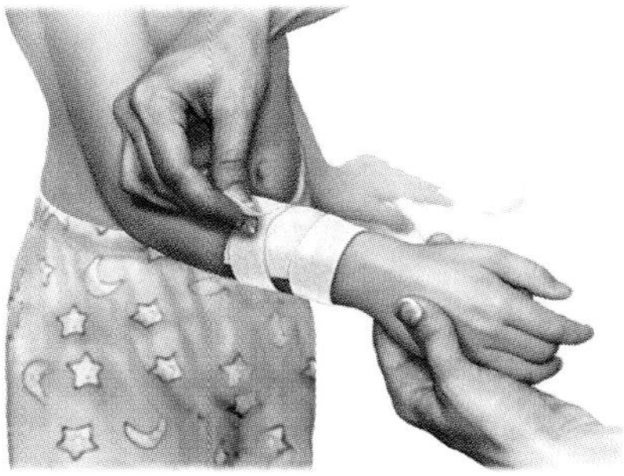

If the cut is likely to get dirty, apply a bandage that won't stick to the injury.

- DO NOT remove a long or deeply embedded object. Seek medical attention.
- DO NOT probe or pick debris from a wound. Seek medical attention.
- DO NOT push exposed body parts back in. Cover them with clean material until medical help arrives.

When to contact a medical professional

Call 911 if:

- The bleeding is severe, spurting, or cannot be stopped (for example, after 15 minutes of pressure).
- The person is seriously injured.

Call your doctor immediately if:

- The wound is large or deep, even if the bleeding is not severe.
- You think the wound might benefit from stitches (the cut is more than a quarter inch deep, on the face, or reaches bone).
- The person has been bitten by a human or animal.
- A cut or puncture is caused by a fishhook or rusty object.
- An object or debris is embedded – DO NOT remove yourself.
- The wound shows signs of infection (warmth and redness in the area, a painful or throbbing sensation, fever, swelling, or pus-like drainage).
- You have not had a tetanus shot within the last 10 years.

Dehydration

Dehydration means your body does not have as much water and fluids as it should. Dehydration can be caused by losing too much fluid, not drinking enough, or both. Vomiting and diarrhea are common causes.

Infants and children are more susceptible to dehydration than adults because of their smaller body weights and higher turnover of water and electrolytes. The elderly and those with illnesses are also at higher risk.

Dehydration is classified as mild, moderate, or severe based on how much of the body's fluid is lost or not replenished. When severe, dehydration is a life-threatening emergency.

Your body may lose too much fluids from:

- Vomiting or diarrhea
- Excessive urine output, such as with uncontrolled diabetes or diuretic use
- Excessive sweating (for example, from exercise)
- Fever

You might not drink enough fluids because of:

- Nausea
- Loss of appetite due to illness
- Sore throat or mouth sores

Dehydration in sick children is often a combination of both – refusing to eat or drink anything while also losing fluid from vomiting, diarrhea, or fever.

Home care

Drinking fluids is usually sufficient for mild dehydration. It is better to have frequent, small amounts of fluid (using a teaspoon or syringe for an infant or child) rather than trying to force large amounts of fluid at one time. Drinking too much fluid at once can bring on more vomiting.

Electrolyte solutions or freezer pops are especially effective. These are available at pharmacies. Sport drinks contain a lot of sugar and can cause or worsen diarrhea. In infants and children, avoid using water as the primary replacement fluid.

Intravenous fluids and hospitalization may be necessary for moderate to severe dehydration. The doctor will try to identify and then treat the cause of the dehydration.

Most cases of stomach viruses (also called viral gastroenteritis) tend to resolve on their own after a few days. See *Diarrhea*.

When to contact a medical professional

Call 911 if you or your child:

- Feels dizzy or lightheaded.
- Is lethargic or confused.

Call your doctor right away if you or your child has any of the following symptoms:

- Not producing tears.
- Sunken eyes.
- Little or no urine output for 8 hours.
- Dry skin that sags back into position slowly when pinched up into a fold (poor skin turgor).

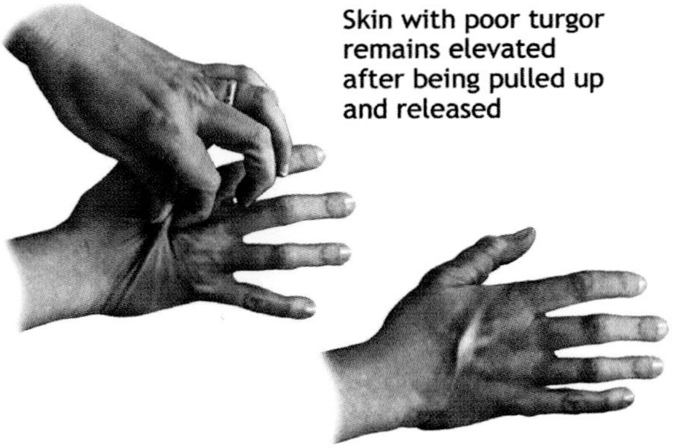
Skin with poor turgor remains elevated after being pulled up and released

- Dry mouth or dry eyes.
- Sunken soft-spot on the top of your infant's head.
- Fast-beating heart.
- Blood in the stool or vomit.
- Your infant is less than 2 months and has diarrhea or vomiting.

Also call your doctor if:

- An illness is combined with the inability to keep down any fluids.
- Vomiting has been going on for longer than 24 hours in an adult or longer than 12 hours in a child.
- Diarrhea has lasted longer than 5 days in an adult or child.
- Your infant or child is much less active than usual or is irritable.
- You or your child have excessive urination, especially if there is a family history of diabetes or you are taking diuretics.

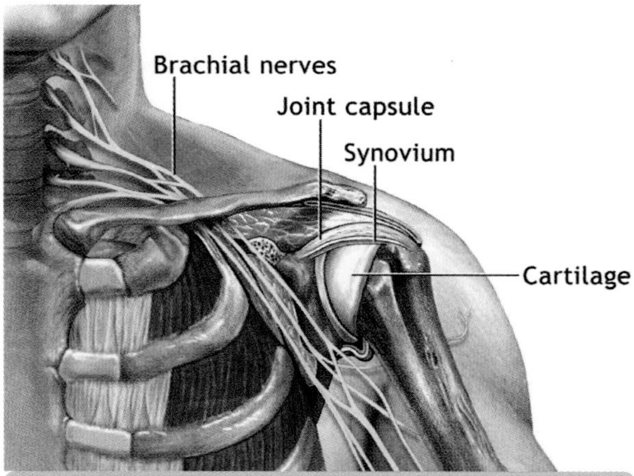

A joint consists of a joint capsule, synovium, synovial fluid, and cartilage. It is supported by ligaments and surrounding muscles.

Prevention

Even when healthy, drink plenty of fluid every day. Drink more when the weather is hot or you are exercising.

Carefully monitor someone who is ill, especially an infant, child, or older adult. If you believe that dehydration is developing, consult a doctor before the person becomes moderately or severely dehydrated. Begin fluid replacement as soon as vomiting and diarrhea start – DO NOT wait for signs of dehydration.

Always encourage the person to drink during an illness, and remember that a person's fluid needs are greater when that person has fever, vomiting, or diarrhea. The easiest signs to monitor are urine output (there should be frequent wet diapers or trips to the bathroom), saliva in the mouth, and tears when crying.

Dislocated bone

Joints are areas where two or more bones come together. If a sudden impact injures a joint, the bones that meet at that joint may become dislocated (not connected). That means the bones are no longer in their normal position. Usually the joint capsule and ligaments tear when a joint becomes dislocated, and often the nerves are injured.

It may be hard to tell a dislocated bone from a broken bone. Both are emergency situations and require the same first-aid treatment. Injuries to the surrounding ligaments generally take 3 to 6 weeks to heal.

Symptoms

A dislocated joint may be:

- Visibly out-of-place, discolored, or misshapen
- Limited in movement
- Swollen or bruised
- Intensely painful, especially if you try to use the joint or bear weight on it

Nursemaid's elbow is a partial dislocation common in toddlers.

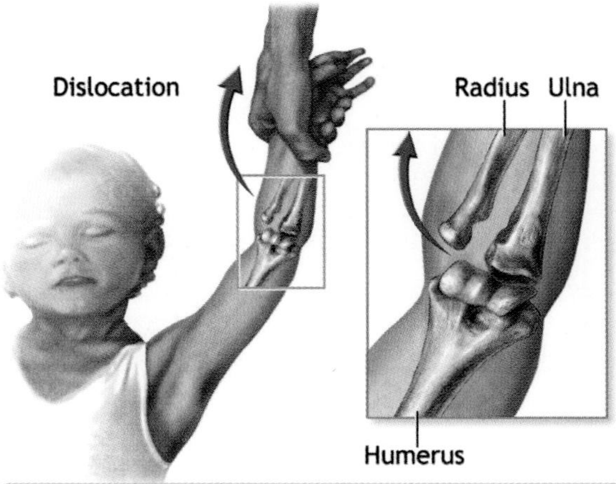

A partial dislocation may be caused by a sudden pull on a child's arm or hand (nursemaid's elbow).

The main symptom is refusal to use the arm. Nursemaid's elbow can be easily treated in a doctor's office without the following first aid steps.

First aid

1. Call 911 before you begin treating someone who may have a dislocation, especially if the accident causing the injury may be life-threatening.

2. If there has been a serious injury, check the person's airway, breathing, and circulation. If necessary, begin rescue breathing, CPR, or bleeding control.

3. Do not move the person if you think that his head, back, or leg has been injured. Keep the person still. Provide reassurance.

4. If the skin is broken, take steps to prevent infection. Do not blow on the wound. Rinse the area gently to remove obvious dirt, but do not scrub or probe. Cover the area with sterile dressings before immobilizing the injury.

5. Splint or sling the injury in the position in which you found it. Do not move the joint. Be sure to immobilize the area above and below the injured joint.

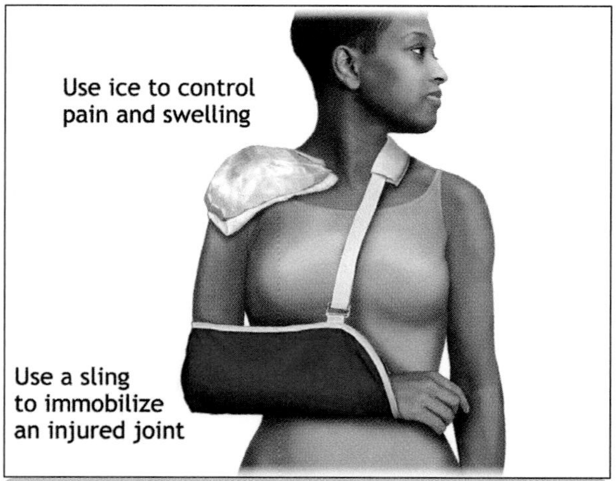

Immobilize the joint with a sling and apply ice.

6. Check the person's blood circulation around the injury by pressing firmly on the skin in the affected area. It should blanch white, then regain color within a couple of seconds.

7. Apply ice packs to ease pain and swelling.

8. Take steps to prevent shock. Unless there is a head, leg, or back injury, lay the person flat, elevate the feet about 12 inches, and cover the person with a coat or blanket.

Do not

- DO NOT move the person unless the injury has been completely immobilized.
- DO NOT move a person with an injured hip, pelvis, or upper leg unless it is absolutely necessary. If you are the only rescuer and the person must be moved, drag him or her by the clothing.
- DO NOT attempt to straighten a misshapen bone or joint or to change its position.
- DO NOT test a misshapen bone or joint for loss of function.
- DO NOT give the person anything by mouth.

When to contact a medical professional

Call 911 if the person has:

- A known or suspected dislocation or broken bone
- Severe bleeding
- An area below the injured joint that is pale, cold, clammy, or blue
- Signs of infection like warmth and redness at the injured site, pus, or a fever
- A bone projecting through the skin

Ear emergencies

Children often stick objects into their ears. These objects can be difficult to remove because the ear canal is a tube of solid bone that is lined with thin, sensitive skin. Any object pressing against the skin can be very painful. In many cases, a doctor will need to use special instruments to examine the ear and safely remove the object.

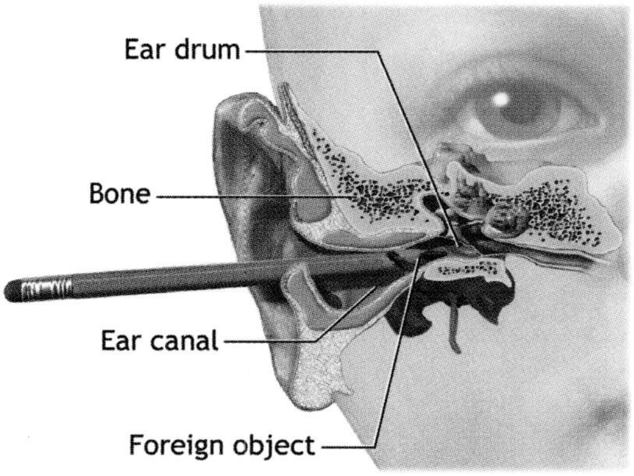

Pain, hearing loss, dizziness, ringing in the ear, and ruptured eardrums can be caused by:

- Inserting cotton swabs, toothpicks, pins, pens, or other objects into the ear.
- Sudden changes in pressure, as from an explosion, blow to the head, flying, scuba diving, falling while water skiing, or being slapped on the head or ear.
- Loud percussions, such as a gun going off.

First aid

Follow the steps below, depending on the type of ear emergency.

OBJECT IN THE EAR

1. Calm and reassure the person.
2. If the object is sticking out and easy to remove, gently remove it by hand or with tweezers. Then, get medical help to make sure the entire object was removed.
3. If you think a small object may be lodged within the ear, but you cannot see it, DO NOT reach inside the ear canal with tweezers. You can do more harm than good.
4. Try using gravity to get the object out by tilting the head to the affected side. DO NOT strike the person's head. Shake it gently in the direction of the ground to try to dislodge the object.
5. If the object doesn't come out, get medical help.

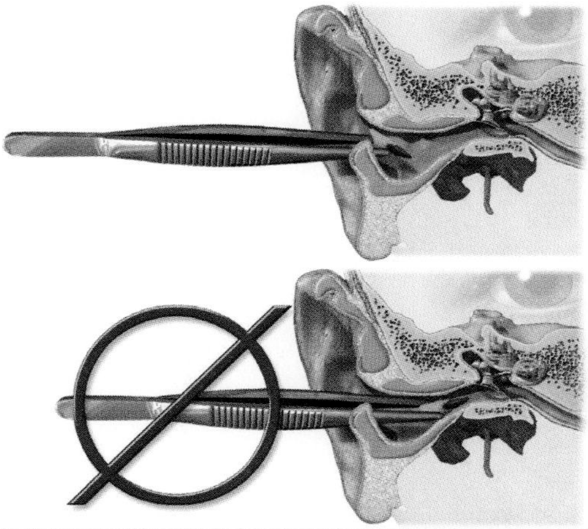

Only use tweezers to remove a foreign object in the ear canal if you can clearly see the object.

INSECT IN THE EAR

1. DO NOT let the person put a finger in the ear, since this may make the insect sting.
2. Turn the person's head so that the affected side is up, and wait to see if the insect flies or crawls out.
3. If this doesn't work, try pouring mineral oil, olive oil, or baby oil into the ear. As you pour the oil, pull the ear lobe gently backward and upward for an adult, or backward and downward for a child. The insect should suffocate and may float out in the oil. AVOID using oil to remove any object other than an insect, since oil can cause other kinds of objects to swell.

RUPTURED EARDRUM

1. The person will have severe pain. Place sterile cotton gently in the outer ear canal to keep the inside of the ear clean.

2. Get medical help.

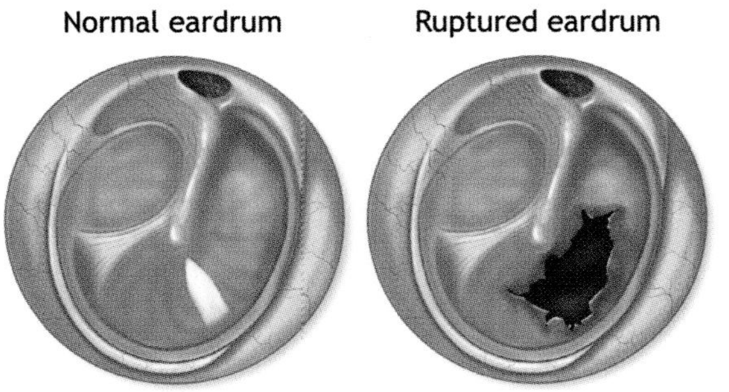

Do not

- DO NOT block any drainage coming from the ear.
- DO NOT try to clean or wash the inside of the ear.
- DO NOT attempt to remove the object by probing with a cotton swab, pin, or any other tool. To do so will risk pushing the object farther into the ear and damaging the middle ear.
- DO NOT reach inside the ear canal with tweezers.

When to contact a medical professional

The following symptoms, which may indicate significant trauma to the ear, should be evaluated by a doctor:

- Pain in the ear
- Ringing sounds
- Hearing loss
- Drainage or blood from the ear
- Recent blow to your ear or head

Prevention

- Never put anything in the ear canal without first consulting a doctor.
- Never thump the head to try to correct an ear problem.
- Teach children not to put things in their ears.
- Avoid cleaning the ear canals altogether.
- Following an ear injury, avoid nose blowing and getting water in the injured ear.
- Treat ear infections promptly.

If you tend to feel pain and pressure when flying, drink lots of fluid before and during the flight. Avoid the use of alcohol, caffeine, or tobacco on the day of the flight. Chew gum, suck on a hard candy, or yawn during take off and landing. Talk to your doctor about taking a decongestant or using a nasal spray before you fly.

Eye emergencies

Eye emergencies include cuts, scratches, objects in the eye, burns, chemical exposure, and blunt injuries to the eye. Since the eye is easily damaged, any of these conditions can lead to vision loss if left untreated.

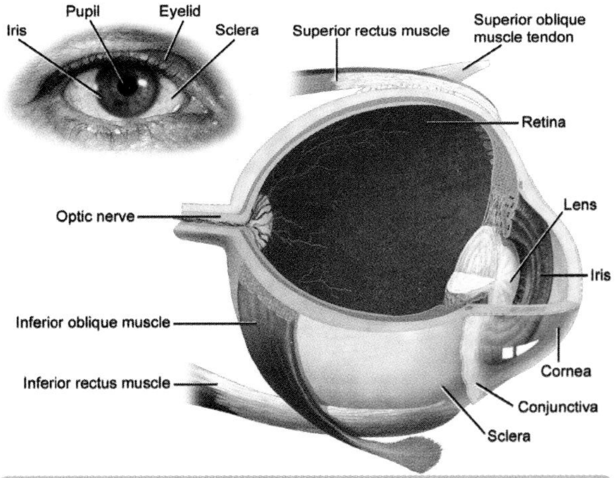

The eye is a sophisticated and delicate organ. Take care of eye emergencies immediately.

It is important to get medical attention for all significant eye injuries and problems. Many eye problems (such as a painful red eye) that are not due to injury still need urgent medical attention.

A chemical injury to the eye can be caused by a work-related accident or by common household products, such as cleaning solutions, garden chemicals, solvents, or many other types of chemicals. Fumes and aerosols can also cause chemical burns.

A black eye is usually caused by direct trauma to the eye or face. Certain types of skull fractures can result in bruising around the eyes, even without direct trauma to the eye. The bruise is caused by bleeding under the skin. The tissue surrounding the eye turns black and blue, then it gradually becomes purple, green, and yellow before the abnormal coloring disappears within 2 weeks. Usually, swelling of the eyelid and tissue around the eye also occurs.

First aid

Take prompt action and follow the steps below if you or someone else has an eye-related injury.

SMALL OBJECT ON THE EYE OR EYELID

The eye will often clear itself of tiny objects, like eyelashes and sand, through blinking and tearing. If not, take these steps:

1. Tell the person not to rub the eye. Wash your hands before examining it.
2. Examine the eye in a well-lighted area. To find the object, have the person look up and down, then side to side.
3. If you can't find the object, grasp the lower eyelid and gently pull down on it to look under the lower eyelid. To look under the upper lid, you can place a cotton-tipped swab on the outside of the upper lid and gently flip the lid over the cotton swab.

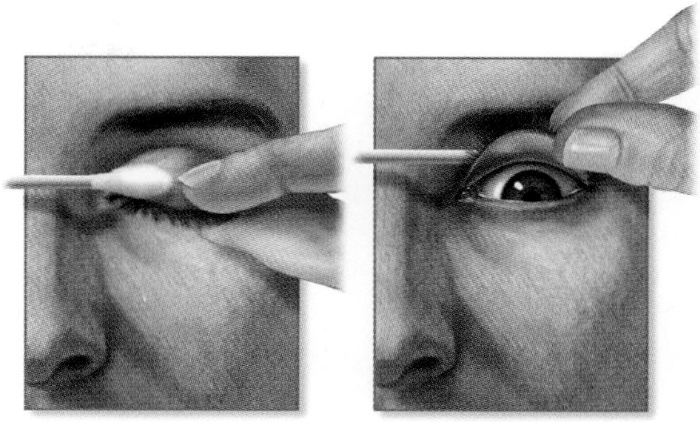

Twist cotton-tipped swab upward — Look downward

4. If the object is on an eyelid, try to gently flush it out with water. If that does not work, try touching a second cotton-tipped swab to the object to remove it.
5. If the object is on the eye, try gently rinsing the eye with water. It may help to use an eye dropper positioned above the outer corner of the eye. DO NOT touch the eye itself with the cotton swab.

A scratchy feeling or other minor discomfort may continue after removing eyelashes and other tiny objects. This will go away within a day or two. If the person continues to have discomfort or blurred vision, get medical help.

OBJECT STUCK OR EMBEDDED IN EYE

1. Leave the object in place. DO NOT try to remove the object. DO NOT touch it or apply any pressure to it.
2. Calm and reassure the person.
3. Wash your hands.
4. Bandage both eyes. If the object is large, place a paper cup or cone over the injured eye and tape it in place. Cover the uninjured eye with gauze or a clean cloth. If the object is small, cover both eyes with a clean cloth or sterile dressing. Even if only one eye is affected, covering both eyes will help prevent eye movement.
5. Get medical help immediately.

CHEMICALS IN THE EYE

1. Flush with cool tap water immediately. Turn the person's head so the injured eye is down and to the side. Holding the eyelid open, allow running water from the faucet to flush the eye for 15 minutes.

2. If both eyes are affected, or if the chemicals are also on other parts of the body, have the person take a shower.

3. If the person is wearing contact lenses and the lenses did not flush out from the running water, have the person try to remove the contacts AFTER the flushing procedure.

4. Cover both eyes (even if only one eye is affected) with a clean dressing, and avoid any rubbing of the eyes. Even if only one eye is affected, covering both eyes will help prevent eye movement.

5. After following the above instructions, seek medical help immediately.

EYE CUTS, SCRATCHES, OR BLOWS

1. If the eyeball has been injured, get medical help immediately.

2. Gently apply cold compresses to reduce swelling and help stop any bleeding. DO NOT apply pressure to control bleeding.

3. If blood is pooling in the eye, cover both of the person's eyes with a clean cloth or sterile dressing, and get medical help.

EYELID CUTS

1. Carefully wash the eye. Apply a thick layer of bacitracin or mupirocin ointment on the eyelid. Place a patch over the eye. Seek medical help immediately.

2. If the cut is bleeding, apply gentle pressure with a clean, dry cloth until the bleeding subsides.

3. Rinse with water, cover with a clean dressing, and place a cold compress on the dressing to reduce pain and swelling.

Do not

- DO NOT press or rub an injured eye.
- DO NOT remove contact lenses unless rapid swelling is occurring, there is a chemical injury and the contacts did not come out with the water flush, or you cannot get prompt medical help.
- DO NOT attempt to remove a foreign body that appears to be embedded in any part of the eye. Get medical help immediately.
- DO NOT use cotton swabs, tweezers, or anything else on the eye itself. Cotton swabs should only be used on the eyelid.
- DO NOT attempt to remove an embedded object.

When to contact a medical professional

Seek emergency medical care if:

- There appears to be any visible scratch, cut, or penetration of your eyeball.
- Any chemical gets into your eye.
- The eye is painful and red.
- Nausea accompanies the eye pain.
- You have any trouble seeing (such as blurry vision).

Prevention

- Supervise children carefully. Teach them how to be safe.
- Always wear protective eye wear when using power tools, hammers, or other striking tools.
- Always wear protective eye wear when working with toxic chemicals.

FAINTING

Fainting is a temporary loss of consciousness due to a drop in blood flow to the brain. The episode is brief (lasting less than a couple of minutes) and is followed by rapid and complete recovery. You may feel lightheaded or dizzy before fainting.

A longer, deeper state of unconsciousness is often called a coma.

When you faint, you not only experience loss of consciousness, but also loss of muscle tone and paleness in your face. You may also feel weak or nauseated just prior to fainting and have the sense that surrounding noises are fading into the background.

Fainting may occur while you are urinating, having a bowel movement (especially if straining), coughing strenuously, or when you have been standing in one place too long. Fainting can also be related to fear, severe pain, or emotional distress.

A sudden drop in blood pressure can cause you to faint. This may happen if you are bleeding or severely dehydrated. It can also happen if you stand up very suddenly from a lying down position.

Certain medications can lead to fainting because of a drop in your blood pressure or other reason. Common drugs that contribute to fainting include those for anxiety, high blood pressure, nasal congestion, and allergies.

Other reasons you may faint include hyperventilation, use of alcohol or drugs, or low blood sugar.

Less common but more serious reasons include heart disease (like abnormal heart rhythm or heart attack) and stroke.

HOME CARE

If you have a history of fainting and have been evaluated medically, follow your doctor's instructions for how to prevent fainting episodes. For example, if you know the situations that cause you to faint, these should be avoided or changed. Avoid sudden changes in posture. Get up from a lying or seated position slowly and gradually. When having blood drawn (if this makes you faint), tell the technician and make sure that you are lying down.

Immediate treatment for fainting includes:

- Check the person's airway and breathing. If necessary, call 911 and begin rescue breathing and CPR.
- Loosen tight clothing around the neck.
- Keep the affected person lying down for at least 10 to 15 minutes, preferably in a cool and quiet space. If the person cannot lie down, have him sit forward and lower his head below the levels of the shoulders, between the knees.
- If the person has vomited, turn him or her to one side to prevent choking
- Elevate the feet above the level of the heart (about 12 inches).

WHEN TO CONTACT A MEDICAL PROFESSIONAL

Call 911 if the person who fainted:

- Fell from a height, especially if injured or bleeding.
- Does not regain consciousness quickly (within a couple of minutes).
- Is pregnant or over 50 years old.
- Has diabetes. (Check medical identification bracelets.)
- Feels chest pain, pressure, or discomfort; pounding or irregular heartbeat; or has loss of speech, visual disturbances, or inability to move one or more limbs.
- Has convulsions, tongue trauma, or loss of bowel control.

Even if it's not an emergency situation, people should be evaluated by a doctor when they have never fainted before, if they are fainting frequently, or they have new symptoms associated with fainting. Call for an appointment to be seen as soon as possible.

HEAD INJURIES

Every year, approximately two million people sustain a head injury. Most of these injuries are minor because the skull provides the brain with considerable protection. The symptoms of minor head injuries usually go away on their own. More than half a million head injuries a year, however, are severe enough to require hospitalization.

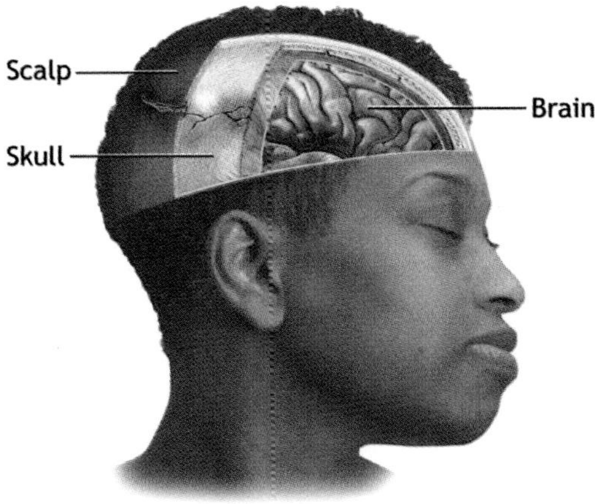

Learning to recognize a serious head injury, and implementing basic first aid, can make the difference in saving someone's life.

SYMPTOMS

The signs of a head injury can occur immediately or develop slowly over several hours. Even if the skull is not fractured, the brain can bang against the inside of the skull and be bruised. (This is called a concussion.) The head may look fine, but complications could result from bleeding inside the skull.

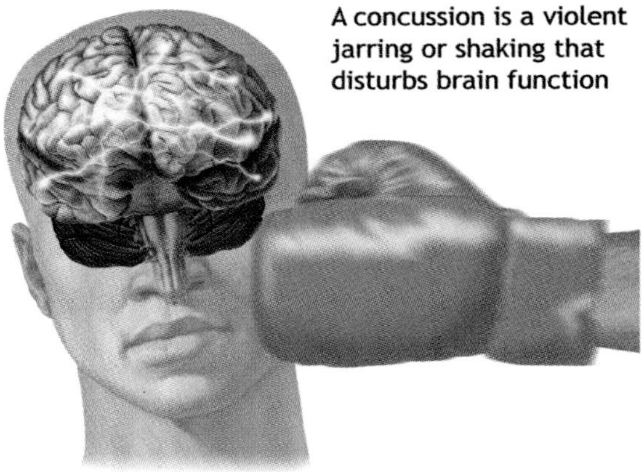

A concussion is a violent jarring or shaking that disturbs brain function

When encountering a person who just had a head injury, try to find out what happened. If he or she cannot tell you, look for clues and ask witnesses. In any serious head trauma, always assume the spinal cord is also injured.

The following symptoms suggest a more serious head injury that requires emergency medical treatment:

- Loss of consciousness, confusion, or drowsiness
- Low breathing rate or drop in blood pressure
- Convulsions
- Fracture in the skull or face, facial bruising, swelling at the site of the injury, or scalp wound
- Fluid drainage from nose, mouth, or ears (may be clear or bloody)
- Severe headache

> **REMEMBER...**
>
> Children often bang their heads, and many of these head injuries can be safely managed at home. Even if your child vomits once, it doesn't necessarily mean that a child needs to go to the hospital. Children often vomit ONCE after a head injury. This may not be a problem, but call a doctor for further guidance.

- Initial improvement followed by worsening symptoms
- Irritability (especially in children), personality changes, or unusual behavior
- Restlessness, clumsiness, lack of coordination
- Slurred speech or blurred vision
- Inability to move one or more limbs
- Stiff neck or vomiting
- Pupil changes
- Inability to hear, see, taste, or smell

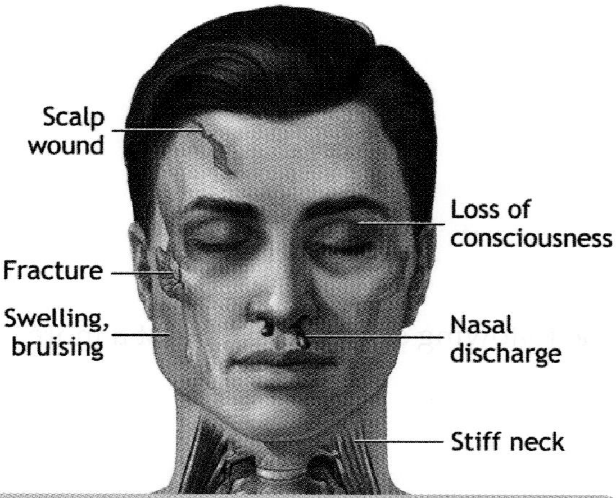

Signs and symptoms of a serious head injury.

First Aid

For a mild head injury, no specific treatment may be needed. However, closely watch the person for any concerning symptoms over the next 24 hours. The symptoms of a serious head injury can be delayed. While the person is sleeping, wake him or her every 2 to 3 hours and ask simple questions to check alertness, such as "What is your name?"

If a child begins to play or run immediately after getting a bump on the head, serious injury is unlikely. However, as with anyone with a head injury, closely watch the child for 24 hours after the incident.

Over-the-counter pain medicine (like acetaminophen or ibuprofen) may be used for a mild headache. DO NOT take aspirin, because it can increase the risk of bleeding.

Get medical help immediately if the person:

- Becomes unusually drowsy
- Develops a severe headache or stiff neck
- Vomits more than once
- Loses consciousness (even if brief)
- Behaves abnormally

For a moderate to severe head injury, take the following steps:

1. Call 911.
2. Check the person's airway, breathing, and circulation. If necessary, begin rescue breathing and CPR.
3. If the person's breathing and heart rate are normal but the person is unconscious, treat as if there is a spinal injury. Stabilize the head and neck by placing your hands on both sides of the person's head, keeping the head in line with the spine and preventing movement. Wait for medical help.
4. Stop any bleeding by firmly pressing a clean cloth on the wound. If the injury is serious, be careful not to move the person's head. If blood soaks through the cloth, DO NOT remove it. Place another cloth over the first one.
5. If you suspect a skull fracture, DO NOT apply direct pressure to the bleeding site, and DO NOT remove any debris from the wound. Cover the wound with sterile gauze dressing.
6. If the person is vomiting, roll the head, neck, and body as one unit to prevent choking. This still protects the spine, which you must always assume is injured in the case of a head injury. (Children often vomit ONCE after a head injury. This may not be a problem, but call a doctor for further guidance.)
7. Apply ice packs to swollen areas.

Do not

- DO NOT wash a head wound that is deep or bleeding a lot.
- DO NOT remove any object sticking out of a wound.
- DO NOT move the person unless absolutely necessary.
- DO NOT shake the person if he or she seems dazed.
- DO NOT remove a helmet if you suspect a serious head injury.
- DO NOT pick up a fallen child with any sign of head injury.
- DO NOT drink alcohol within 48 hours of a serious head injury.

When to contact a medical professional

Call 911 if:

- There is severe head or facial bleeding.
- The person is confused, drowsy, lethargic, or unconscious.
- The person stops breathing.
- You suspect a serious head or neck injury or the person develops any symptoms of a serious head injury.

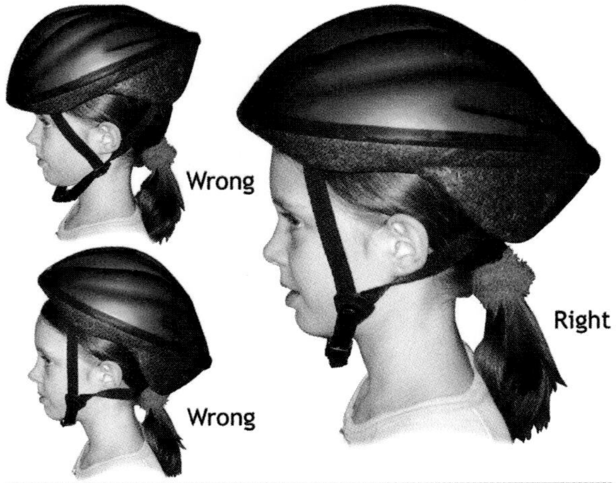

Use safety equipment during activities that could result in a head injury, like bicycle riding. It is important to wear helmets and other equipment correctly.

Heat emergencies

Heat emergencies fall into three categories of increasing severity: heat cramps, heat exhaustion, and heatstroke.

Heat illnesses are easily preventable by taking precautions in hot weather.

Children, elderly, and obese people have a higher risk of developing heat illness. People taking certain medications or drinking alcohol also have a higher risk. However, even a top athlete in superb condition can succumb to heat illness if he or she ignores the warning signs.

If the problem isn't addressed, heat cramps (caused by loss of salt from heavy sweating) can lead to heat exhaustion (caused by dehydration), which can progress to heatstroke. Heatstroke, the most serious of the three, can cause shock, brain damage, organ failure, and even death.

Symptoms

The early symptoms of heat illness include:

- Profuse sweating
- Fatigue
- Thirst
- Muscle cramps

Later symptoms of heat exhaustion include:

- Headache
- Dizziness and light-headedness
- Weakness
- Nausea and vomiting
- Cool, moist skin
- Dark urine

The symptoms of heatstroke include:

- Fever (temperature above 104°F)
- Irrational behavior
- Extreme confusion

- Dry, hot, and red skin
- Rapid, shallow breathing
- Rapid, weak pulse
- Seizures
- Unconsciousness

First aid

1. Have the person lie down in a cool place. Elevate the person's feet about 12 inches.

2. Apply cool, wet cloths (or cool water directly) to the person's skin and use a fan to lower body temperature. Place cold compresses on the person's neck, groin, and armpits.

3. If alert, give the person beverages to sip (such as Gatorade), or make a salted drink by adding a teaspoon of salt per quart of water. Give a half cup every 15 minutes. Cool water will do if salt beverages are not available.

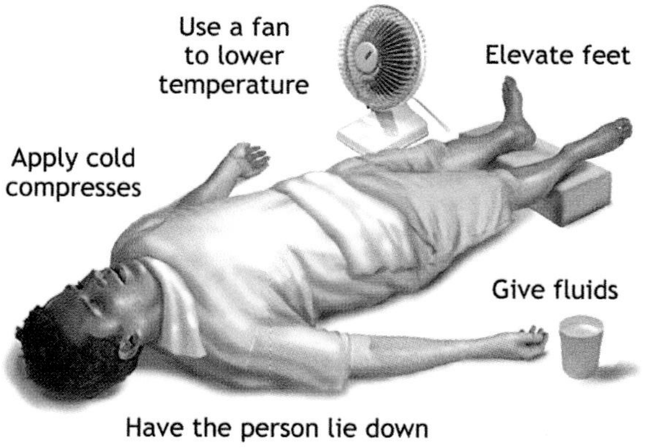
Use a fan to lower temperature
Elevate feet
Apply cold compresses
Give fluids
Have the person lie down

4. For muscle cramps, give beverages as above and massage affected muscles gently, but firmly, until they relax.

5. If the person shows signs of shock (bluish lips and fingernails and decreased alertness), starts having seizures, or loses consciousness, call 911 and administer first aid accordingly.

Do not

- DO NOT underestimate the seriousness of heat illness, especially if the person is a child, elderly, or injured.
- DO NOT give the person medications that are used to treat fever (such as aspirin or acetaminophen). They will not help, and they may be harmful.
- DO NOT give the person salt tablets.
- DO NOT give the person liquids that contain alcohol or caffeine. They will interfere with the body's ability to control its internal temperature.
- DO NOT use alcohol rubs on the person's skin.
- DO NOT give the person anything by mouth (not even salted drinks) if the person is vomiting or unconscious.

When to contact a medical professional

Call 911 if:

- The person loses consciousness at any time.
- There is any other change in the person's alertness (for example, confusion or seizures).
- The person has a fever over 102°F.
- Other symptoms of heat stroke are present (like rapid pulse or rapid breathing).
- The person's condition does not improve, or worsens despite treatment.

Prevention

- Wear loose-fitting, lightweight clothing in hot weather.
- Rest frequently and seek shade when possible.
- Avoid exercise or strenuous physical activity outside during hot or humid weather.
- Drink plenty of fluids every day. Drink more fluids before, during, and after physical activity.

- Be especially careful to avoid overheating if you are taking drugs that impair heat regulation, or if you are overweight or elderly.
- Be careful of hot cars in the summer. Allow the car to cool off before getting in.

Hypothermia

Hypothermia is dangerously low body temperature, below 95°F (35°C).

People most likely to experience hypothermia include:

- Very old or very young
- Chronically ill, especially with heart or circulation problems
- Malnourished
- Overly tired
- Under the influence of alcohol or drugs

Hypothermia occurs when more heat is lost than the body can generate. It is usually caused by extended exposure to the cold.

Common causes include:

- Being outside without enough protective clothing in winter.
- Falling overboard from a boat into cold water.
- Wearing wet clothing in windy or cold weather.
- Heavy exertion, not drinking enough fluids, or not eating enough in cold weather.

Symptoms

As people develop hypothermia, their abilities to think and move are often lost slowly. In fact, they may even be unaware that they need emergency treatment. Someone with hypothermia also is likely to have frostbite.

The symptoms include:

- Drowsiness
- Weakness and loss of coordination
- Pale and cold skin
- Confusion
- Uncontrollable shivering (although at extremely low body temperatures, shivering may stop)
- Slowed breathing or heart rate

Lethargy, cardiac arrest, shock, and coma can set in without prompt treatment. Hypothermia can be fatal.

First aid

1. If any symptoms of hypothermia are present, especially confusion or changes in mental status, immediately call 911.

2. If the person is unconscious, check airway, breathing, and circulation. If necessary, begin rescue breathing or CPR. If the person is breathing less than 6 breaths per minute, begin rescue breathing.

3. Take the person inside to room temperature and cover him or her with warm blankets. If going indoors is not possible, get the person out of the wind and use a blanket to provide insulation from the cold ground. Cover the person's head and neck to help retain body heat.

4. Once inside, remove any wet or constricting clothes and replace them with dry clothing.

5. Warm the person. If necessary, use your own body heat to aid the warming. Apply warm compresses to the neck, chest wall, and groin. If the person is alert and can easily swallow, give warm, sweetened, nonalcoholic fluids to aid the warming.

6. Stay with the person until medical help arrives.

Do not

- DO NOT assume that someone found lying motionless in the cold is already dead.

- DO NOT use direct heat (such as hot water, a heating pad, or a heat lamp) to warm the person.
- DO NOT give the person alcohol!

When to contact a medical professional

Call 911 anytime you suspect someone has hypothermia. Give first aid while awaiting emergency assistance.

Prevention

Before you spend time outside in the cold, DO NOT drink alcohol or smoke. Drink plenty of fluid and get adequate food and rest.

Wear proper clothing in cold temperatures to protect your body. These include:

- Mittens (not gloves)
- Wind-proof, water-resistant, many-layered clothing
- Two pairs of socks (cotton next to skin, then wool)
- Scarf and hat that cover the ears (to avoid major heat loss through the top of your head)

Avoid:

- Extremely cold temperature, especially with high winds
- Wet clothes
- Poor circulation, which is more likely from age, tight clothing or boots, cramped positions, fatigue, certain medications, smoking, alcohol, and diseases that affect the blood vessels (such as diabetes)

Nosebleeds

Nosebleeds are very common. The nose contains many tiny blood vessels that bleed easily. Air moving through the nose can dry and irritate the membranes lining the inside of the nose, forming crusts. These crusts bleed when irritated by rubbing, picking, or blowing the nose.

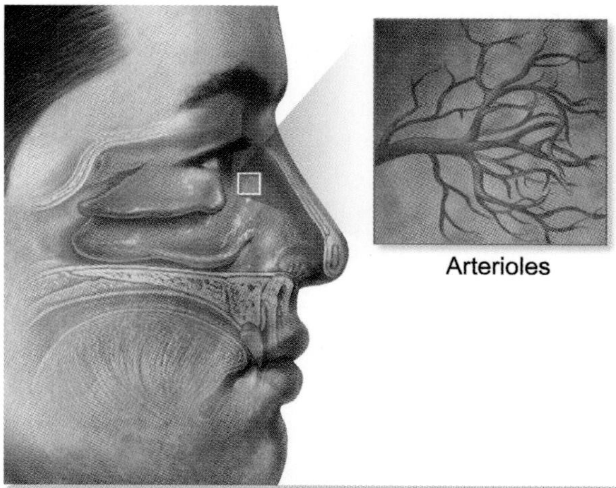

The nose is a very vascular area, meaning that it contains many tiny blood vessels (arterioles).

The lining of the nose is more likely to become dry and irritated from low humidity, allergies, colds, or sinusitis. Thus, nosebleeds occur more frequently in the winter when viruses are common and heated indoor air dries out the nostrils. A foreign object in the nose or direct impact to the nose can also cause a nosebleed.

If you have a deviated septum, you may be prone to frequent nosebleeds.

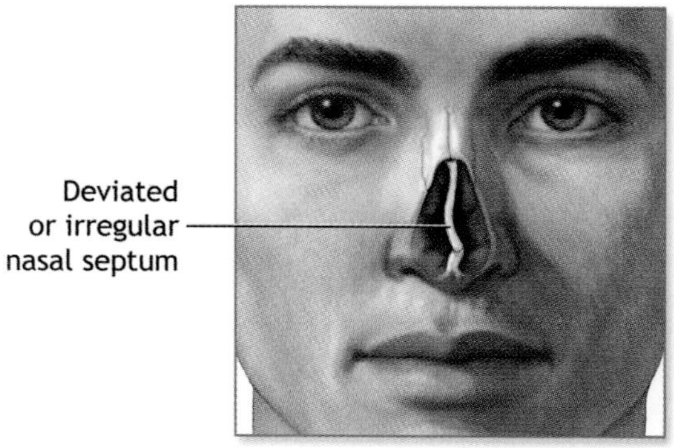

Occasionally, nosebleeds may indicate other disorders such as bleeding disorders or high blood pressure.

Blood thinners such as Coumadin or aspirin may cause or worsen nosebleeds.

Home care

Sit down and gently squeeze the soft portion of the nose between your thumb and finger (so that the nostrils are closed) for about 5-10 minutes. Lean forward to avoid swallowing the blood and breathe through your mouth. Wait at least 5 minutes before checking if the bleeding has stopped. Almost all nose bleeds can be controlled in this way if sufficient time is allowed for the bleeding to stop.

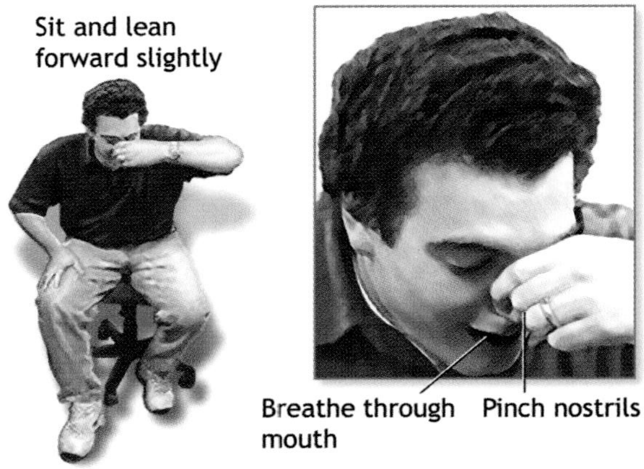

It may help to apply cold compresses or ice across the bridge of the nose. DO NOT pack the inside of the nose with gauze.

When to contact a medical professional

Get emergency care if:

- The bleeding does not stop after 20 minutes.
- A nosebleed occurs after an injury to the head – this may indicate a skull fracture. X-rays should be taken no matter how trivial the blow seemed to be at the time.
- Your nose may be broken (for example, it is misshapen after a blow or injury).

Call your doctor if you or your child has repeated nosebleeds, particularly if they are becoming more frequent and are not associated with a cold or other minor irritation.

Prevention

A cooler house and a vaporizer, to return humidity to the air, help many people with frequent nosebleeds. Nasal saline spray can help prevent nosebleeds, especially during the winter months.

Poisoning

For a POISON EMERGENCY call:

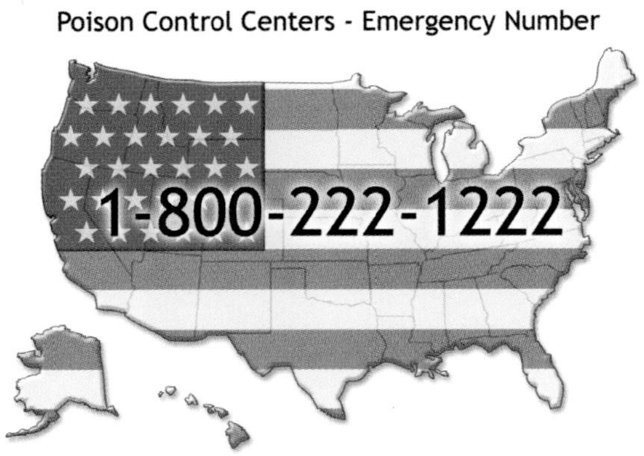

Poison Control Centers - Emergency Number
1-800-222-1222

This national hotline number will let you talk to experts in poisoning. This is a free and confidential service. All local poison control centers in the U.S. use this national number. You should call if you have any questions about poisoning or poison prevention. It does NOT need to be an emergency. You can call for any reason, 24 hours a day, 7 days a week.

Scrape

A scrape is an area where the skin is rubbed off, usually from falling down or hitting something. Scrapes are usually not serious, but can be painful. There may be mild bleeding.

When to contact a medical professional

Call your doctor if:

- The scrape contains deeply embedded debris.
- The scrape is very large.
- The scrape looks like it may be infected.

Signs of infection include warmth or red streaks at the injured site, pus, or a fever.

- You have not had a tetanus shot within 10 years.

First Aid

A scrape is often dirty. Even if you don't see visible dirt, the scrape can get infected. Make sure to clean the area thoroughly.

1. Wash your hands.
2. Wash the cut thoroughly with mild soap and water. (This is important, even when children cry and protest.)
3. Large pieces of dirt or debris should be removed with tweezers.
4. If available, apply antibiotic ointment.
5. If a small scrape is likely to get rubbed or dirty, apply a non-adhesive bandage. Otherwise let it air dry.
6. Larger scrapes, or scrapes that bleed more, should be covered with a gauze bandage. Ice can help reduce swelling. Do not apply ice directly to the skin.

Shock

Shock is a life-threatening condition that occurs when the body is not getting enough blood flow. This can damage multiple organs. Shock requires IMMEDIATE medical treatment and can get worse very rapidly.

Shock can be caused by any condition that reduces blood flow, including:

- Heart problems (such as heart attack or heart failure)
- Low blood volume (as with heavy bleeding or dehydration)
- Changes in blood vessels (as with infection or severe allergic reactions)

Shock is often associated with heavy external or internal bleeding from a serious injury. Spinal injuries can also cause shock.

Symptoms

A person in shock has extremely low blood pressure. Depending on the specific cause and type of shock, symptoms will include one or more of the following:

- Anxiety or agitation
- Confusion
- Pale, cool, clammy skin
- Low or no urine output
- Bluish lips and fingernails
- Dizziness, light-headedness, or faintness
- Profuse sweating, moist skin
- Rapid but weak pulse
- Shallow breathing
- Chest pain
- Unconsciousness

First Aid

- Call 911 for immediate medical help.
- Check the person's airway, breathing, and circulation. If necessary, begin rescue breathing and CPR.
- Even if the person is able to breathe on his or her own, continue to check rate of breathing at least every 5 minutes until help arrives.
- If the person is conscious and DOES NOT have an injury to the head, leg, neck, or spine, place the person in the shock position. Lay the person on the back and elevate the legs about 12 inches. DO NOT elevate the head. If raising the legs will cause pain or potential harm, leave the person lying flat.
- Give appropriate first aid for any wounds, injuries, or illnesses.
- Keep the person warm and comfortable. Loosen tight clothing.

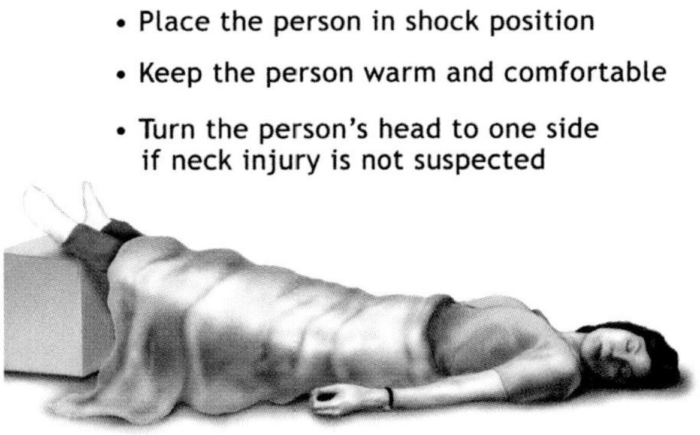

• Place the person in shock position
• Keep the person warm and comfortable
• Turn the person's head to one side if neck injury is not suspected

IF THE PERSON VOMITS OR DROOLS

- Turn the head to one side so he or she will not choke. Do this as long as there is NO suspicion of spinal injury.
- If a spinal injury is suspected, "log roll" him or her instead. Keep the person's head, neck and back in line and roll him or her as a unit.

Do not

- DO NOT give the person anything by mouth, including anything to eat or drink.
- DO NOT move the person with a known or suspected spinal injury.
- DO NOT wait for milder shock symptoms to worsen before calling for emergency medical help.

When to contact a medical professional

Call 911 any time a person has symptoms of shock. Stay with the person and follow the First Aid steps until medical help arrives.

Prevention

Learn ways to prevent heart disease, falls, injuries, dehydration, and other causes of shock. If you have a known allergy (for example, to insect bites or stings), carry an epinephrine pen. Your doctor will teach you how and when to use it.

Once someone is already in shock, the sooner shock is treated, the less damage there may be to the person's vital organs (like the kidney, liver, and brain). Early first aid and emergency medical help can save a life.

Spinal injuries

Your spinal cord contains the nerves that carry messages between your brain and body. The cord passes through your neck and back. A spinal cord injury is very serious because it can cause paralysis below the site of the injury.

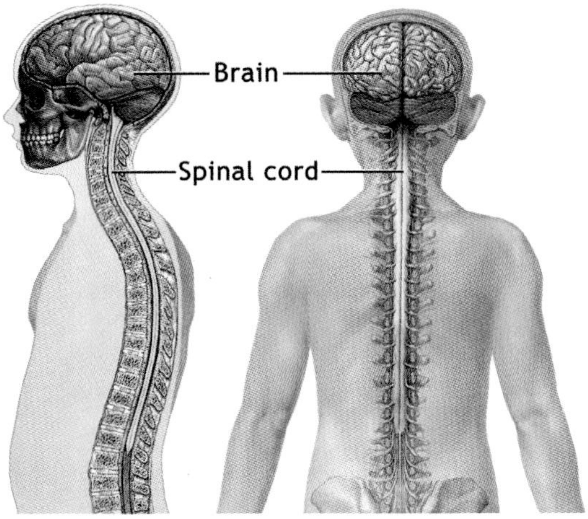

When someone has a spinal injury, additional movement may cause further damage to the nerves in the cord and can sometimes mean the difference between life and death.

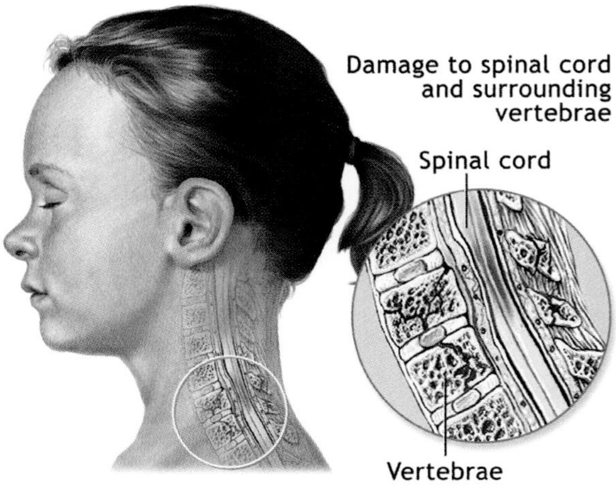

Moving a person with a neck injury may cause further damage to the nerves and spinal cord.

If you think someone could possibly have a spinal injury, DO NOT move the injured person even a little bit, unless it is absolutely necessary (like getting someone out of a burning car).

If you are in doubt about whether a person has a spinal injury, assume that he or she DOES have one.

Symptoms

- Major blow to the head or chest, car accident, fall from a great height
- Head held in unusual position
- Numbness or tingling that radiates down an arm or leg
- Weakness
- Difficulty walking
- Paralysis of arms or legs
- No bladder or bowel control
- Shock (pale, clammy skin; bluish lips and fingernails; acting dazed or semi-conscious)
- Unconscious
- Stiff neck, headache, or neck pain

First Aid

The main goal is to keep the person immobile and safe until medical help arrives.

1. You or someone else should call 911.
2. Hold the person's head and neck in the position in which they were found. DO NOT attempt to reposition the neck. Do not allow the neck to bend or twist.

IF THE PERSON IS UNRESPONSIVE

1. Check the person's breathing and circulation. If necessary, begin rescue breathing and CPR.
2. DO NOT tilt the head back when attempting to open the airway. Instead, place your fingers on the jaw on each side of the head. Lift the jaw forward.

IF YOU NEED TO ROLL THE PERSON

Do not roll the person over unless the person is vomiting or choking on blood, or you need to check for breathing.

1. Two people are needed.
2. One person should be stationed at the head, the other at the person's side.

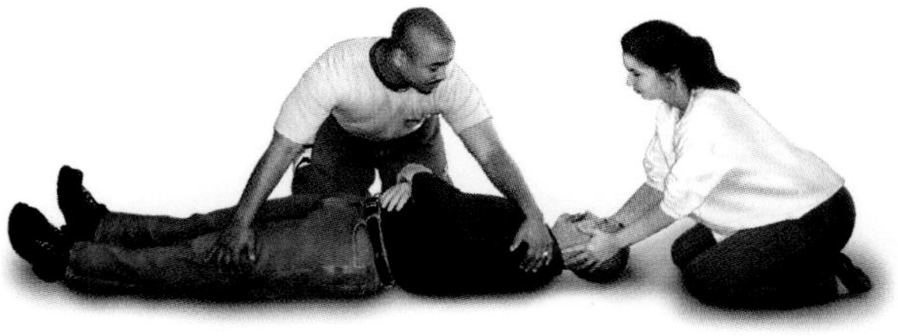

3. Keep the person's head, neck, and back in line with each other while you roll him or her onto one side.

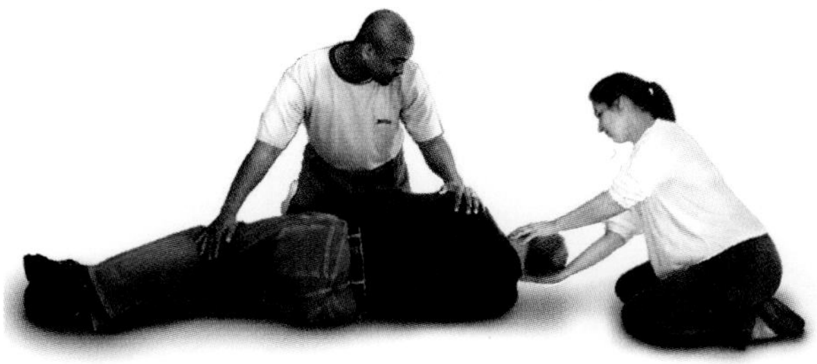

Do not

- DO NOT bend, twist, or lift the person's head or body.
- DO NOT attempt to move the person before medical help arrives unless it is absolutely necessary.
- DO NOT remove a helmet if a spinal injury is suspected.

Prevention

- Wear seat belts.
- Avoid drinking alcohol and driving.

- Avoid diving into pools, lakes, rivers and surf, particularly if you cannot determine the depth of the water, or if the water is not clear.
- Avoid motorcycles and all-terrain vehicles.
- Avoid "spearing" (tackling or diving into a person with your head).

Splinters

To remove a splinter:

1. Wash your hands with soap and water.
2. Use tweezers to grab the splinter. Carefully pull it out at the same angle it went in.

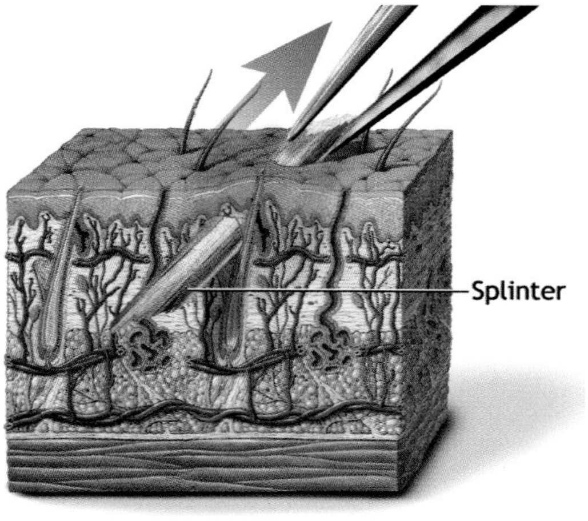

3. If the splinter is under the skin or hard to grab: Sterilize a pin or needle by soaking it in rubbing alcohol or placing the tip in a flame. Wash your hands with soap. Use the pin to gently remove skin over the splinter. Then use the tip of the pin to lift the end of the splinter out. You will probably still need to use tweezers as in step 2.
4. Wash the area with soap and water after the splinter is out. Pat it dry. (Don't rub.) Apply antibiotic ointment. Bandage the cut only if it is likely to get dirty. It will heal faster if exposed to the air.

See your doctor if there is inflammation or pus, or if the splinter is deeply embedded. Also, seek medical attention if the splinter is close to your eye.

Sprains

A sprain is an injury to the ligaments around a joint. Ligaments are strong, flexible fibers that hold bones together. When a ligament is stretched too far or tears, the joint will become painful and swell.

Sprains are caused when a joint is forced to move into an unnatural position. For example, "twisting" one's ankle causes a sprain to the ligaments around the ankle.

First aid

1. Apply ice immediately to help reduce swelling. Wrap the ice in cloth – DO NOT place ice directly on the skin.
2. Try NOT to move the affected area. To help you do this, bandage the affected area firmly, but not tightly. ACE bandages work well. Use a splint if necessary.
3. Keep the swollen joint elevated above the level of the heart, even while sleeping.
4. Rest the affected joint for several days.

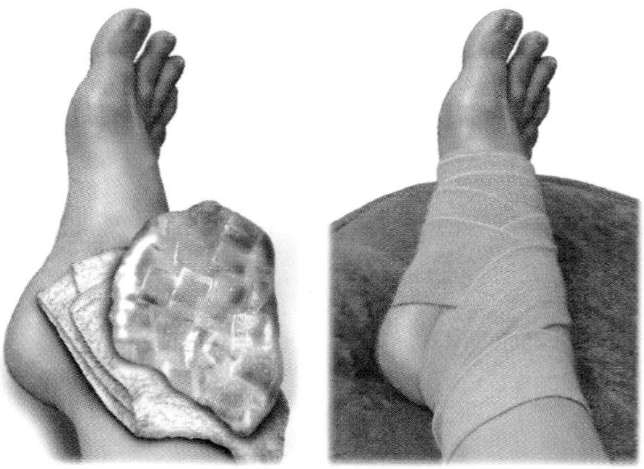

Remember the word "R.I.C.E." when treating an ankle sprain: rest, ice, compression, and elevation.

Ankle anatomy and ankle sprain

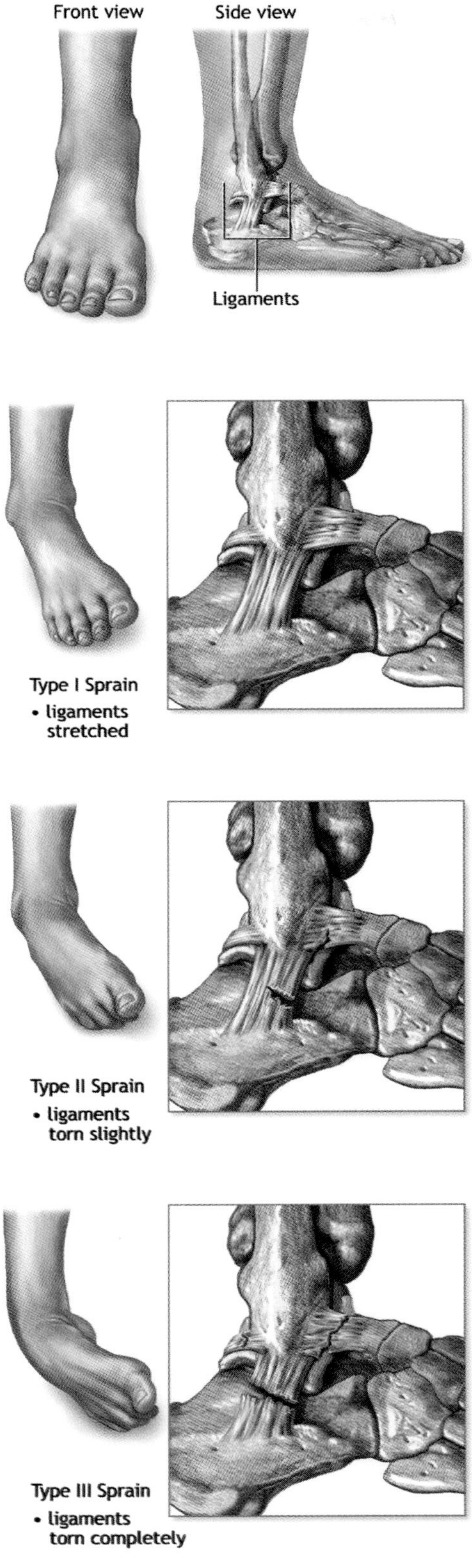

Aspirin, ibuprofen, or other pain relievers can help. DO NOT give aspirin to children.

Keep pressure off the injured area until the pain subsides (usually 7 to 10 days for mild sprains and 3 to 5 weeks for severe sprains). You may require crutches when walking.

When to contact a medical professional

Go to the hospital right away or call 911 if:

- You suspect a broken bone.
- The joint appears to be deformed.
- You have a serious injury or the pain is severe.
- There is an audible popping sound and immediate difficulty using the joint.

Call your doctor if:

- Swelling does not go down within 2 days.
- You have symptoms of infection – the area becomes redder, more painful, or warm, or you have a fever over 100°F.
- The pain does not go away after several weeks.

Two questions to ask yourself if you hurt your ankle

Are you able to put weight on your ankle immediately after the injury? Are you able to take 4 steps on the injured ankle pretty soon after you hurt it?

If the answer to these questions is "yes," there is a good chance you don't have a fracture and a trip to the ER may not be necessary to treat your ankle sprain. Call your doctor for further evaluation.

Prevention

- Wear protective footwear for activities that place stress on your ankle and other joints.
- Make sure that shoes fit your feet properly.

- Avoid high-heeled shoes.
- Always warm-up and stretch prior to exercise and sports.
- Avoid sports and activities for which you are not conditioned.

Strains

A strain is when a muscle becomes overstretched and tears. This painful injury, also called a "pulled muscle," can be caused by an accident, improper use of a muscle, or overuse of a muscle.

Symptoms

- Pain and difficulty moving the injured muscle
- Discolored and bruised skin
- Swelling

First aid

- Apply ice immediately to reduce swelling. Wrap the ice in cloth – avoid using ice directly on the skin. Apply ice for 10 to 15 minutes every 1 hour for the first day. Then, every 3 to 4 hours.
- Use ice for the first 3 days. After that, either heat or ice may be helpful.

Common locations of muscles strains in the leg

Hamstring muscles
(back of your thigh)

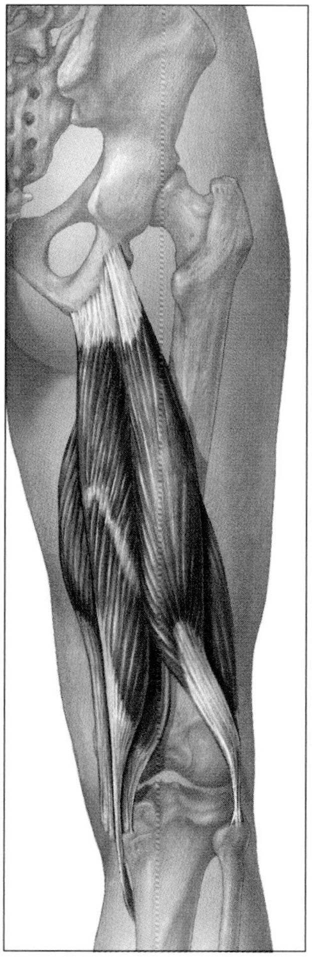

Quadricep muscles
(front of your thigh)

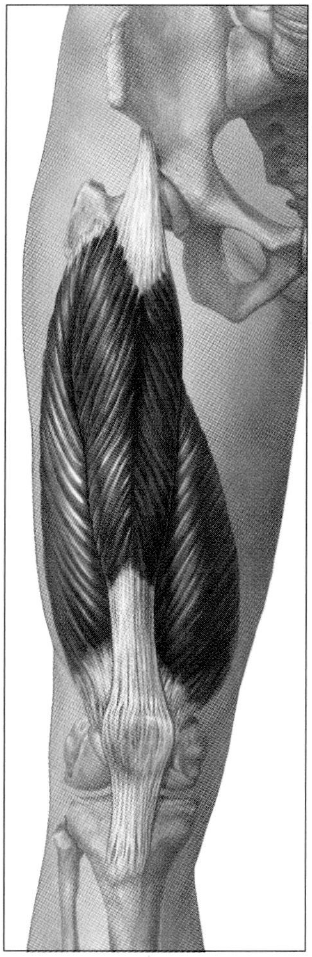

Groin muscles
(inner part of your thigh)

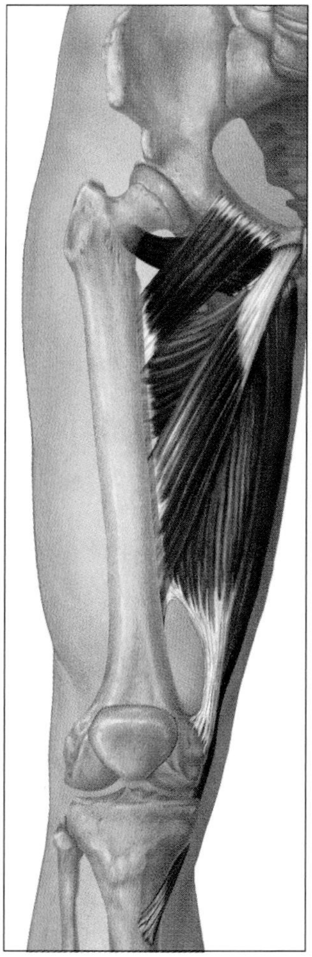

- Rest the pulled muscle for at least a day. If possible, keep the pulled muscle elevated above the level of the heart.
- Avoid using a strained muscle while it is still painful. When the pain subsides, start activity slowly and in moderation.

When to contact a medical professional

- You are unable to move the muscle.
- The injury is bleeding.
- The pain does not go away after several weeks.

Prevention

- Warm-up properly before exercise and sports. **See stretching exercises below**.
- Keep your muscles strong and flexible.

Triceps (back of arm) stretch

Bring an elbow across your body, towards the opposite shoulder, or raise your arm over your head and bend your elbow. Hold for 10-20 seconds, then switch sides.

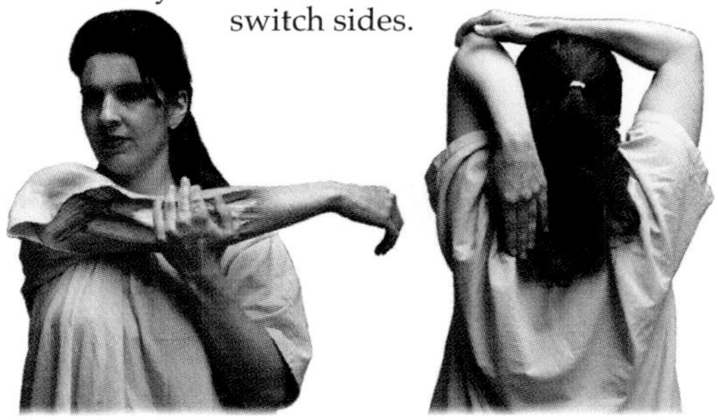

Chest and upper arm stretch

Clasp your hands behind your back with your palms facing up. Pull your hands down and press your shoulder blades together. Your chest should stick out. Hold for 10-20 seconds.

You should feel the stretch in your upper arms and chest.

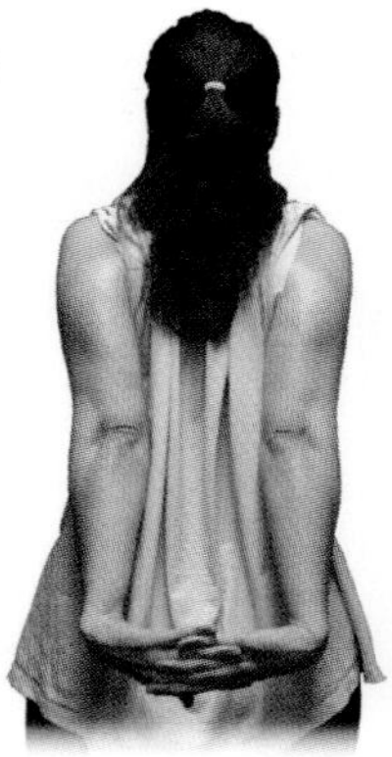

Quadricep stretch

Hold on to something for balance. Standing on one leg, grasp the foot of the other leg. Keep your knee pointing down. Pull up with light pressure. You do NOT need to pull up all the way to your buttocks.

Hold your foot behind you for 10-20 seconds, then switch sides. You should feel the stretch in the front of the thigh.

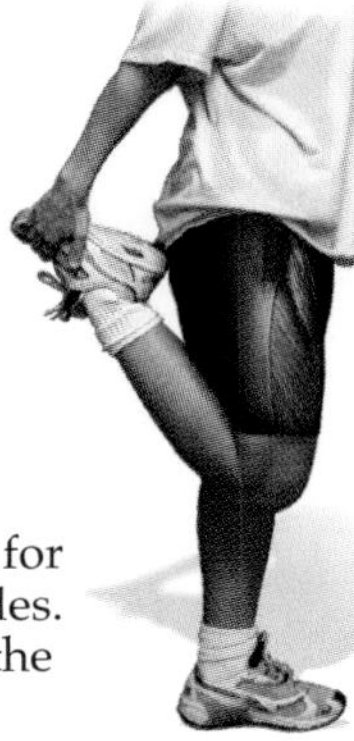

Hamstring stretch

Extend one leg in front of you with the foot flexed. Bend your other knee and lean back slightly. Your pelvis should be tilted forward. Keep your upper body upright as you hold the stretch for 10-20 seconds, then switch sides.

You should feel the stretch up the back of your extended leg (all the way up your calf and thigh).

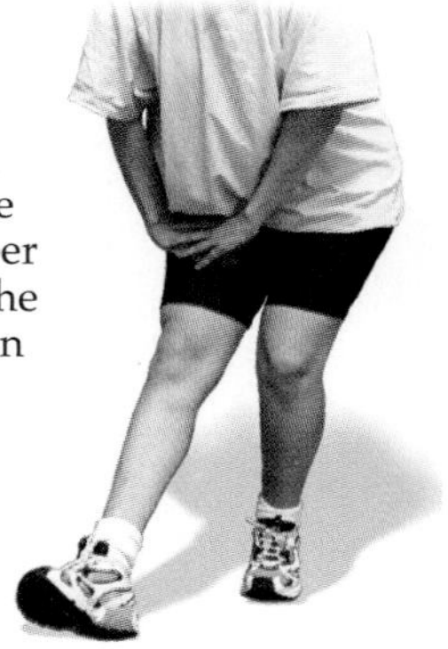

Groin stretch

Stand with your legs wide apart. Shift your weight to one side, bending your knee. Do not let your knee bend beyond your ankle. You should feel the stretch in your opposite leg, which remains extended. Both of your feet stay flat on the ground.

Hold for 10-20 seconds, then lean to the other side.

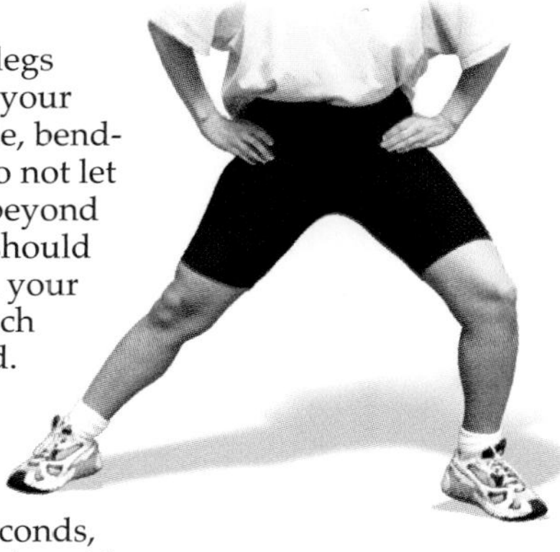

Hip stretch

Stand with one foot in front of you and your weight equally distributed between them. Bend both knees and lift your back heel off the ground. Bring your pelvis forward so your back is flat.

Hold for 10-20 seconds, then repeat on the other side. You should feel the stretch in the front of your hip and into your abdomen.

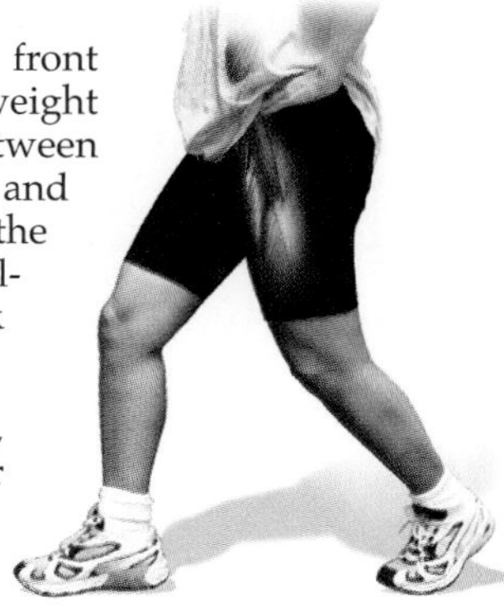

Sunburn

Sunburn is from over-exposure to the harmful ultraviolet rays of the sun. While the symptoms are usually temporary (such as red skin that is painful to the touch), the skin damage is often permanent and can have serious long-term health effects, including skin cancer.

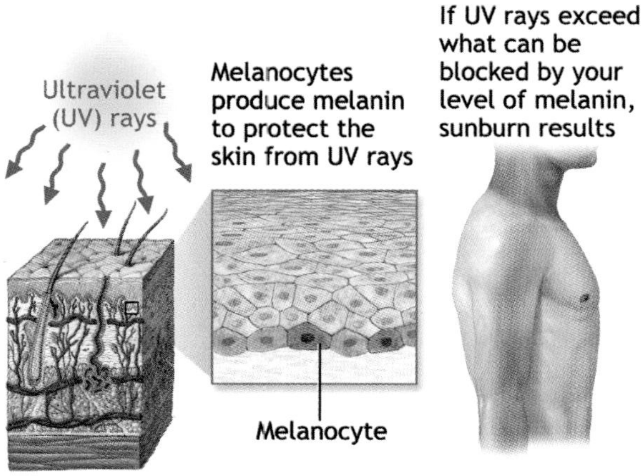
Ultraviolet (UV) rays
Melanocytes produce melanin to protect the skin from UV rays
If UV rays exceed what can be blocked by your level of melanin, sunburn results
Melanocyte

Keep in mind:

- Unprotected sun exposure causes premature aging of the skin.
- Sun exposure can cause first and second degree burns.
- Skin cancer usually appears in adulthood, but is caused by sun exposure and sunburns that began as early as childhood. You can help prevent skin cancer by protecting your skin and your children's skin from the harmful rays of the sun.

Examine your skin

As an adult, make sure you check your skin regularly for cancer. See *Skin Self-Exam* in the Screening and Checkups chapter for more information.

Factors that make sunburn more likely:

- Infants and children are especially sensitive to the burning effects of the sun.
- People with fair skin are more likely to get sunburn. But even dark and black skin can burn and should be protected.
- The sun's rays are strongest during the hours of 10:00 a.m. to 2:00 p.m. The sun's rays are also stronger at higher altitudes and lower latitudes (closer to the tropics). Reflection off water, sand, or snow can intensify the sun's burning rays.
- Sun lamps can cause severe sunburn.
- Some medications (such as the antibiotic doxycycline) can make you more susceptible to sunburn.

Symptoms

The first signs of a sunburn may not appear for a few hours. The full effect to your skin may not appear for 24 hours or longer. Possible symptoms include:

- Red, tender skin that is warm to touch.
- Blisters that develop hours to days later.
- Severe reactions (sometimes called "sun poisoning"), including fever, chills, nausea, or rash.
- Skin peeling on sunburned areas several days after the sunburn.

First Aid

- Try taking a cool bath or shower. Or place wet, cold wash cloths on the burn for 10 to 15 minutes, several times a day. You can mix baking soda in the water to help relieve the pain. (Small children may become easily chilled, so keep the water tepid.)
- Apply a soothing lotion to the skin.
- Aloe gel is a common household remedy for sunburns. Aloe contains active compounds that help stop pain and inflammation of the skin.
- An over-the-counter pain medication, such as acetaminophen or ibuprofen may be helpful. DO NOT give aspirin to children.

Do not

- DO NOT apply petroleum jelly, benzocaine, lidocaine, or butter to the sunburn. They make the symptoms worse and can prevent healing.
- DO NOT wash burned skin with harsh soap.

When to contact a medical professional

Call immediately if there are signs of shock, heat exhaustion, dehydration, or other serious reaction. These signs include:

- Feeling faint or dizzy
- Rapid pulse or rapid breathing
- Extreme thirst, no urine output, or sunken eyes
- Pale, clammy, or cool skin
- Nausea, fever, chills, or rash
- Your eyes hurt and are sensitive to light
- Severe, painful blisters

Prevention

- Avoid sun exposure during hours of peak sun ray intensity.
- Apply generous amounts of sunscreen with a sun protection factor (SPF) of at least 30. Pay special attention to your face, nose, ears, and shoulders. The higher the SPF, the greater the protection.
- Apply sunscreen 30 minutes prior to sun exposure to allow penetration. Re-apply after swimming and every 2 hours while you are outdoors.
- Wear sun hats. There is also SPF clothing and swimwear available.
- Wear sunglasses with UV protection.
- Use a lip balm with sunscreen.

Tooth - broken or knocked out

Save any tooth that has been knocked out for possible reimplantation. Bring it to your dentist as soon as possible. The longer you wait, the less chance there is for successful reimplantation. Handle the tooth only by the crown (chewing edge).

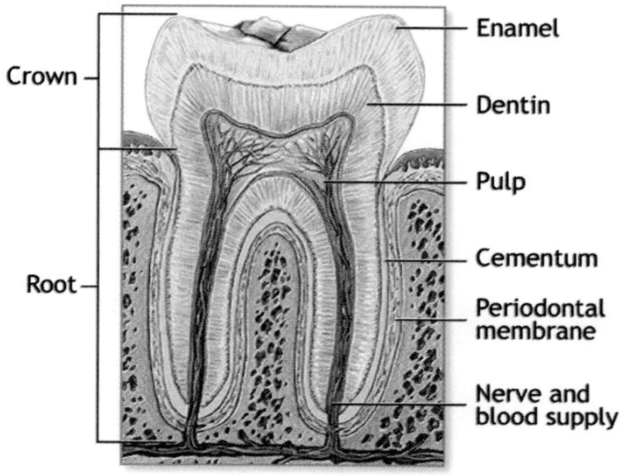

Use one of the following options to transport the tooth:

1. Try to replace the tooth in the socket, to the level of adjacent teeth. Bite down gently on gauze or a wet tea bag to help keep it in place. The surrounding teeth can be used as anchors. Care must be taken not to swallow the tooth.

2. If the tooth cannot be replaced in the socket, place it in a container and cover with a small amount of whole milk or saliva. The tooth can also be carried between lower lip and lower gum or under the tongue.

3. The Save-A-Tooth storage device can be purchased at many pharmacies. It contains a travel case and fluid solution. Consider buying one for your home first aid kit.

For additional first aid, follow these steps:

1. Apply a cold compress to the mouth and gums for pain.

2. Apply direct pressure, using gauze, to control bleeding.

3. Get dental help immediately. The sooner dental attention is received, the better the chances are for successful reimplantation.

Teeth that have been badly fractured may expose nerve tissue inside the tooth. In this case, immediate attention is needed to avoid infection, abscess, and pain.

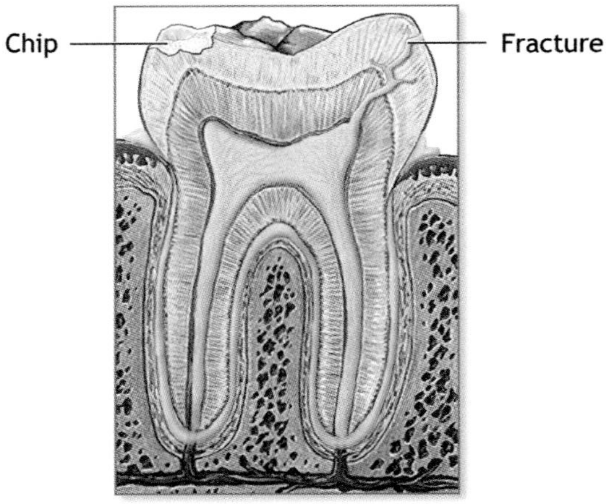

Simple chips or fractures may be tended to on a non-emergency basis, but should still be fixed to avoid sharp edges that can cut the lips or tongue, and for cosmetic reasons.

Do not

1. DO NOT handle the roots of the tooth. Handle only the chewing edge – the crown portion of the tooth.

2. DO NOT scrape the root of the tooth to remove dirt.

When to contact a medical professional

See a dentist immediately if:

- A permanent tooth has been knocked out.
- A tooth has been partially fractured and pain and swelling results.

In the case of simple tooth fractures, a non-emergency dental appointment can be made.

After a major accident, if you are not able to bring your upper and lower teeth together, the jaw may be broken. This requires immediate attention. You may call a dentist, but also seek help at a hospital.

Prevention

- Wear a mouth guard when playing any contact sport.
- Avoid fights.
- Avoid hard foods, such as bones, stale bread, and tough bagels.
- Always wear a seatbelt.

Teeth in children and adults

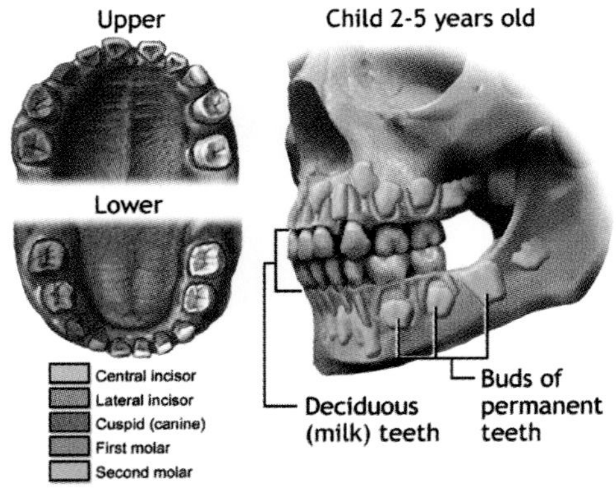

Children have 20 "baby" teeth.

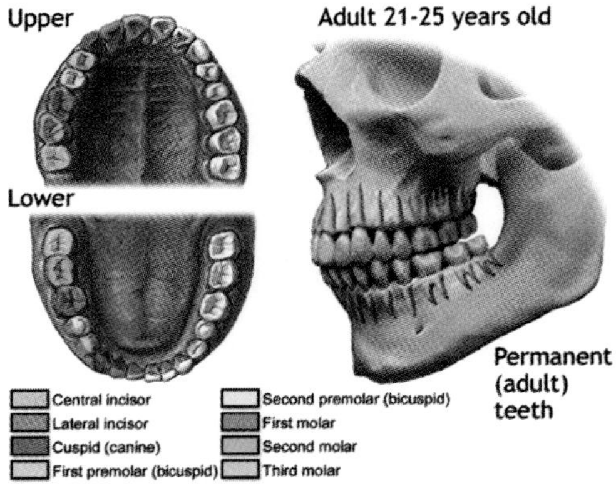

Adults have 32 permanent teeth.

Unconsciousness

Unconsciousness is when a person is unable to respond to people and other stimuli around him or her. Often, this is called a coma or being in a comatose state.

Other changes in awareness can occur without becoming unconscious. Medically, these are called "Altered Mental Status" or "Changed Mental Status." They include sudden confusion, disorientation, or stupor.

Unconsciousness and any other SUDDEN change in mental status must be treated as a medical emergency.

If someone is awake but less alert than usual, ask a few simple questions – What is your name? What is the date? How old are you? If the person doesn't know or answers incorrectly, then his or her mental status is diminished.

Being asleep is not the same thing as being unconscious. A sleeping person will respond to loud noises or gentle shaking – an unconscious person will not.

An unconscious person cannot cough or clear his or her throat. This can lead to death if the airway becomes obstructed.

First aid

1. Call or instruct someone to call 911.

2. Check the person's airway, breathing, and circulation frequently. If necessary, begin rescue breathing and CPR.

3. If the person is breathing, and a spinal injury is NOT suspected, and he is lying on his back, carefully roll him toward you onto his side. Bend the top leg so both hip and knee are at right angles. Gently tilt the head back to keep the airway open. If breathing or circulation stops at any time, roll the person on to his back and begin CPR.

4. If a spinal injury is suspected, leave the person as he was found (as long as he is breathing freely). If spinal injury is suspected and the person vomits, "log roll" the person to his side. Support the neck and back to keep head and body in the same position while you roll.

Recovery position

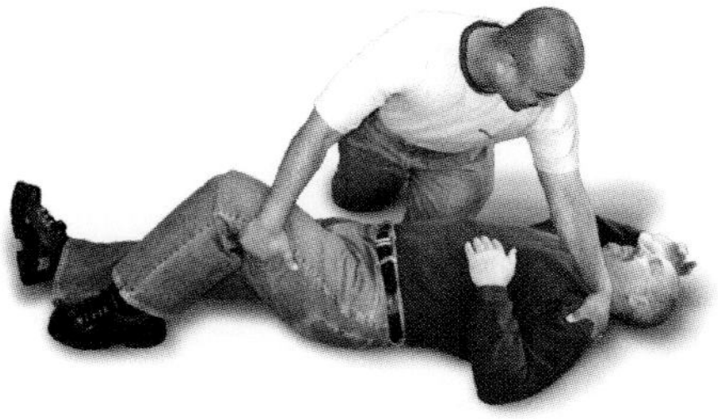

Carefully roll the person towards you.

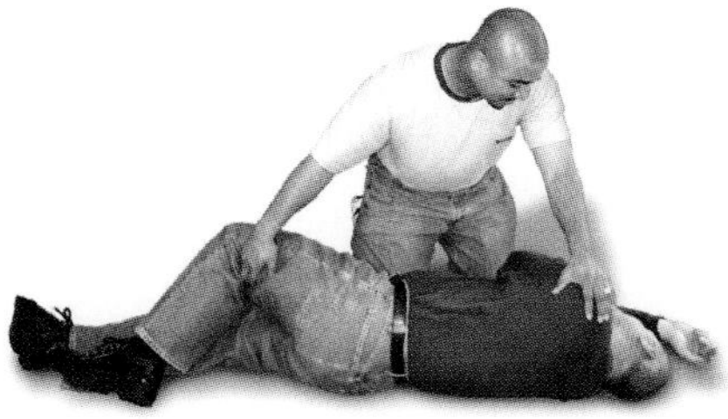

Bend the person's top leg so his/her hip and knee are at right angles.

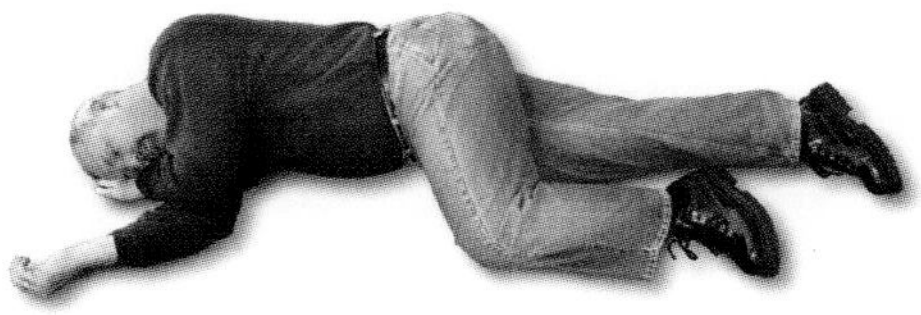

Recovery position supports the head, keeps the airway open, and doesn't stress joints.

5. Keep the person warm until medical help arrives.
6. If you witness a person fainting, try to prevent him or her from falling. Lie the person flat on the floor and elevate the feet about 12 inches.
7. If fainting is likely due to low blood sugar, have the person eat or drink something sweet when he or she fully regains consciousness.

Do not

- DO NOT give an unconscious person any food or drink.
- DO NOT leave the person alone.
- DO NOT place a pillow under the head of an unconscious person.
- DO NOT slap an unconscious person's face or splash water on the face to try to revive him.

When to contact a medical professional

Call 911 if the person:

- Is not breathing.
- Does not regain consciousness quickly (within a couple of minutes).
- Fell from a height or has been injured, especially if bleeding.
- Has diabetes.
- Is pregnant or is over 50 years old.
- Feels chest pain, chest pressure, chest discomfort, or has a pounding or irregular heartbeat.
- Can't speak, has vision problems, or can't move a limb.
- Has convulsions, tongue trauma, or loss of bowel control.

Prevention

- People with known medical conditions, such as diabetes, should always wear a medical alert tag or bracelet.
- Avoid situations where your blood sugar level gets too low.
- Avoid standing in one place too long without moving, especially if prone to fainting.
- If you feel like you are about to faint, lie down or sit with your head bent forward between you knees.

Whiplash

Whiplash is when the soft tissues of the neck are injured by a sudden jerking or "whipping" of the head. This type of motion strains the muscles and ligaments of the neck beyond their normal range of motion.

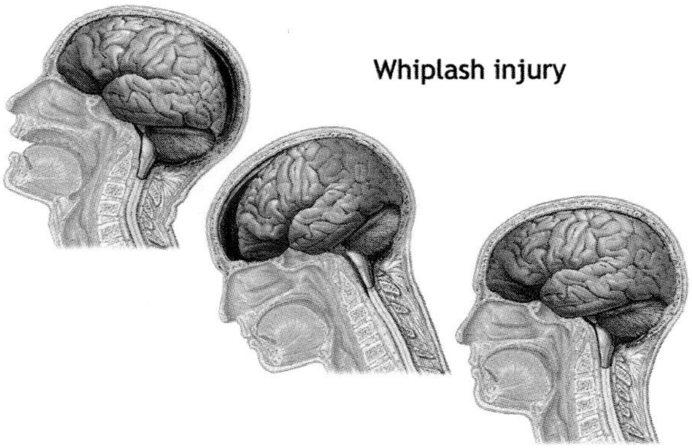

When a vehicle stops suddenly in a crash or is struck from behind, a seat belt will keep a person's body from being thrown forward. But the head may snap forward, then backward, causing whiplash.

In addition to car accidents, whiplash can be caused by roller coasters and other amusement park rides, sports injuries, or being punched or shaken. (Whiplash is one of the hallmarks of shaken baby syndrome.)

Symptoms

You may feel pain and stiffness in your neck for the first few days following a whiplash injury. Then you feel better, but the pain and stiffness may come back several days later.

The discomfort you feel may involve surrounding muscle groups in your head, chest, shoulders, and arms.

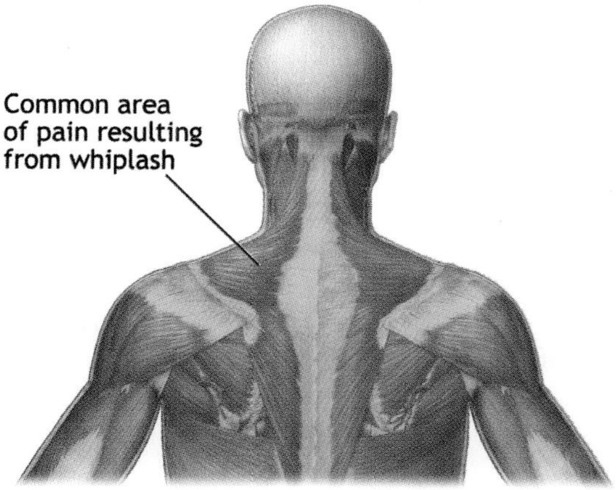

First aid

- Try over-the-counter pain relievers like aspirin, acetaminophen, or ibuprofen.
- For at least 2 to 3 weeks, avoid activities that bring on or worsen your pain and stiffness. Don't lift or carry anything heavy or participate in sports.
- If you have pain when you move your head or the pain involves your shoulders or arms, your doctor may recommend a soft neck collar or short-term prescription drug to relax the muscles.

When to contact a medical professional

Call your doctor if:

- Neck pain and stiffness comes back after it had resolved.
- The pain spreads to your shoulders or arms.
- You have pain when you move your head.

Prevention

Headrests in your car can reduce the severity of neck pain from a car accident. Make sure that the headrest is positioned properly for your height.

If you do get whiplash, learn proper stretching exercises once your neck has healed. This reduces the chance that neck pain or stiffness will come back.

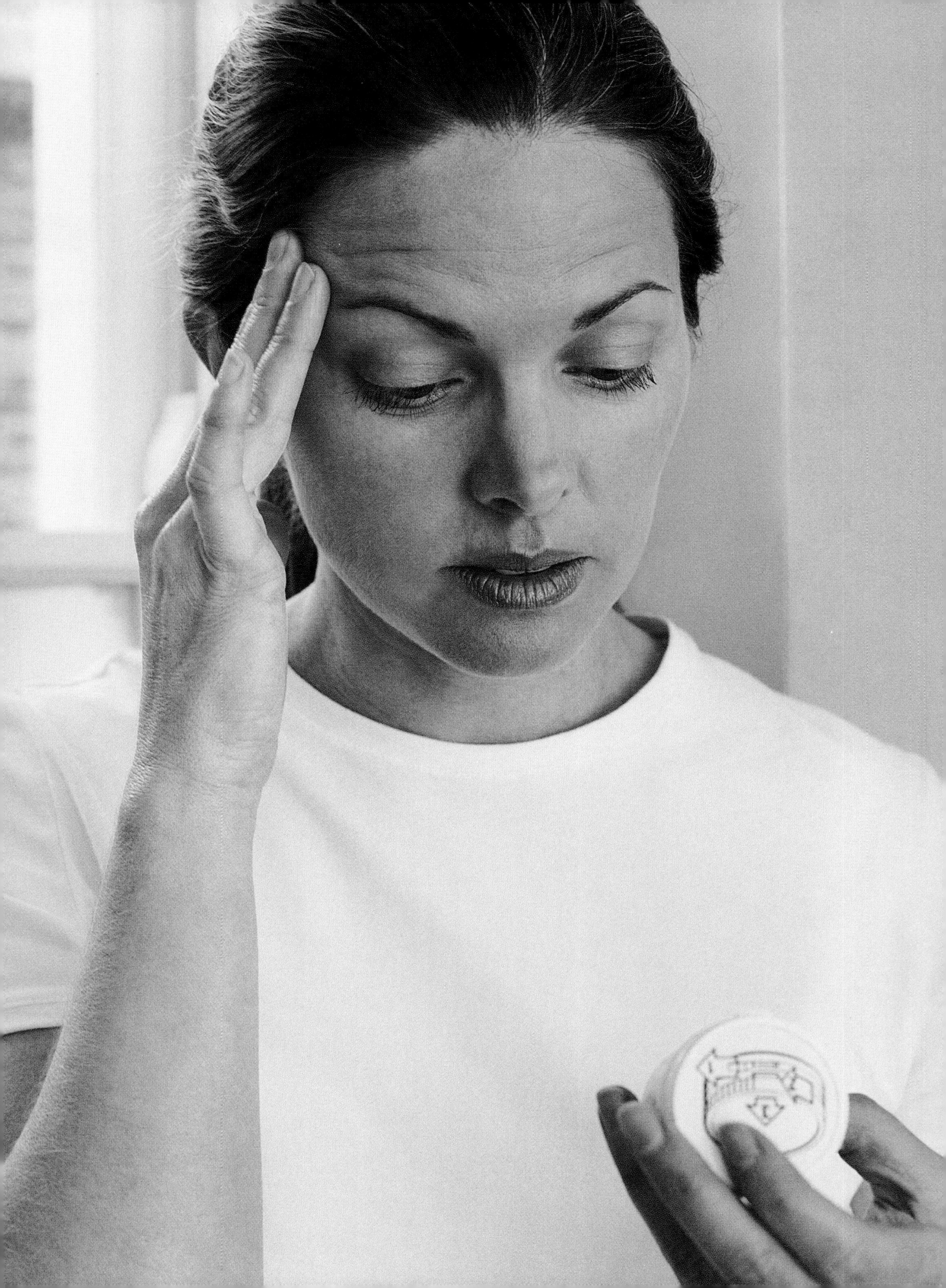

SYMPTOMS AND CONDITIONS

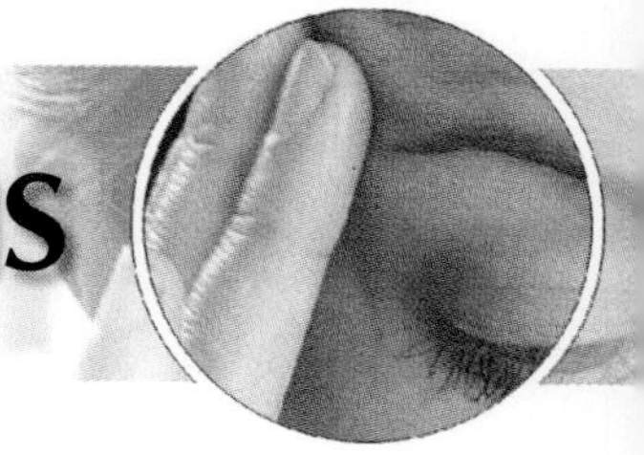

ABDOMINAL PAIN

Abdominal pain is pain that you feel anywhere between your chest and groin. This is often referred to as the stomach region or belly.

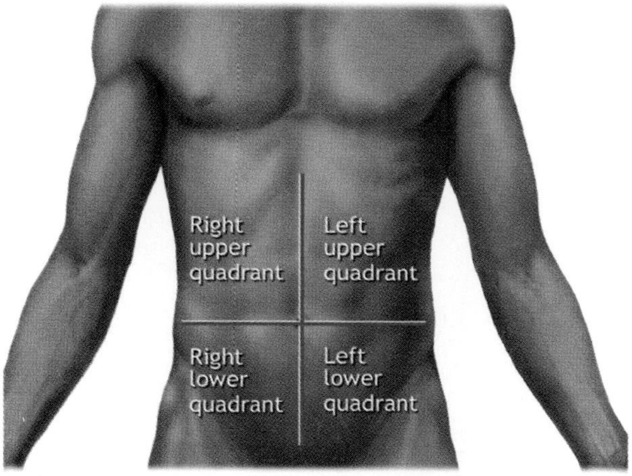

The abdomen (belly region) can be divided into four quadrants to describe the location of pain.

The intensity of the pain does not always reflect the seriousness of the condition causing the pain. Severe abdominal pain can be from mild conditions, such as gas or the cramping of viral gastroenteritis. On the other hand, relatively mild pain or no pain may be present with life-threatening conditions, such as cancer of the colon or early appendicitis.

Many different conditions can cause abdominal pain. The key is to know when you must seek medical care right away. In many cases you can simply wait, use home care remedies, and call your doctor at a later time only if the symptoms persist.

In infants, prolonged unexplained crying (often called "colic") may be caused by abdominal pain that may end with the passage of gas or stool. Colic is often worse in the evening. Cuddling and rocking the child may bring some relief.

HOME CARE

For mild pains:

- Sip water or other clear fluids.
- Avoid solid food for the first few hours. If there has been vomiting, wait 6 hours. Then, eat small amounts of mild foods.
- If the pain is high up in your abdomen and occurs after meals, antacids may provide some relief, especially if you feel heartburn or indigestion. Avoid citrus, high-fat foods, fried or greasy foods, tomato products, caffeine, alcohol, and carbonated beverages. You may also try H2 blockers (Tagamet, Pepcid, or Zantac) available over the counter. If any of these medicines worsen your pain, CALL your doctor right away.
- AVOID aspirin, ibuprofen, and narcotic pain medications unless your health care provider prescribes them. If you know that your pain is not related to your liver, you can try acetaminophen (Tylenol).

WHEN TO CONTACT A MEDICAL PROFESSIONAL

Call 911 if you:

- Have sudden, sharp abdominal pain
- Have chest, neck, or shoulder pain
- Are vomiting blood or have blood in your stool (especially if maroon or dark, tarry black)
- Have a rigid, hard abdomen that is tender to touch

- Are unable to pass stool, especially if you are also vomiting

Call your doctor if you have:

- Bloating that persists for more than 2 days
- Diarrhea for more than 5 days
- Abdominal discomfort that lasts one week or longer
- Fever (over 100°F for adults or 100.4°F for children) with your pain
- A burning sensation when you urinate or frequent urination
- Pain in your shoulder blades and nausea
- Pain with menstruation
- Pain that develops during pregnancy (or possible pregnancy)
- Pain that worsens when you take antacids or eat something
- Prolonged poor appetite
- Unexplained weight loss

Should I go to the emergency room?

Many cases of abdominal pain are NOT emergencies. (See When to Contact a Medical Professional in this article.) Remember that people with non-urgent problems often have to wait several hours or longer before being seen at an emergency room.

Prevention

- Eat small meals more frequently.
- Make sure that your meals are well-balanced and high in fiber. Eat plenty of fruits and vegetables.
- Limit foods that produce gas.
- Drink plenty of water each day.
- Exercise regularly.

For prevention of symptoms from heartburn or gastroesophageal reflux disease:

Serious causes of abdominal pain

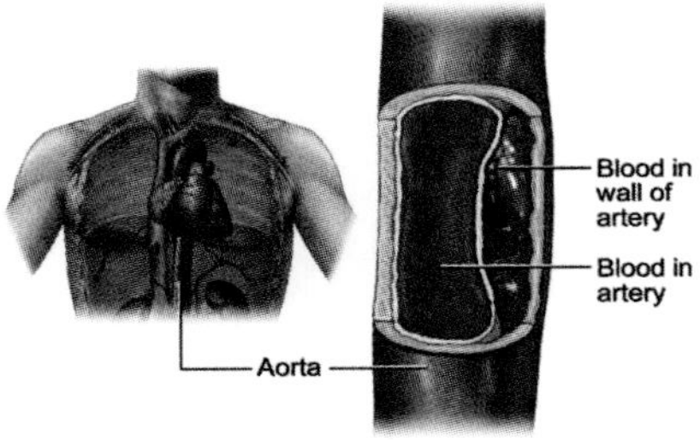

Aortic dissection

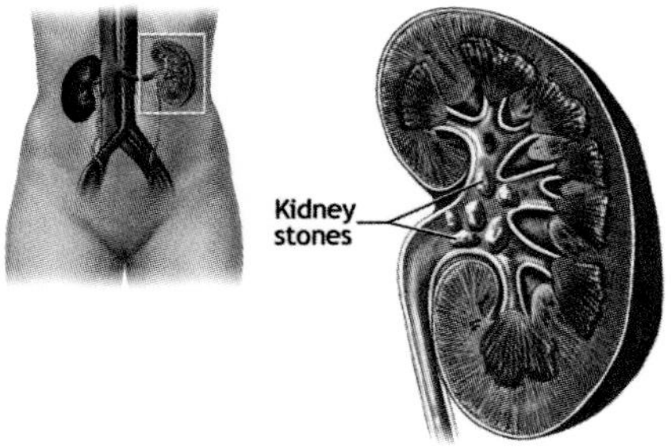

Kidney stones

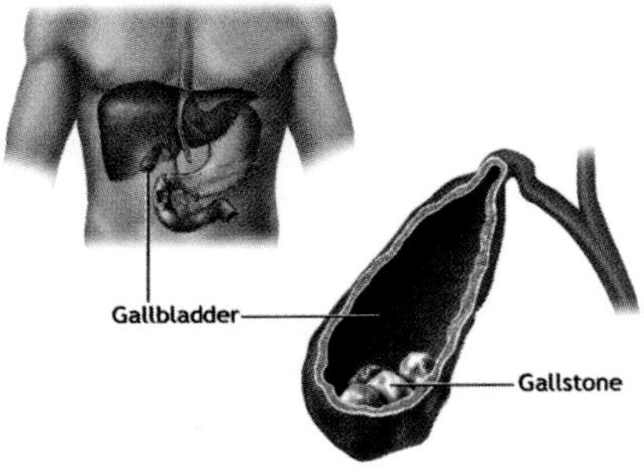

Gallstones

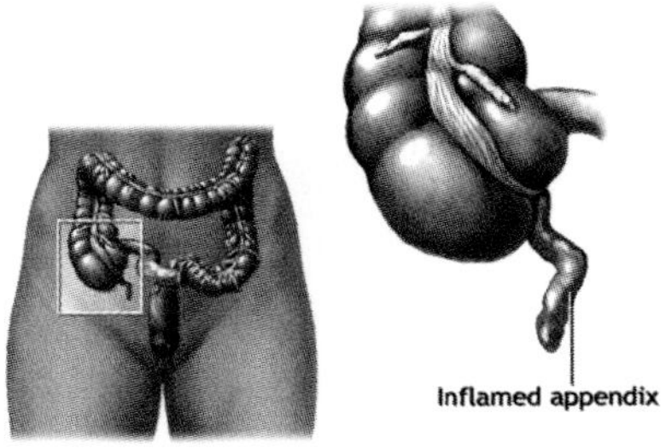

Appendicitis

- Quit smoking.
- Lose weight if you need to.
- Finish eating at least 2 hours before you go to bed.
- After eating, stay upright for at least 30 minutes.
- Elevate the head of your bed.

Acne

Acne is a skin condition characterized by whiteheads, blackheads, and inflamed red pimples ("zits").

Facial acne

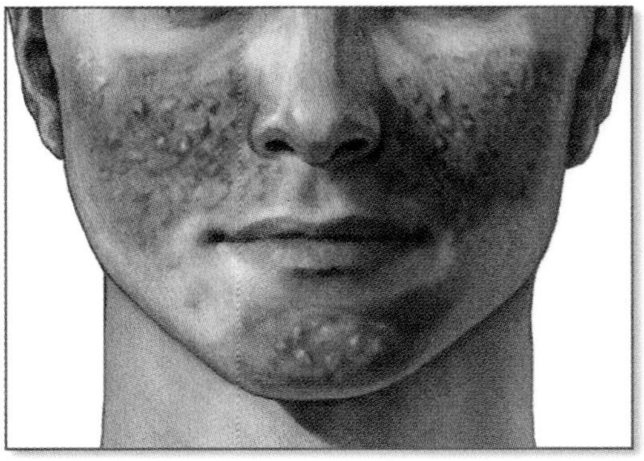

The condition occurs when tiny holes on the surface of the skin, called pores, become plugged. Each pore is an opening to a canal called a follicle, which contains a hair and an oil gland.

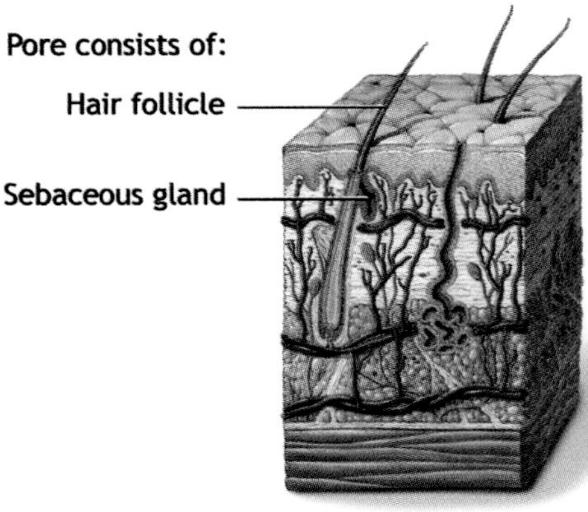

Enlarged cut-section of skin

Normally, the oil glands help keep the skin lubricated and help remove old skin cells. When glands produce too much oil, the pores can become blocked, accumulating dirt, debris, and bacteria. The blockage or plug is often called a comedone.

The top of the plug may be white (whitehead) or dark (blackhead). If the comedone ruptures, the material inside, including oil and bacteria, can spread to the surrounding area and cause an inflammatory reaction. If the inflammation is deep in your skin, the pimples may enlarge to form firm, painful cysts.

Acne commonly appears on the face and shoulders, but may also occur on the trunk, arms, legs, and buttocks.

Acne is most common in teenagers, but it can happen at an age, even as an infant. Three out of four teenagers have acne to some extent, probably caused by hormonal changes that stimulate oil production. It may persist into a person's 30's and 40's.

Acne tends to run in families and can be triggered by:

- Hormonal changes related to menstrual periods, pregnancy, birth control pills, or stress
- Greasy or oily cosmetic and hair products
- Certain drugs (such as steroids, testosterone, estrogen, and phenytoin)
- High levels of humidity and sweating

Despite the popular belief that chocolate, nuts, and other foods cause acne, this does not seem to be true.

Home care

Take the following self-care steps to lessen the effects of acne:

- Clean your skin gently with a mild, nondrying soap (like Dove, Neutrogena, or Basics). Remove all dirt or make-up. Wash once or twice a day, including after exercising. However, avoid excessive or repeated skin washing.

- Shampoo your hair daily, especially if it's oily. Comb or pull your hair back to keep the hair out of your face. Avoid tight headbands.
- Try not to squeeze, scratch, pick, or rub the pimples. Although it might be tempting to do this, it can lead to scarring and skin infections.
- Avoid touching your face with your hands or fingers.
- Avoid greasy cosmetics or creams. Look for water-based or "non-comedogenic" formulas. Take make-up off at night.

If these steps do not clear up the blemishes to an acceptable level, try over-the-counter acne medications. These creams and lotions are applied directly to the skin. They may contain benzoyl peroxide, sulfur, resorcinol, or salicylic acid. They work by killing bacteria, drying up the oil, and causing your skin to peel.

If the pimples are still a problem, a dermatologist can prescribe stronger medications and discuss other options with you.

Remember...

When treating acne, start with the most gentle treatments first. Self-care steps often work. But if they don't, see your doctor or dermatologist about medication. Even then, simpler is better. Newer medications tend to be much more expensive – and are NOT necessarily better.

Allergies

Your body's immune system is designed to attack harmful substances, like bacteria and viruses. But in the case of allergies, your body launches an assault on substances that are basically harmless – such as pollen, mold, dust mites, pet dander, food, latex, or medications.

Just about any substance that you inhale, swallow, or touch can cause allergy symptoms. If you are allergic to something in the air, you may develop sneezing, congestion, and itchy eyes.

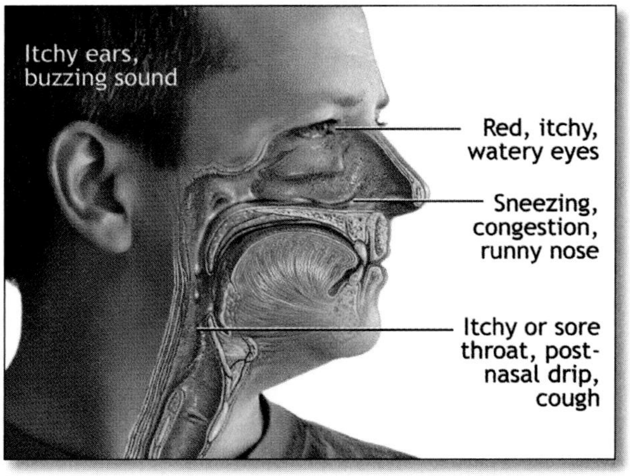

Allergies can also cause skin-related symptoms (such as hives, eczema, and rashes) and even gastrointestinal problems.

In addition, allergies can aggravate or trigger other conditions, such as asthma, sinusitis, and ear infections. When allergies cause inflammation in your nasal passages, the opening to your sinuses can become blocked, leading to sinus inflammation and pain. Similarly, if allergies cause inflammation in your ear canal, the ears don't drain properly, which can lead to ear infections.

Your first step towards feeling better on a daily basis is to avoid the things that cause your allergic reactions.

Avoid allergy triggers

Here is a list of common culprits and how to avoid them:

- **Pollen** – Obviously, pollen is hard to avoid, but you can probably minimize some of your exposure. Stay indoors on high pollen days, or wear a face mask while doing outdoor activities like yard work. Have someone without allergies cut the grass. Take a shower after coming indoors. Change your clothes and wash them. Don't dry clothing on an outdoor clothesline. Keep doors and windows closed, and use the air conditioner if you can. (This applies while you're riding in a car as well.)

- **Dust mites** – Encase mattresses, box springs, and pillows with mite-proof covers. Wash bedding once a week in hot water. Replace upholstered furniture with wooden, leather, or vinyl alternatives. Try to keep the indoor humidity level lower than 50%. Remove clutter and stuffed animals from bedrooms. Wipe dust with a damp cloth and vacuum (using a HEPA filter) weekly. Replace wall-to-wall carpet with hardwood or other flooring – though costly, this can significantly reduce dust mite populations in your home.

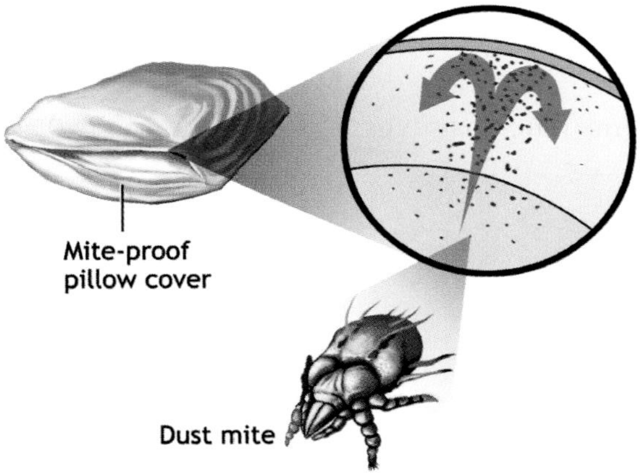

- **Mold spores** – Keep doors and windows closed, use the air conditioner, and try to keep the indoor humidity less than 50%. Keep sinks and tubs dry and clean, and fix leaky pipes. Clean the refrigerator tray when necessary. Use an exhaust fan in the bathroom while showering. Avoid putting damp clothes into a basket or hamper.
- **Pet dander** – The most important step is to try to keep your pet out of the bedroom, or at least off beds and linens. Since you lie in a bed all night long, you definitely don't want allergens accumulating on your bedding. Try to keep pets off upholstered furniture and carpets. If you have a central air conditioning system, consider installing a HEPA filter to remove airborne pet dander. Vacuum cleaners with HEPA filters may help. If these measures don't work, you may have to consider finding your pet a new home.
- **Tobacco or wood smoke** – Don't allow smoking in the house or car. Encourage family members and friends to stop smoking around you. Avoid using fireplaces. If you need to burn wood, use an air-tight woodburning stove.

Role of your immune system

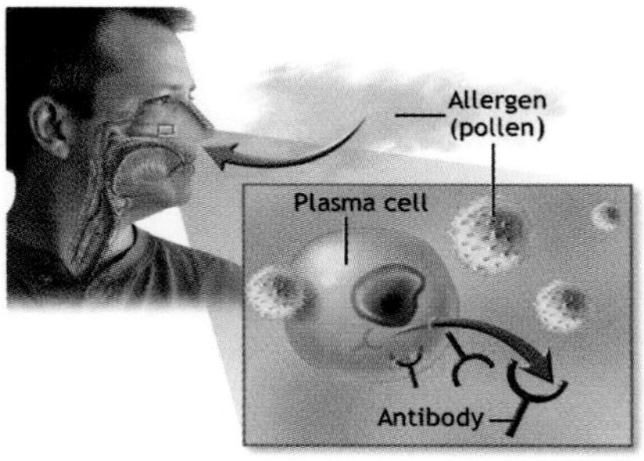

The first time you breathe in pollen, your body identifies it as a "foreign invader". Plasma cells make large amounts of antibodies against it.

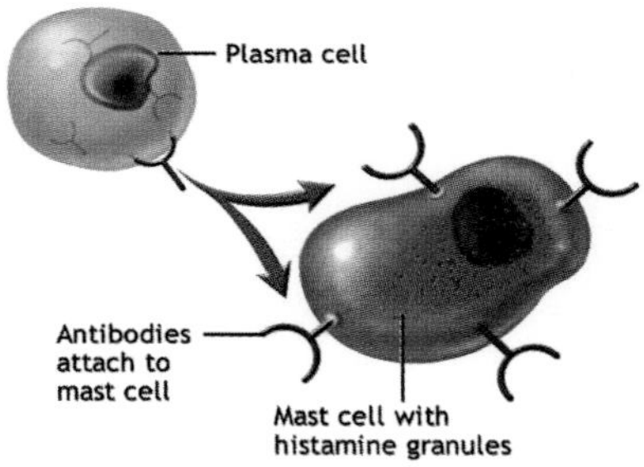

The antibodies attach to mast cells. Your body is now "primed" and ready for future pollen encounters.

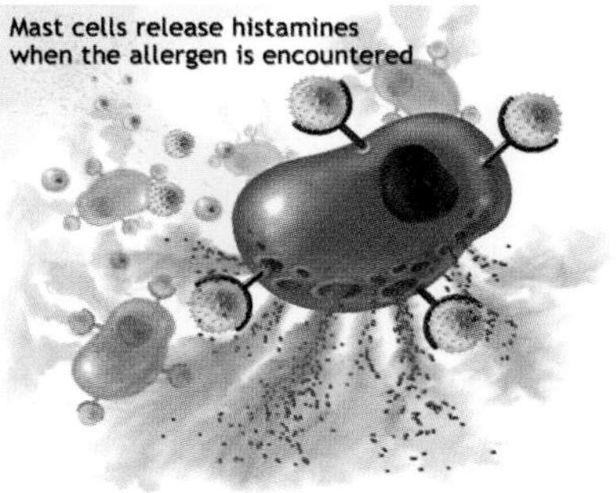

The next time you breathe in pollen, the antibodies "grab" the pollen and signal the mast cells to release chemicals that cause sneezing and a runny nose to remove the pollen.

Non-prescription medication

If you still have symptoms despite your efforts to avoid allergy triggers, try non-prescription (over-the-counter) medication. Antihistamines are a main ingredient in most allergy medications. The main goal of these drugs is to stop the histamine reaction that causes swelling, itching, and mucus production during an allergic reaction.

However, many non-prescription antihistamines have drawbacks. They relieve mild or moderate symptoms but are short-acting and can cause drowsiness. In fact, diphenhydramine can impair a person's motor skills as much as alcohol! These antihistamines can also blunt learning in children (even in the absence of drowsiness).

Fortunately, there are good alternatives. One long-acting antihistamine called loratadine (Alavert, Claritin) does NOT tend to cause drowsiness or interfere with learning. Loratadine was formerly a prescription medicine that is now available over-the-counter.

Cromolyn sodium nasal spray is an anti-inflammatory medication that can be used to treat and sometimes prevent hay fever symptoms. It works by preventing the release of histamine. Cromolyn nasal spray is available over-the-counter and is gentle and effective. It usually takes a few days to start working. Eyedrop versions are available for itchy, bloodshot eyes.

Medicines that cause drowsiness

Many over-the-counter allergy medicines cause drowsiness. This can affect children's learning abilities, and make it unsafe for adults to drive or operate heavy machinery. (It is like being drunk.) There is good news, however. You can now get non-sedating antihistamines over-the counter, without a prescription. Look for loratadine as the main ingredient.

When to contact a medical professional

Talk to your doctor about allergy control and treatment options if:

- Your allergy symptoms significantly interfere with your life
- You or anyone in your family has had a life-threatening allergic reaction in the past

A doctor can also conduct tests to pinpoint what causes your allergies. The results of your allergy tests tell you what substances you need to avoid.

Alzheimer's disease

Alzheimer's disease (AD), one form of dementia, is a progressive, degenerative brain disease. It impairs memory, thinking, and behavior.

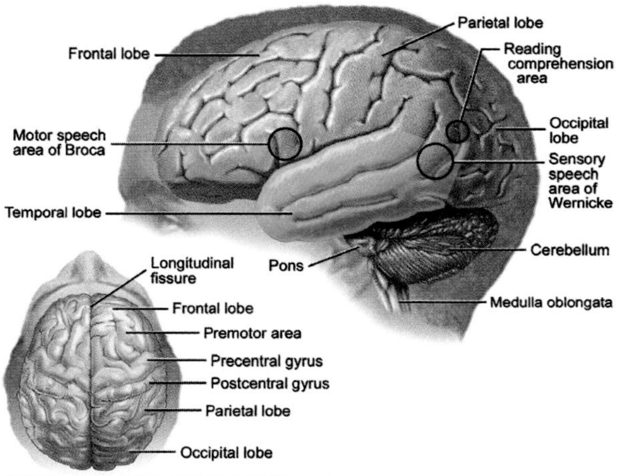

Specific areas of the brain control functions such as speech, reading comprehension, memory, and muscular coordination and movement.

As many as 4 million Americans currently have AD. The older you get, the greater your risk of developing AD, although it is not a part of normal aging. Family history is another common risk factor.

Symptoms

In the early stages, the symptoms of AD may be subtle and resemble signs that people mistakenly attribute to "natural aging." Symptoms often include:

- Repeating statements
- Misplacing items
- Having trouble finding names for familiar objects
- Getting lost on familiar routes
- Personality changes
- Losing interest in things previously enjoyed
- Difficulty performing tasks that take some thought, but used to come easily, like balancing a checkbook, playing complex games (such as bridge), and learning new information or routines

In a more advanced stage, symptoms are more obvious:

- Forgetting details about current events
- Forgetting events in your own life history, losing awareness of who you are
- Problems choosing proper clothing
- Hallucinations, arguments, striking out, and violent behavior
- Delusions, depression, agitation
- Difficulty performing basic tasks like preparing meals and driving

At end stages of AD, a person can no longer survive without assistance. Most people in this stage no longer:

- Understand language
- Recognize family members
- Perform basic activities of daily living such as eating, dressing, and bathing

Home care

The most promising treatments include lifestyle changes, medications, and antioxidant supplements like vitamin E and ginkgo biloba.

The following steps can help people with AD:

- Walk regularly with a caregiver or other reliable companion. This can improve communication skills and prevent wandering.
- Use bright light therapy to reduce insomnia and wandering.
- Listen to calming music. This may reduce wandering and restlessness, boost brain chemicals, ease anxiety, enhance sleep, and improve behavior.

Areas of the brain examined by MRI

Alzheimer's disease usually has symptoms that can be diagnosed by taking a person's history and a physical exam. A MRI scan may also be ordered.

In the early stages of the disease, brain image scans may be normal. In later stages, MRI scans may show a decrease in the size of the brain's cortex or of the area of the brain responsible for memory (the hippocampus).

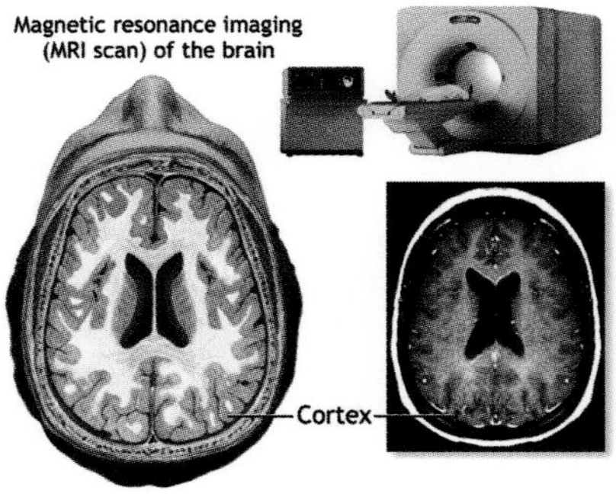

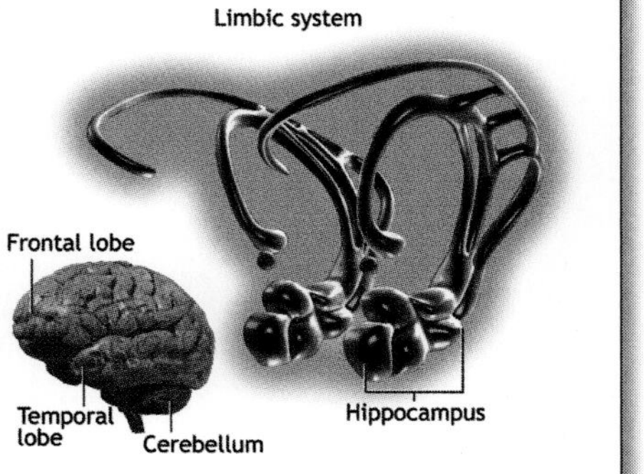

- Get a pet dog.
- Practice relaxation techniques.
- Receive regular massages. This is relaxing and provides social interactions.

If you are considering any drugs or supplements, you MUST talk to your doctor first. Remember that herbs and supplements available over the counter are NOT regulated by the FDA.

Someone with AD will need support in the home as the disease worsens. Family members or other caregivers can help by trying to understand how the person with AD perceives his or her world. Simplify the patient's surroundings. Give frequent reminders, notes, lists of routine tasks, or directions for daily activities. Give the person with AD a chance to talk about their challenges and participate in their own care.

Eventually, 24-hour monitoring and assistance may be necessary to provide a safe environment, control aggressive or agitated behavior, and meet physiologic needs. This may include in-home care, nursing homes, or adult day care.

ANKLE PAIN

Ankle pain is often due to an ankle sprain. A sprain is an injury to the ligaments that connect bones to one another.

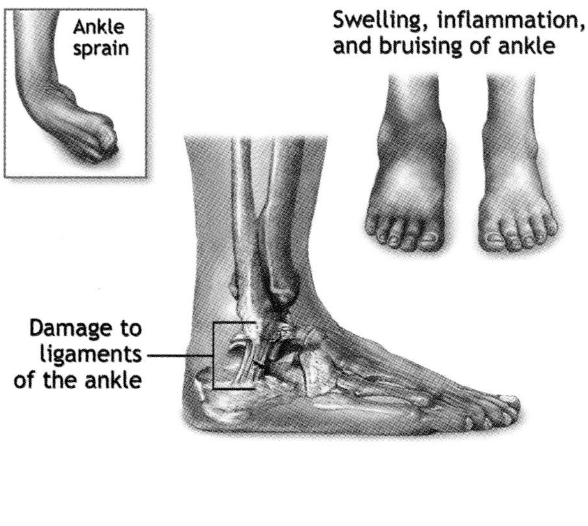

In most cases, the ankle is twisted inward, and there are tiny tears in the ligaments that may make the ankle somewhat unstable. This tearing leads to swelling and bruising, making it difficult to bear weight on the joint.

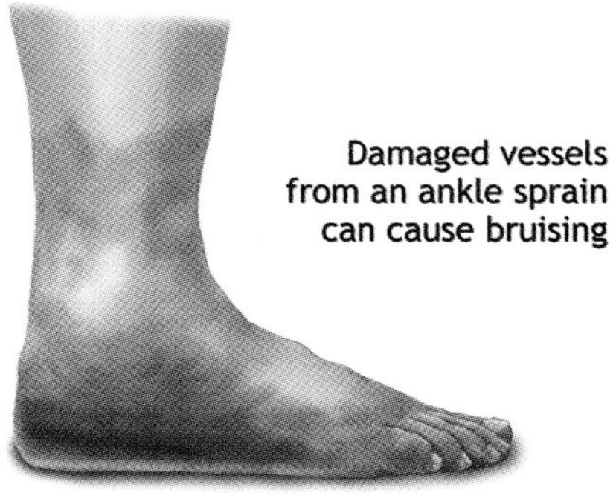

Damaged vessels from an ankle sprain can cause bruising

Once an ankle is sprained, the injury may take a few weeks to many months to fully heal. Often, the injured ankle remains a little weaker and less stable than the uninjured one. A proper recovery program can prevent this problem.

Other structures in the ankle that can be damaged and cause pain are tendons (join muscles to bone), cartilage (cushion joints), and blood vessels. Adjacent areas can cause pain to be referred to the ankle – these include the foot, lower leg, knee, and even hip.

In addition to ankle sprains and other injuries, ankle pain can be caused by arthritis, gout, pseudogout, and infection.

HOME CARE

- If you feel pain in your ankle, rest it for several days. Try NOT to move the affected area.
- If your ankle is unstable, support it, especially during standing or walking. ACE bandages work well. If this does not provide enough support, you may need to be fit for a brace. Crutches or a cane can help take the weight off a sore or unsteady ankle.

- For swelling, keep your foot elevated above the level of the heart, even while sleeping. Ice the area right away. Apply ice for 10-15 minutes every hour for the first day. Then, every 3-4 hours for 2 more days.

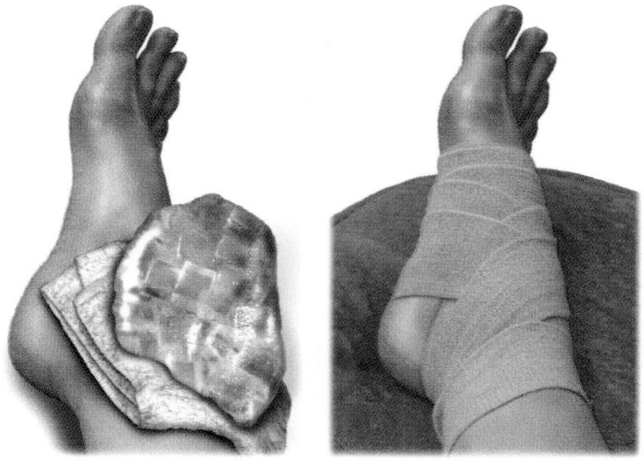

Remember the word "**R.I.C.E.**" when treating an ankle sprain: rest, ice, compression and elevation.

- Try acetaminophen or ibuprofen for pain and swelling.

Even after the pain subsides, you will need to keep pressure off of it for up to 10 days for a mild sprain and up to 5 weeks for a more severe sprain.

For arthritis of the ankle, take medication exactly as prescribed. When the pain and swelling start to decrease, gently begin to exercise the joint again. Swimming is good, followed by stretching. Walking can be added later. Exercises can be done several times a day; but DO NOT overdo it. Pain is a message from your body to stop.

When to contact a medical professional

Go to the hospital or call 911 if:

- You have severe pain when NOT bearing weight.
- You suspect a broken bone.
- The joint appears deformed.
- There is an audible popping sound and immediate difficulty using the joint.

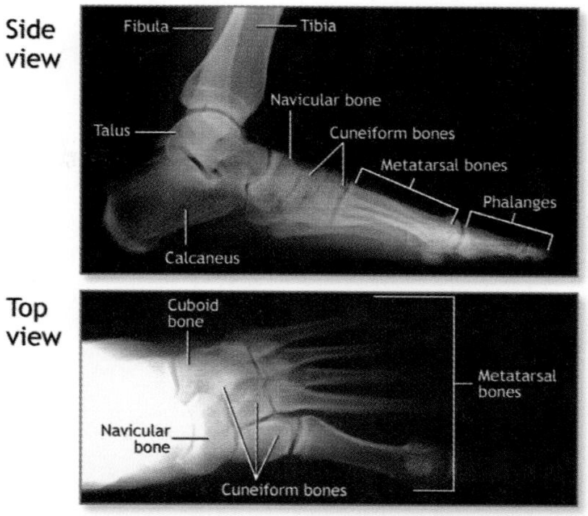

Your doctor may take an x-ray to check for broken bones or fractures. This foot x-ray is normal.

Call your doctor if:

- Swelling does not go down within 2-3 days.
- You have symptoms of infection – the area becomes red, more painful, or warm, or you have a fever over 100°F.
- The pain does not go away after several weeks.

Prevention

- Lose weight if you are overweight. Extra pounds put strain on your ankles.
- Warm-up before exercising. Stretch the muscles and tendons that anchor the ankle.
- Avoid sports and activities for which you are not properly conditioned.
- Make sure that shoes fit you properly. Avoid high-heeled shoes.
- If you are prone to ankle pain or twisting your ankle during certain activities, use ankle support braces. These include air-casts, ACE bandages, or lace-up ankle supports.

Athlete's foot

Athlete's foot is an infection of the feet caused by fungus. The medical term is tinea pedis. Once you have athlete's foot, it may last for a short or long time and may come back after treatment, especially if you are not careful.

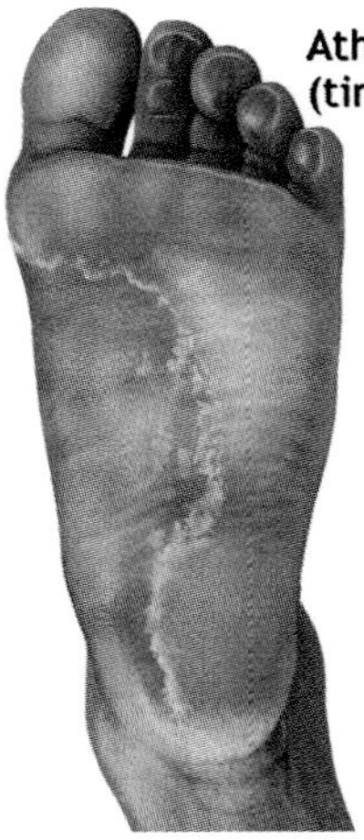

Athlete's foot is contagious, and can be passed through direct contact, or contact with items such as shoes, stockings, and shower or pool surfaces.

The most common symptom is cracked, flaking, peeling skin between the toes. The affected area is usually red and itchy. You may feel burning or stinging, and there may be blisters, oozing, or crusting. In addition to the toes, the symptoms can also occur on the heels, palms, and between the fingers.

If the fungus spreads to your nails, they can become discolored, thick, and even crumble.

Home care

Over-the-counter antifungal powders or creams can help control the infection. These generally contain miconazole, clotrimazole, or tolnaftate. Continue using the medicine for 1-2 weeks after the infection has cleared from your feet to prevent the infection from returning.

In addition:

- Keep your feet clean and dry, especially between your toes.
- Wash your feet thoroughly with soap and water and dry the area very carefully and completely. Try to do this at least twice a day.
- Wear clean, cotton socks and change your socks and shoes as often as necessary to keep your feet dry.

You need to know

It is important to treat athlete's foot early. Why? Because you need to prevent it from spreading into your nails. Once that happens, it becomes much harder to control.

When to contact a medical professional

Call your doctor right away if:

- Your foot is swollen and warm to the touch, especially if there are red streaks. These are signs of a possible bacterial infection. Other signs include pus or other discharge and fever.
- You have diabetes and develop athlete's foot.

Also call your doctor if athlete's foot symptoms do not go away within one month of using self-care measures.

Prevention

To prevent athlete's foot, follow these measures:

- Dry your feet thoroughly after bathing or swimming.
- Wear sandals or flip-flops at a public shower or pool.
- Change your socks often to keep your feet dry. This should be done at least once a day.

- Use antifungal or drying powders to prevent athlete's foot if you are susceptible to getting it, or you frequent areas where athlete's foot fungus is common (like public showers).
- Wear shoes that are well ventilated and, preferably, made of natural material such as leather. It may help to alternate shoes each day, so they can dry completely between wearings. Avoid plastic-lined shoes.

Back pain

If you are like most people, you will have at least one backache in your life. While such pain or discomfort can happen anywhere in your back, the most common area affected is your low back. This is because the low back supports most of your body's weight.

Low back pain is the #2 reason that Americans see their doctor – second only to colds and flus. Many back-related injuries happen at work. But you can change that. There are many things you can do to lower your chances of getting back pain.

Most back problems will get better on their own. The key is to know when you need to seek medical help and when self-care measures alone will allow you to get better.

You'll usually first feel back pain just after you lift a heavy object, move suddenly, sit in one position for a long time, or have an injury or accident. But prior to that moment in time, the structures in your back may be losing strength or integrity.

Home care

Many people will feel better within one week after the start of back pain. After another 4-6 weeks, the back pain will likely be completely gone. To get better quickly, take the right steps when you first get pain.

A common misconception about back pain is that you need to rest and avoid activity for a long time. In fact, **bed rest is NOT recommended**.

If you have no indication of a serious underlying cause for your back pain (like loss of bowel or bladder control, weakness, weight loss, or fever), then you should reduce physical activity only for the first couple of days. Gradually resume your usual activities after that. Here are some tips for how to handle pain early on:

- Stop normal physical activity for the first few days. This helps calm your symptoms and reduce inflammation.
- Apply heat or ice to the painful area. Try ice for the first 48-72 hours, then use heat after that.
- Take over-the-counter pain relievers such as ibuprofen (Advil, Motrin IB) or acetaminophen (Tylenol).

While sleeping, try lying in a curled-up, fetal position with a pillow between your legs.

Various causes of back pain

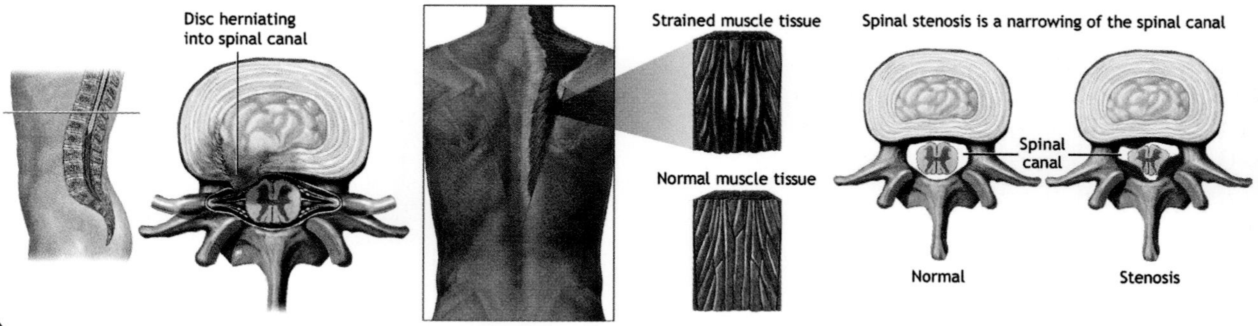

If you usually sleep on your back, place a pillow or rolled towel under your knees to relieve pressure.

Do not perform activities that involve heavy lifting or twisting of your back for the first 6 weeks after the pain begins. After 2-3 weeks, you should gradually resume exercise.

Begin with light cardiovascular training. Walking, riding a stationary bicycle, and swimming are great examples. Such aerobic activities can help blood flow to your back and promote healing. They also strengthen muscles in your stomach and back.

Stretching and strengthening exercises are important in the long run. However, starting these exercises too soon after an injury can make your pain worse. A physical therapist can help you determine when to begin stretching and strengthening exercises and how to do so.

AVOID the following exercises during initial recovery unless your doctor or physical therapist says it is okay:

- Jogging
- Football
- Golf
- Ballet
- Weight lifting
- Leg lifts when lying on your stomach
- Sit-ups with straight legs (rather than bent knees)

When to contact a medical professional

Call 911 if you have lost bowel or bladder control. Otherwise, call your doctor if you have:

- Unexplained fever with back pain.
- Back pain after a severe blow or fall.
- Redness or swelling on the back or spine.
- Pain traveling down your legs below the knee.
- Weakness or numbness in your buttocks, thigh, leg, or pelvis.
- Burning with urination or blood in your urine.
- Worse pain when you lie down or pain that awakens you at night.
- Very sharp pain.

Also call if:

- You have been losing weight unintentionally
- You use steroids or intravenous drugs.
- You have never had or been evaluated for back pain before.
- You have had back pain before but this episode is distinctly different.

How to lift

To prevent back pain, it is also very important to learn to lift and bend properly. Follow these tips:

- If an object is too heavy or awkward, get help.
- Spread your feet apart to give a wide base of support.
- Stand as close to the object you are lifting as possible.
- Bend at your knees, not at your waist. Use your leg muscles to lift.
- Tighten your stomach muscles as you lift the object up or lower it down.
- Hold the object as close to your body as you can.

- This episode of back pain has lasted longer than four weeks.

Prevention

Exercise is important for preventing future back pain. Through exercise you can:

- Improve your posture
- Strengthen your back and improve flexibility
- Lose weight
- Avoid falls

A complete exercise program should include aerobic activity (like walking, swimming, or riding a stationary bicycle) as well as stretching and strength training.

To prevent back pain, it is also very important to learn to lift and bend properly. Follow these tips:

- If an object is too heavy or awkward, get help.
- Spread your feet apart to give a wide base of support.
- Stand as close to the object you are lifting as possible.
- Bend at your knees, not at your waist.
- Tighten your stomach muscles as you lift the object up or lower it down.
- Hold the object as close to your body as you can.
- Lift using your leg muscles.
- As you stand up with the object, DO NOT bend forward.
- DO NOT twist while you are bending for the object, lifting it up, or carrying it.

Other measures to take to prevent back pain include:

- Avoid standing for long periods of time. If you must for your work, try using a stool. Alternate resting each foot on it.
- DO NOT wear high heels. Use cushioned soles when walking.
- When sitting for work, especially if using a computer, make sure that your chair has a straight back with adjustable seat and back, armrests, and a swivel seat.
- Use a stool under your feet while sitting so that your knees are higher than your hips.
- Place a small pillow or rolled towel behind your lower back while sitting or driving for long periods of time.
- If you drive long distance, stop and walk around every hour. Bring your seat as far forward as possible to avoid bending. Don't lift heavy objects just after a ride.
- Quit smoking.
- Lose weight.
- Learn to relax. Try methods like yoga, tai chi, or massage.

Do I need back surgery?

Most people experience back pain at least once in their life. It may come as a relief to know that back pain almost always resolves by following simple self-care measures. Once in awhile, however, surgery may be considered if your back pain is due to pressure on a spinal nerve and it doesn't get better with self care. Such pressure can be caused by a herniated disk, spinal stenosis, or sciatica.

Even a back surgeon will tell you that treatment without surgery is best whenever possible. Back surgery has risks and complications. And it doesn't always work. In addition, you must take the same steps to recover from the operation as you would to treat back pain. But after surgery, it often takes longer to recuperate.

Remember that when you hear the words "slipped disk" or "herniated disk", surgery is NOT inevitable, despite this popular misconception. In fact, 90% of people with a herniated disk are treated successfully without surgery.

Bedsores (Pressure Ulcers)

A pressure ulcer is an area of skin that breaks down when you stay in one position for too long without shifting your weight. This often happens if you use a wheelchair or you are bedridden, even for a short period of time (for example, after surgery or an injury). The constant pressure against the skin reduces the blood supply to that area, and the affected tissue dies.

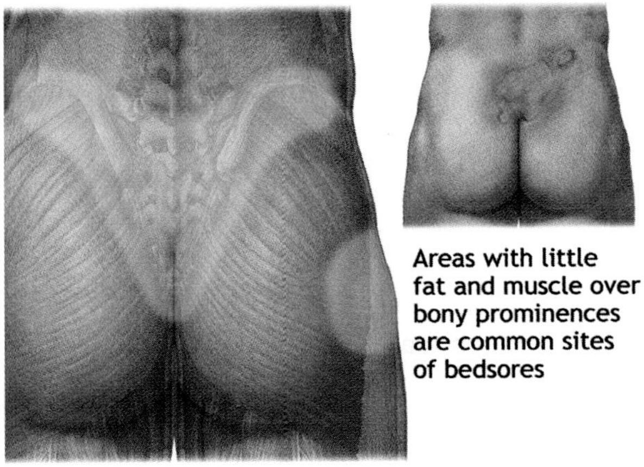

Areas with little fat and muscle over bony prominences are common sites of bedsores

A pressure ulcer starts as reddened skin but gets progressively worse, forming a blister, then an open sore, and finally a crater. The most common places for pressure ulcers are over bony prominences (bones close to the skin) like the elbow, heels, hips, ankles, shoulders, back, and the back of the head.

When to contact a medical professional

Contact your health care provider if an area of the skin blisters or forms an open sore. Contact the provider immediately if there are any signs of an infection. An infection can spread to the rest of the body and cause serious problems. Signs of an infected ulcer include:

- A foul odor from the ulcer
- Redness and tenderness around the ulcer
- Skin close to the ulcer is warm and swollen

Fever, weakness, and confusion are signs that the infection may have spread to the blood or elsewhere in the body.

Prevention

If bedridden or immobile with diabetes, circulation problems, incontinence, or mental disabilities, you should be checked for pressure sores every day. Look for reddened areas that, when pressed, do not turn white. Also look for blisters, sores, or craters. In addition, take the following steps:

- Change position at least every two hours to relieve pressure.
- Use items that can help reduce pressure – pillows, sheepskin, foam padding, and powders from medical supply stores.
- Eat healthy, well-balanced meals.
- Exercise daily, including range-of-motion exercises for immobile patients.
- Keep skin clean and dry. Incontinent people need to take extra steps to limit moisture.

Bedwetting

Children develop complete control over their bladders at different ages. Nighttime dryness is usually the last stage of toilet learning. When children wet the bed more than twice per month after age 5 or 6, we call it bedwetting or enuresis.

Children who were dry for at least 6 months and then started wetting again have secondary enuresis. The key here is to find what changed. It might be physical, emotional, or just a change in sleep.

When the child has never been dry, that is called primary enuresis. The cause is usually making more urine overnight than the bladder can hold and being a deep sleeper. The child's brain has not learned to respond to the signal that the bladder is full. It is not the child's or the parent's fault.

Bedwetting runs strongly in families. More than 5 million children in the U.S. wet the bed.

Home care

Doing nothing or punishing the child are both common responses to bedwetting. Neither helps. Waking the child once each night may give dry sheets and improve self-esteem, but won't speed the end of bedwetting. Without taking steps to solve the bedwetting, about 85 percent of children wetting this year will still be wetting next year. With the proper help, most children can be dry within 12 weeks.

Some children just need to drink less than 2 ounces in the 2 hours before bed to decrease the amount of urine made. If the wetting doesn't improve within 2 weeks, though, continuing this won't help.

Some children respond to star charts. Getting a star for dry nights can help the sleeping brain be alert for the bladder's signal. Again, if the wetting doesn't improve within 2 weeks, continuing won't help. Gently telling the child as he is falling asleep to be ready later for his bladder's signal may be useful.

Many children will stop wetting with just 30 minutes more sleep each night.

Most will be dry within 12 weeks with a bedwetting alarm that wakes the parents (and then they wake the child) when the bladder is full. Here, you will often NOT see a response within the first two weeks.

Prescription medications such as DDAVP are available to treat bedwetting by forcing the body to make less urine at night. They are easy to use and have quick results. They can be used short term for an important sleepover. To help outgrow bedwetting, however, they must be continued for at least 6 months beyond achieving dryness, and they are expensive.

With secondary enuresis, it is important to look for the cause before treating.

When to contact a medical professional

Be sure to mention bedwetting to your child's health care provider. Children should have a physical exam and a urine test to rule out urinary tract infection or other causes.

> **The bottom line**
>
> Bedwetting is far more common than most people recognize. It's not your fault or the child's. With home treatment, most children can look forward to dry nights within 12 weeks.

Breast lump

Normal breast tissue is present in both males and females of all ages. This tissue responds to hormonal changes and, therefore, certain lumps can come and go.

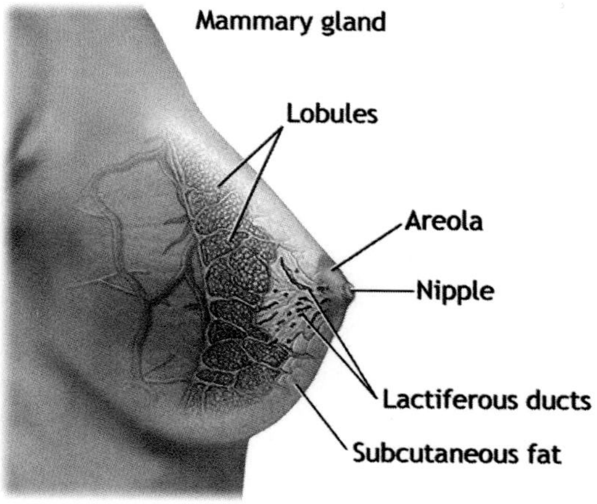

Breast lumps may appear at all ages:

- Infants may have breast lumps related to estrogen from the mother. The lump generally goes away on its own as the estrogen clears from the baby's body. It can happen to boys and girls.
- Young girls often develop "breast buds" that appear just before the beginning of puberty. These bumps may be tender. They are common around age 9, but may happen as early as age 6.

- Teenage boys may develop breast enlargement and lumps because of hormonal changes in mid-puberty. Although this may distress the teen, the lumps or enlargement generally go away on their own over a period of months.
- Breast lumps in an adult woman raises concern for breast cancer, even though most lumps turn out to be not cancerous.

Lumps in a woman are often caused by fibrocystic changes, fibroadenomas, and cysts.

Fibrocystic changes can occur in either or both breasts. These changes occur in many women (especially during the reproductive years) and are considered a normal variation of breast tissue. Having fibrocystic breasts does not increase your risk for breast cancer. It does, however, make it more difficult to interpret lumps that you or your doctor find on exam. Many women feel tenderness in addition to the lumps and bumps associated with fibrocystic breasts.

Fibroadenomas are non-cancerous lumps that feel rubbery and are easily moveable within the breast tissue. Like fibrocystic changes, they occur most often during the reproductive years. Usually, they are not tender and, except in rare cases, do not become cancerous later. A doctor may feel fairly certain from an exam that a particular lump is a fibroadenoma. The only way to be sure, however, is to remove or biopsy them.

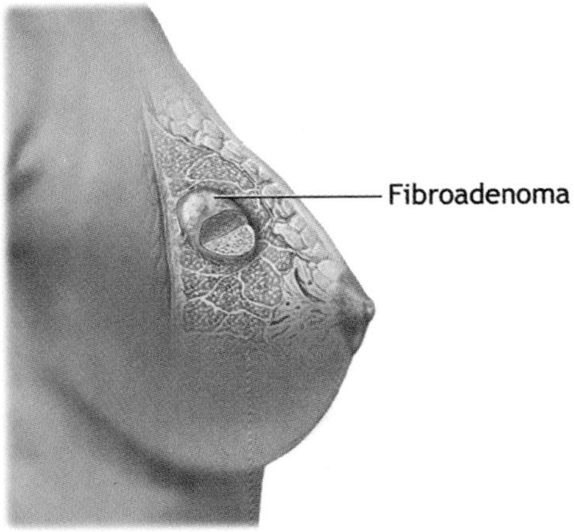

Cysts are fluid-filled sacs that often feel like soft grapes. These can sometimes be tender, especially just before your menstrual period. Cysts may be drained in the doctor's office. If the fluid removed is clear or greenish, and the lump disappears completely after it is drained, no further treatment is needed. If the fluid is bloody, it is sent to the lab to look for cancer cells. If the lump doesn't disappear, or recurs, it is usually removed surgically.

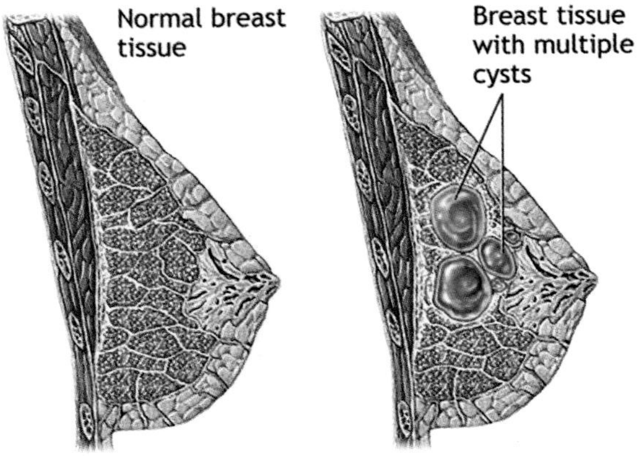

Inside look at normal vs. cystic breast tissue.

Home care

Treatment of a breast lump depends on the cause. Solid breast lumps are often removed surgically, or at least a biopsy is taken. The biopsy is to check whether it is cancerous or not. Cysts can be drained. Breast infections require antibiotics.

For fibrocystic changes, birth control pills are often helpful. Other women are helped by:

- Avoiding caffeine and chocolate.
- Taking vitamin E, vitamin B complex, or evening primrose oil supplements.
- Limiting fat and increasing fiber in the diet.

When to contact a medical professional

Call your doctor if:

- You find a new breast lump during your monthly self-exam.

- You have bruising on your breast but did not experience any injury.
- You have nipple discharge, especially if bloody or pinkish (blood tinged).
- The skin on your breast appears dimpled or wrinkled (like the peel of an orange).
- Your nipple is inverted (turned inward) but normally is not inverted.

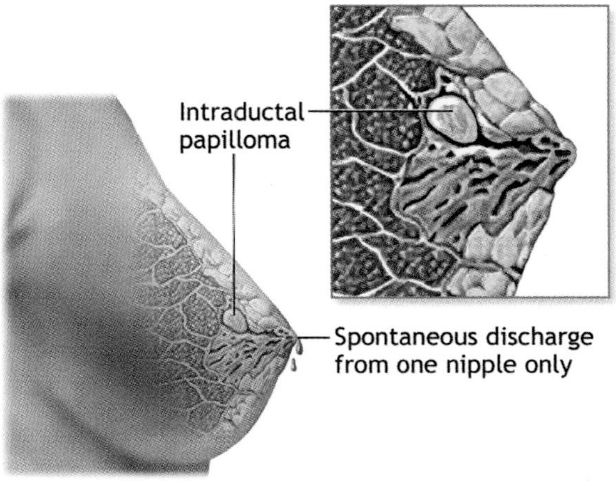

Fluid discharge from the nipple may be caused by a small growth inside a milk duct called an intraductal papilloma. Although it is harmless, any watery nipple discharge should be evaluated by your provider.

Prevention

Breast cancer screening is an important way to find breast cancer early, when it is most easily treated and cured:

- If you are over age 20, consider doing a monthly breast self-exam. See *Breast Self-Exam*. Talk to your provider about the pros and cons.
- If you are over age 20, have a complete breast exam by your provider at least every 3 years – every year if you are over 40.
- If you are over age 50, get a yearly screening mammogram. Women between ages 40 and 50 should have mammograms at least every other year.

Having fibrocystic breast tissue, mastitis, or breast tenderness related to PMS does NOT put you at greater risk for breast cancer. Hav-

Breast lump biopsy

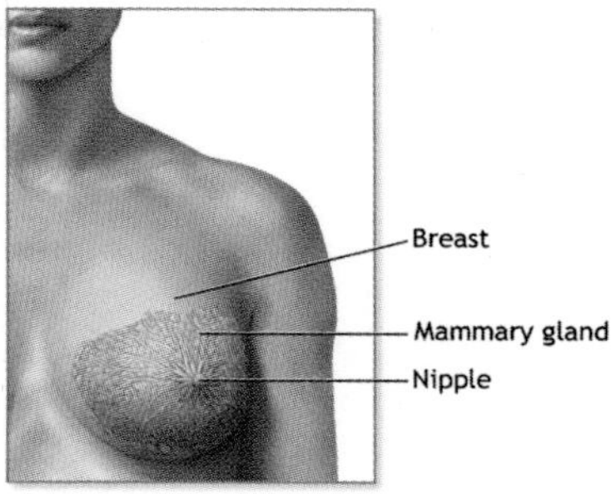

The female breast is composed mainly of fatty tissue interspersed with fibrous tissue.

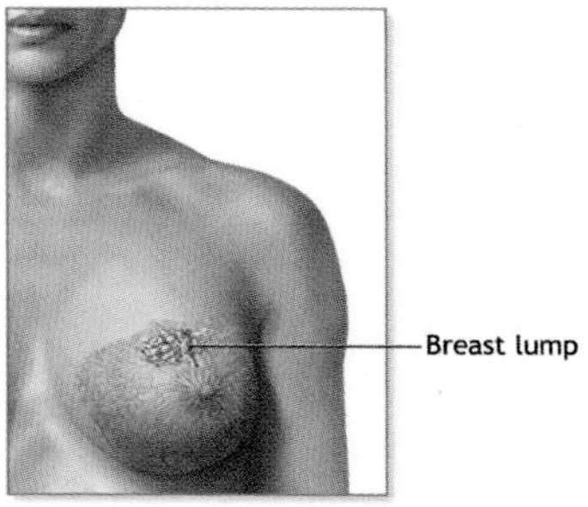

Early detection of a lump is very important.

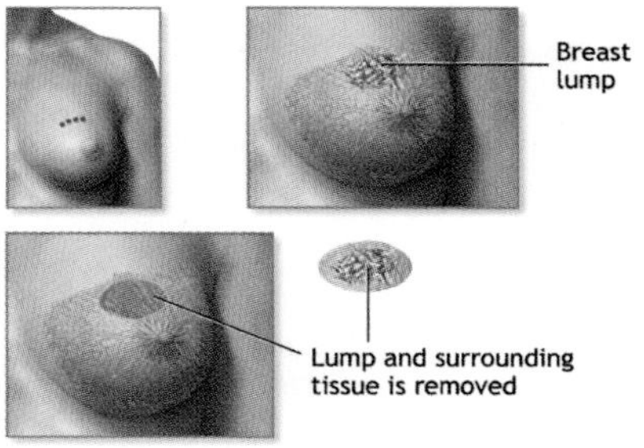

A biopsy may be performed to remove the breast lump. The tissue will be examined by a laboratory to determine if it is cancerous or not.

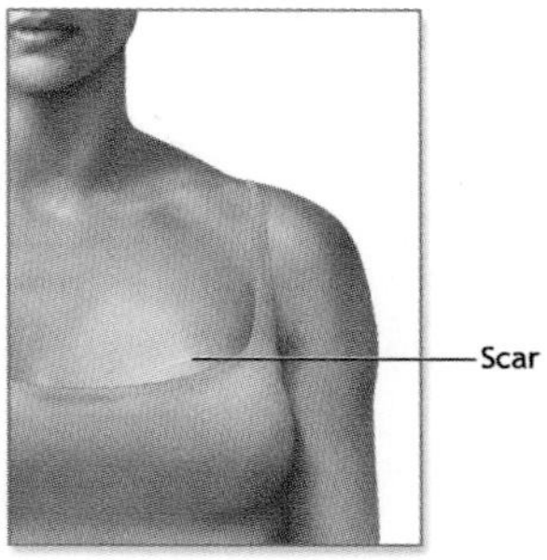

The incision for a breast lump biopsy is usually 3-4 centimeters long and should heal within a couple of weeks, leaving only a small scar.

ing fibrocystic breasts does, however, make your self-exam more confusing since there are many lumps and bumps.

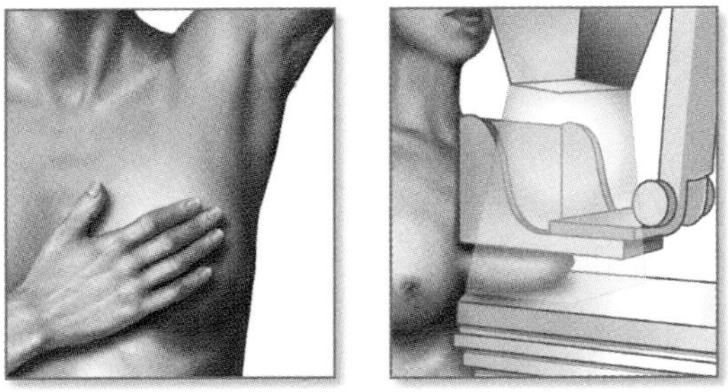

Breast lumps may be found in several ways, such as self-exam, health care provider exam, or mammography

To prevent breast cancer:

- Exercise regularly
- Reduce fat intake
- Eat lots of fruits, vegetables, and other high fiber foods
- Limit alcoholic beverages to no more than 1 to 1½ per day.

Breast pain or tenderness

There are many possible causes for breast pain. For example, hormonal fluctuations related to menstruation or pregnancy are often responsible for breast tenderness.

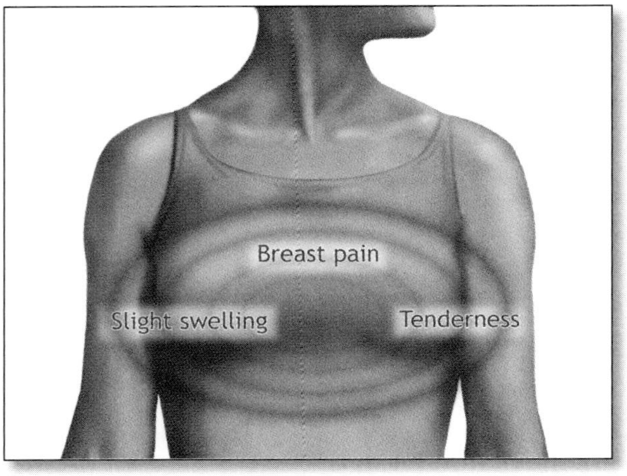

Some degree of swelling and tenderness just before your period is normal. The question is how tolerable (or intolerable) the discomfort is to you.

Although many women with pain in one or both breasts understandably fear breast cancer, breast pain is NOT a common symptom of cancer.

Soon after childbirth, your breasts may become engorged with milk. This can be very painful and is usually accompanied by swelling. If you have an area of redness, call your health care provider.

Other common causes of breast pain include:

- Fibrocystic breast changes
- Mastitis – a blocked and infected milk duct that may have some redness, usually associated with breastfeeding
- Premenstrual syndrome (PMS)
- Alcoholism with liver damage
- Injury

Fibrocystic breast tissue is a common condition. It involves breast lumps and bumps throughout the breast tissue that tend to be more tender just before your menstrual period.

Home care

For tips on how to manage pain from fibrocystic breasts, see *Breast Lumps*.

When to contact a medical professional

Call your doctor if you have:

- Discharge from your nipples, especially blood or pus
- Given birth within the last week and your breasts are swollen or hard
- Signs of a breast infection, including localized redness, pus, or fever

- Noticed a new lump associated with the pain that does not go away after your menstrual period
- Persistent, unexplained breast pain

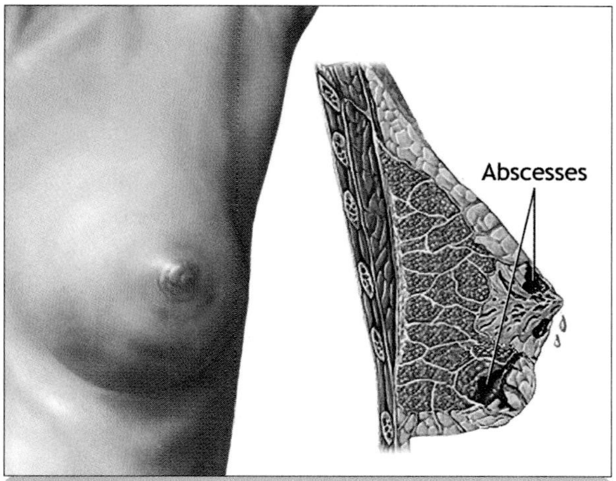

A breast abscess will require antibiotic treatment. Look for signs of infection like localized redness, nipple discharge, and fever.

Bronchitis

Bronchitis is an inflammation of the main air passages to the lungs. Bronchitis may be sudden (acute) and short-lived, or chronic, meaning that it lasts a long time and often recurs. To be classified as chronic, you must have a cough with mucus most days of the month for three months out of the year.

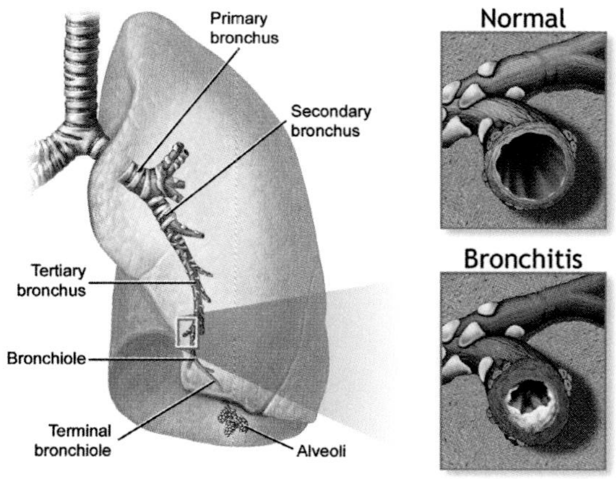

Acute bronchitis generally follows a viral respiratory infection. Initially, it affects your nose, sinuses, and throat and then spreads to the large bronchial airway passages. Sometimes, you may get what is called a secondary bacterial infection. This means that bacteria infect the airways, in addition to the virus. The already inflamed area is one in which bacteria like to grow.

People at risk for acute bronchitis include:

- Elderly, infants, and young children
- Smokers
- People with heart or lung disease

Chronic bronchitis is a long-term condition of excessive mucus with a productive cough. This ongoing condition is inflammation but not infection. It blocks air flow in and out of the lungs.

Chronic bronchitis, like emphysema, is also known as chronic obstructive pulmonary disease. As these lung conditions progress over time, you become increasingly short of breath, have difficulty walking or exerting yourself physically, and may need oxygen on a regular basis.

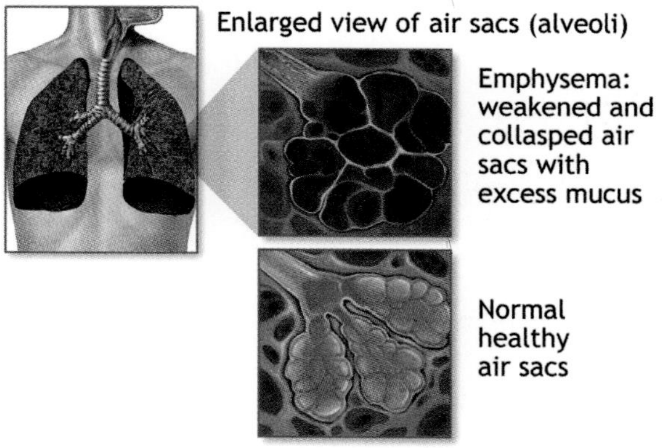

Cigarette smoke is the chief cause of chronic bronchitis, including long-term exposure to second-hand smoke.

Symptoms

The symptoms of either type of bronchitis include:

- Cough that produces mucus; if yellow-green in color, you are more likely to have a bacterial infection

- Shortness of breath worsened by exertion or mild activity
- Wheezing
- Fatigue
- Fever – usually low
- Chest discomfort

Even after acute bronchitis has cleared, you may have a dry, nagging cough that lingers for several weeks.

Additional symptoms of chronic bronchitis include:

- Frequent respiratory infections (such as colds or the flu)
- Ankle, feet, and leg swelling
- Blue-tinged lips from low levels of oxygen

Home care

For acute bronchitis from a virus, you DO NOT need antibiotics. The infection will generally clear on its own within one week. Take the following steps for some relief:

- Take aspirin or acetaminophen (Tylenol) if you have a fever. DO NOT give children aspirin.
- Rest.
- Drink plenty of fluids.
- Use a humidifier or steam in the bathroom.
- DO NOT smoke.

Key point

Antibiotics are usually NOT helpful for bronchitis! Nonetheless, when people are diagnosed with bronchitis, they often get a prescription for antibiotics. Instead of calling your doctor right away, try the self-care measures outlined here.

If your symptoms do not improve, your doctor may prescribe an inhaler to open your airways. If your doctor thinks that you have a secondary *bacterial* infection, antibiotics will be prescribed.

For chronic bronchitis, the most important step you can take is to QUIT smoking. If caught early enough, you can reverse the damage to your lungs. Other important steps include:

- Limit your exposure to pollutants and other lung irritants.
- Get a flu vaccine each year and a pneumococcal vaccine one time.
- Attend a respiratory training program that includes physical activity and breathing exercises. Your doctor can recommend a medically appropriate and well-supervised program. If it is early in your disease process, you can likely exercise on your own; talk to your doctor about safety.

Your doctor will usually prescribe inhaled medicines for chronic bronchitis. If you have low oxygen levels, home oxygen will be used.

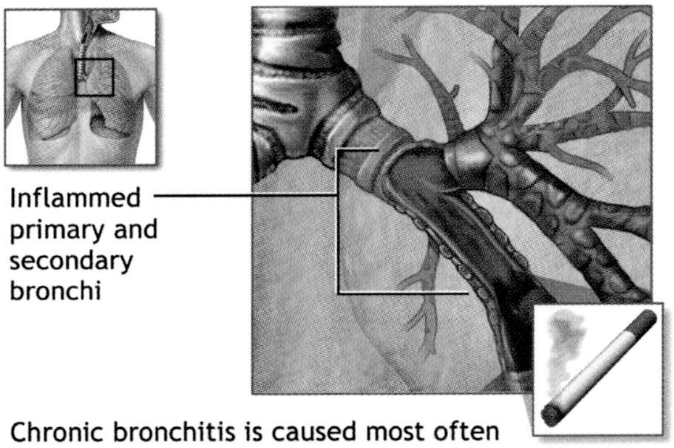

Chronic bronchitis is caused most often by exposure to airborne pollutants such as cigarette smoke

The most important action you can take to combat chronic bronchitis is to quit smoking.

When to contact a medical professional

Call your doctor if

- You are coughing up blood.

- You have a high fever or shaking chills.
- You have a low-grade fever for three or more days.
- You have thick, greenish mucus, especially if it has a bad smell.
- You feel short of breath or have chest pain.
- You have an underlying chronic illness, like heart or lung disease.
- You have a cough most days of the month or you have a frequently recurring cough.

Bunions

A bunion is when your big toe points toward the second toe. This causes a bump on the edge of your foot, at the joint of your big toe.

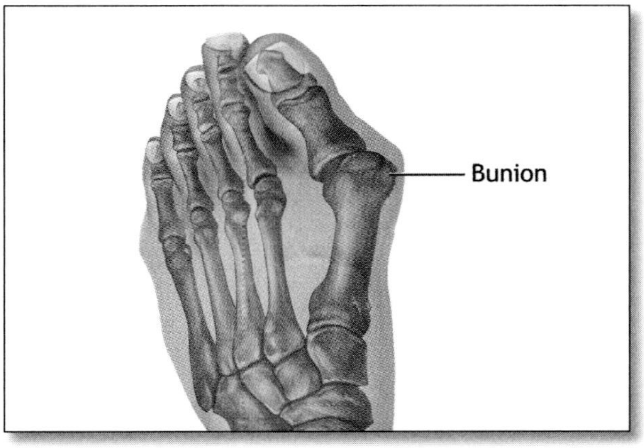

Bunions are often caused by narrow-toed, high-heeled shoes. These compress the big toe and push it toward the second toe. The condition may become painful as extra bone and a fluid-filled sac grow at the base of the big toe. This leads to swelling and pain. Bunions occur more frequently in women and sometimes run in families.

Home care

When a bunion first begins to develop, take good care of your feet and wear wide-toed shoes. This often solves the problem and prevents the need for any further treatment. It may help to wear felt or foam pads on the foot to protect the bunion, or devices to separate the first and second toes at night. These are available at drugstores. You can also try cutting a hole in a pair of old, comfortable shoes to wear around the house.

Chest pain

Many people with chest pain fear a heart attack. However, there are many possible causes of chest pain. Some causes are mildly inconvenient, while other causes are serious, even life-threatening. Any organ or tissue in your chest can be the source of pain, including your heart, lungs, esophagus, muscles, ribs, tendons, or nerves.

Angina is a type of heart-related chest pain. This pain occurs because your heart is not getting enough blood and oxygen. Angina pain can be similar to the pain of a heart attack.

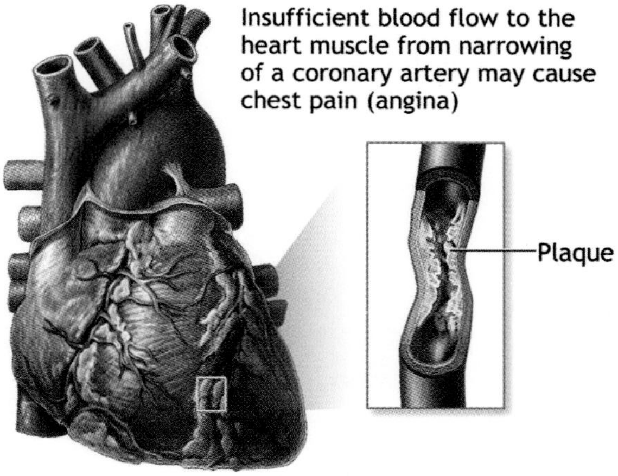

Insufficient blood flow to the heart muscle from narrowing of a coronary artery may cause chest pain (angina)
Plaque

Angina is called stable angina when your chest pain begins at a predictable level of activity. (For example, when you walk up a steep hill.) However, if your chest pain happens unexpectedly after light activity or occurs at rest, this is called unstable angina. This is a more dangerous form of angina and you need to be seen in an emergency room right away.

Other causes of chest pain include:

- Asthma, which is generally accompanied by shortness of breath, wheezing, or cough.

- Pneumonia, a blood clot to the lung (pulmonary embolism), the collapse of a small area of a lung (pneumothorax), or inflammation of the lining around the lung (pleurisy). In these cases, the chest pain often worsens when you take a deep breath or cough and usually feels sharp.
- Strain or inflammation of the muscles and tendons between the ribs.
- Anxiety and rapid breathing.

Chest pain can also be related to problems with your digestive system. These include stomach ulcer, gallbladder disease, gallstones, indigestion, heartburn, or gastroesophageal reflux (when acid from your stomach backs up into your esophagus).

Ulcer pain burns if your stomach is empty and feels better with food. Gallbladder pain often gets worse after a meal, especially a fatty meal.

In children, most chest pain is not caused by the heart.

Home care

If injury, over-exertion, or coughing have caused muscle strain, your chest wall is often tender or painful when you press a finger at the location of the pain. This can often be treated at home. Try acetaminophen or ibuprofen, ice, heat, and rest.

If you know you have asthma or angina, follow the instructions of your doctor and take your medications regularly to avoid flare-ups.

When to contact a medical professional

Call 911 if:

- You have sudden crushing, squeezing, tightening, or pressure in your chest.
- Pain radiates to your jaw, left arm, or between your shoulder blades.
- You have nausea, dizziness, sweating, a racing heart, or shortness of breath.
- You know you have angina and your chest discomfort is suddenly more intense, brought on by lighter activity, or lasts longer than usual.
- Your angina symptoms occur at rest.
- You have sudden sharp chest pain with shortness of breath, especially after a long trip, a stretch of bedrest (for example, following an operation), or other lack of movement that can lead to a blood clot in your leg.

Know that your risk of heart attack is greater if you have a family history of heart disease, you smoke or use cocaine, or you have high cholesterol, high blood pressure, or diabetes.

Call your doctor if:

- You have a fever or a cough that produces yellow-green phlegm.
- Chest-wall pain persists for longer than 3 to 5 days.

> **Key point**
>
> Although you may fear a heart attack, there are many potential causes of chest pain. Understanding the different types of chest discomfort may save you an unnecessary trip to your doctor or ER.

Prevention

Make healthy lifestyle choices to prevent chest pain from heart disease:

- Achieve and maintain normal weight.
- Control high blood pressure, high cholesterol, and diabetes.
- Avoid cigarette smoking and second-hand smoke.
- Eat a diet low in saturated and hydrogenated fats and cholesterol, and high in starches, fiber, fruits, and vegetables.
- Exercise 3 hours per week or more (such as 30 minutes per day, 6 days per week).
- Reduce stress.

Chickenpox

Chickenpox is one of the classic childhood diseases, and one of the most contagious. The affected child or adult may develop hundreds of itchy, fluid-filled blisters that burst and form crusts. Chickenpox is caused by a virus.

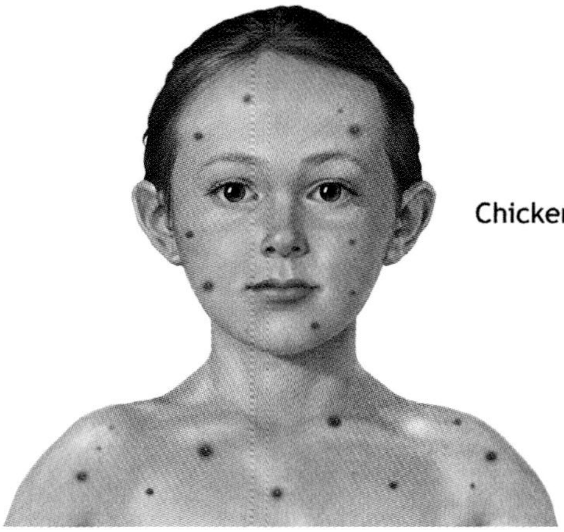

In a typical scenario, a young child is covered in pox and out of school for a week. The first half of the week the child feels miserable from intense itching; the second half from boredom. Since the introduction of the chickenpox vaccine, classic chickenpox is much less common.

When someone becomes infected, the pox usually appear 10 to 21 days later. People become contagious 1 to 2 days **before** breaking out with pox. They remain contagious while uncrusted blisters are present.

Once you catch chickenpox, the virus usually remains in your body for your lifetime, kept in check by the immune system. About 1 in 10 adults will experience shingles when the virus re-emerges during a period of stress.

Most cases of chickenpox occur in children younger than ten. The disease is usually mild, although serious complications sometimes occur. Adults and older children usually get sicker than younger children do.

The pox are worse in children who have other skin problems, such as eczema or a recent sunburn.

Complications are more common in those who are immunocompromised from an illness or medicines like chemotherapy. Some of the worst cases of chickenpox have been seen in children who have taken steroids (for example, for asthma) during the incubation period, before they have any symptoms.

Symptoms

Most children with chickenpox act sick with vague symptoms, such as a fever, headache, tummy ache, or loss of appetite, for a day or two before breaking out in the classic pox rash. These symptoms last 2 to 4 days after breaking out.

The average child develops 250 to 500 small, itchy, fluid-filled blisters over red spots on the skin ("dew drops on a rose petal"). The blisters often appear first on the face, trunk, or scalp and spread from there. After a day or two, the blisters become cloudy and then scab. Meanwhile, new crops of blisters spring up in groups. The pox often appear in the mouth, in the vagina, and on the eyelids. Children with skin problems such as eczema may get more than 1,500 pox.

Most pox will not leave scars unless they become contaminated with bacteria from scratching.

Some children who have had the vaccine will still develop a mild case of chickenpox. They usually recover much quicker and only have a few pox. These often do not follow the classic descriptions of the disease.

Home care

In most cases, it is enough to keep children comfortable while their own bodies fight the illness. Oatmeal baths in lukewarm water provide a crusty, comforting coating on the skin. An oral antihistamine can help to ease the itching, as can topical lotions such as Calamine. Trim the fingernails short to reduce secondary infections and scarring.

Safe antiviral medicines have been developed. To be effective, they usually must be started within the first 24 hours of the rash. For most otherwise healthy children, the benefits of these medicines may not outweigh the costs.

However, for those with skin conditions (such as eczema or recent sunburn), lung conditions (such as asthma), or those who have recently taken steroids, the antiviral medicines may be very important. The same is true for adolescents and children who must take aspirin on an ongoing basis.

Some doctors also give antiviral medicines to people in the same household who subsequently come down with chickenpox. Because of their increased exposure, they would normally experience a more severe case of chickenpox.

DO NOT USE ASPIRIN for someone who may have chickenpox.

When to contact a medical professional

Call your health care provider if you think that your child has chickenpox or if your child is over 12 months of age and has not been vaccinated against chickenpox.

Prevention

Because chickenpox is airborne and very contagious before the rash appears, it is difficult to avoid. It is possible to catch chickenpox from someone on a different aisle in the supermarket, who doesn't even know they have chickenpox!

A chickenpox vaccine is part of the routine immunization schedule. It is about 100% effective against moderate or severe illness, and 85-90% effective against mild chickenpox. Parents often express concern that the immunity from the vaccine might not last. The chickenpox vaccine, though, is the only routine vaccine that does not require a booster.

Talk to your doctor if you think your child might be at high risk for complications and might have been exposed. Immediate preventive measures may be important.

Colic and crying in infants

Almost all babies go through a fussy period. When crying lasts for longer than about three hours a day and is not caused by a medical problem (such as a hernia or infection), it is called colic. This phenomenon occurs in almost all babies. The only thing that differs is the degree.

Colic usually strikes toward the end of a long day, when your baby is just about at the age when your sleep deprivation has really begun to set in. Your baby stops being the quiet, peaceful, miracle baby and begins screaming every evening. It is no wonder that parents can become frustrated, discouraged, and depressed.

The child with colic tends to be unusually sensitive to stimulation. Some babies experience greater discomfort from intestinal gas. Some cry from hunger, others from overfeeding. Some breastfed babies are intolerant of foods in their mothers' diets. Some bottle-fed babies are intolerant of the proteins in formula. Fear, frustration, or even excitement can lead to abdominal discomfort and colic. When other people around them are worried, anxious, or depressed, babies may cry more, which in turn makes those around them *even more* worried, anxious, or depressed.

About 20% of babies cry enough to meet the definition of colic. The timing varies, but colic usually affects babies beginning at about 3 weeks of age and peaking somewhere between 4-6 weeks of age.

Colic will not last forever! After about 6 weeks of age, it usually begins improving, slowly but surely, and is generally gone by

12 weeks of age. When colic is still going strong at 12 weeks, it's important to consider another diagnosis (such as reflux).

Symptoms

Colic frequently, but not always, begins at about the same time every day. For most infants the most intense fussiness is in the evening. The attack often begins suddenly. The legs may be drawn up and the belly distended. The hands may be clenched. The episode may last for minutes or hours. It often winds down when the baby is exhausted, or when gas or stool is passed.

In spite of apparent abdominal pain, colicky infants eat well and gain weight normally.

Home care

Helping a child with colic is primarily a matter of experimentation and observation. If you can identify and eliminate a trigger for the colic, that is best. Even if you can't, learn which measures most comfort your baby.

POSSIBLE TRIGGERS

- **Foods** - Avoid stimulants such as caffeine and chocolate. Try eliminating diary products and nuts for a few weeks, as these may be causing allergic reactions in the baby. Other foods may also irritate the baby.
- **Formula** - Switching formulas is NOT helpful for most babies, but is very important for some.
- **Medicine** - Some medicines Mom may be taking can also lead to crying.
- **Feeding** - If a bottle feeding takes less than 20 minutes, the hole in the nipple may be too large. Avoid overfeeding the infant or feeding too quickly.

TIPS FOR COMFORTING THE BABY

Different children are comforted by different measures. Some prefer to be swaddled in a warm blanket; others prefer to be free. Try many different things, and pay attention to what seems to help, even just a little bit.

- Holding your child is one of the most effective measures. The more hours held, even early in the day when they are not fussy, the less time they will be fussy in the evening. This will not spoil your child. Body carriers can be a great way to do this.
- As babies cry, they swallow more air, creating more gas and perhaps more abdominal pain, which causes more crying. This vicious cycle can be difficult to break. Gentle rocking can be very calming. This is directly comforting and seems to help them pass gas. When you get tired, an infant swing is a good alternative for babies at least 3 weeks old with good head control.
- Singing lullabies to your baby can be powerfully soothing. It is no accident that lullabies have developed in almost every culture. The noise of a vacuum or clothes dryer is soothing to many babies.
- Holding your child in an upright position may help. This aids gas movement and reduces heartburn. A warm towel or warm water bottle on the abdomen can help. Some babies prefer to lie on their tummies, while awake, while someone gives them a backrub. The gentle pressure on the abdomen may help. (To avoid SIDS, DO NOT put babies on their tummies to **sleep**.)
- Some babies are only happy when they are sucking on something. A pacifier can be like a miracle in these cases.
- The concentration of breast milk changes during a feeding. The "foremilk" at the beginning is plentiful but low in calories and fat. The "hindmilk" at the end of emptying each breast is far richer. Sometimes you can reduce colic by allowing the baby to finish the first breast before offering the second. If the baby still seems uncomfortable or eating too much, then offering only one breast (as often as desired) over a 2-3 hour period might give the baby more hindmilk, which is richer and sometimes more soothing.
- Some children seem to do best when they are riding in a car. If your child is one of

these, you might try a device developed by a pediatrician to imitate car motion and sound.

- Simethicone drops, a defoaming agent that reduces intestinal gas, may help. It is not absorbed into the body and is therefore quite safe. Sometimes doctors will prescribe stronger medicines for severe colic (but this should only be done after a physical exam).

Take breaks. Each of you can take charge and relieve the other. Time for oneself is an important part of the new family dynamic. You will be able to pay more loving attention to your baby when you've had a chance to get refreshed.

When to contact a medical professional

Call your health care provider if you have concerns. The most important thing to keep in mind is not to misdiagnose a serious condition and call it colic. If your baby's behavior or crying pattern changes suddenly or if the crying is associated with fever, forceful vomiting, diarrhea, bloody stools, or other abnormal activity or symptoms, call your doctor immediately.

Do not be afraid to seek help immediately if you feel overwhelmed and are afraid that you may hurt your baby.

> **Good to know**
>
> Contrary to popular belief, changing your baby's formula might help relieve colic. Talk to your doctor about switching the type of formula. Food allergies are possible at a very young age. Switching from a milk or soy based formula to one that is hypoallergenic can make a big difference.

Prevention

A fussy period is likely no matter what prevention techniques are undertaken. However, good feeding techniques (as advised by a lactation consultant, if you are breastfeeding), good burping, and early identification of possible allergies in the baby's or mother's diet may help prevent colic. Try different comfort techniques *before* colic develops to identify your baby's particular needs and desires. This can help stop the fussy period from becoming so intense.

Common cold

The common cold generally involves a runny nose, nasal congestion, and sneezing. You may also have a sore throat, cough, headache, or other symptoms. Over 200 viruses can cause a cold.

Symptoms of a cold:

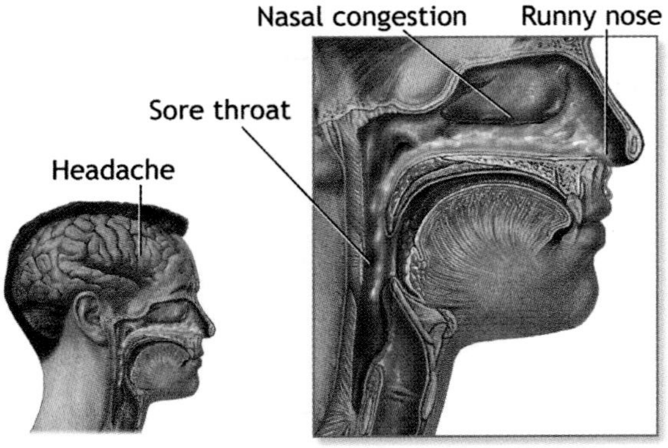

We call it the "common cold" for good reason. There are over *one billion* colds in the United States each year. You and your children will probably have more colds than any other type of illness. Children average 3 to 8 colds per year. They continue getting them throughout childhood. Parents often get them from the kids. It's the most common reason that children miss school and parents miss work.

Children usually get colds from other children. When a new strain is introduced into a school or day care, it quickly travels through the class.

When someone has a cold, their runny nose is teeming with cold viruses. Sneezing, nose-blowing, and nose-wiping spread the virus. You can catch a cold by inhaling the virus if you are sitting close to someone who sneezes, or by touching your nose, eyes, or mouth after you have touched something contaminated by the virus.

People are most contagious for the first 2 to 3 days of a cold, and usually not contagious at all by day 7 to 10.

Symptoms

Adults and older children with colds generally have minimal or no fever. Young children, however, often run a fever around 100-102°F.

Once you have "caught" a cold, the symptoms usually begin in 2 or 3 days, though it may take a week. Typically, an irritated nose or scratchy throat is the first sign, followed within hours by sneezing and a watery nasal discharge.

Within one to three days, the nasal secretions usually become thicker and perhaps yellow or green. This is a normal part of the common cold and not a reason for antibiotics.

For children with asthma, colds are the most common trigger of asthma symptoms.

Colds are a common precursor of ear infections. However, children's eardrums are usually congested during a cold, and it's possible to have fluid buildup without a true bacterial infection.

The entire cold is usually over all by itself in about 7 days, with perhaps a few lingering symptoms (such as cough) for another week. If it lasts longer, consider another problem, such as a sinus infection or allergies.

Home care

Try over-the-counter cold remedies to relieve your symptoms. These won't actually shorten the length of a cold, but can help you feel better. Meanwhile, get rest. Drink plenty of fluids. And don't force a child with a cold to eat.

Antibiotics should NOT be used to treat a common cold. They will NOT help and may make the situation worse! Thick yellow or green nasal discharge is not a reason for antibiotics, unless it lasts for 10 to 14 days without improving. (In this case, it may be sinusitis.)

Chicken soup has been used for treating common colds at least since the 12th century. It may really help. The heat, fluid, and salt may help you fight the infection.

Key points

When you have a cold, you are most contagious for the first 2 to 3 days but can spread the virus for up to 7 to 10 days. Wash your hands often to try to avoid spreading to others.

Also, antibiotics DO NOT work for the common cold. Read this article for more information about preventing the spread of colds and the best ways to treat them.

When to contact a medical professional

Try home care measures first. Call your health care provider if:

- The symptoms worsen or do not improve after 7 to 10 days
- Breathing difficulty develops
- Specific symptoms deserve a call (for example, see the article on fever)

Prevention

It might seem overwhelming to try to prevent colds, but you can do it. Children average 3 to 8 colds per year. It is certainly better to get 3 than 8!

Here are 5 proven ways to reduce exposure to germs:

- **Switch day care:** Using a day care of 6 or fewer children dramatically reduces germ contact.

- **Wash hands:** Children and adults should wash hands at key moments – after nose-wiping, after diapering or toileting, before eating, and before food preparation.
- **Use instant hand sanitizers:** Talk about convenient! A little dab will kill 99.99% of germs without any water or towels. It uses alcohol to destroy germs. It is an antiseptic, not an antibiotic, so resistance can't develop. And it's fun. Many kids think it's a treat to use it!
- **Disinfect:** Clean commonly touched surfaces (sink handles, sleeping mats) with an EPA-approved disinfectant.
- **Use paper towels**... instead of shared cloth towels.

Here are seven ways to support the immune system:

- **Avoid unnecessary antibiotics:** The more people use antibiotics, the more likely they are to get sick with longer, more stubborn infections caused by more resistant organisms in the future.
- **Breastfeed:** Breast milk is known to protect against respiratory tract infections, even years after breastfeeding is done. Kids who don't breastfeed average 5 times more ear infections.
- **Avoid second-hand smoke:** Keep as far away from it as possible! It is responsible for many health problems, including millions of colds.
- **Get enough sleep:** Late bedtimes and poor sleep leave people vulnerable.
- **Drink water:** Your body needs fluids for the immune system to function properly.
- **Eat yogurt:** The beneficial bacteria in some active yogurt cultures help prevent colds.
- **Take zinc:** Children and adults who are zinc-deficient get more infections and stay sick longer.

Constipation

Constipation refers to infrequent or hard stools, or difficulty passing stools. Constipation may involve pain during the passage of a bowel movement, inability to pass a bowel movement after straining or pushing for more than 10 minutes, or no bowel movements after more than 3 days. Infants who are still exclusively breastfed may go 7 days without a stool.

Constipation is a relative term. Normal patterns of bowel elimination vary widely from person to person and you may not have a bowel movement every day. While some healthy people have consistently soft or near-runny stools, others have consistently firm stools, but no difficulty passing them.

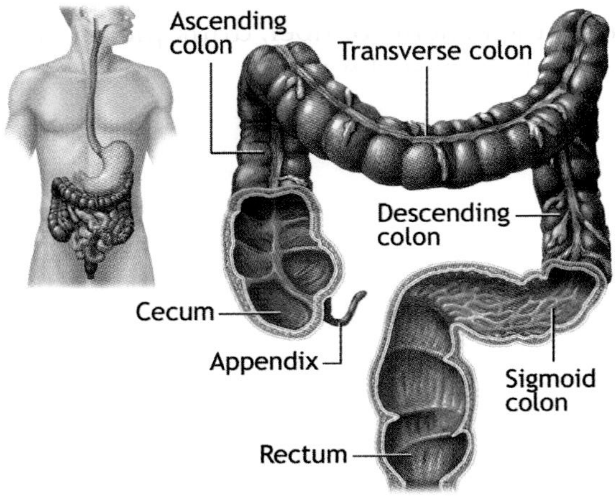

At the end of the digestive system, the body reabsorbs water in the colon. From there, the remaining waste (feces) passes through the rectum and is eliminated from the body.

Constipation is most often caused by a low-fiber diet, lack of physical activity, not drinking enough water, or delay in going to the bathroom when you have the urge to defecate. Stress and travel can also contribute to constipation or other changes in bowel habits.

Constipation in children often occurs if they hold back bowel movements when they aren't ready for toilet training or are afraid of it.

Home care

Children and adults should get enough fiber in their diet. Vegetables, fresh fruits, dried fruits, and whole wheat, bran, or oatmeal cereals are excellent sources of fiber.

Fiber

Food sources of fiber include whole wheat, bran, fresh or dried fruits, and vegetables

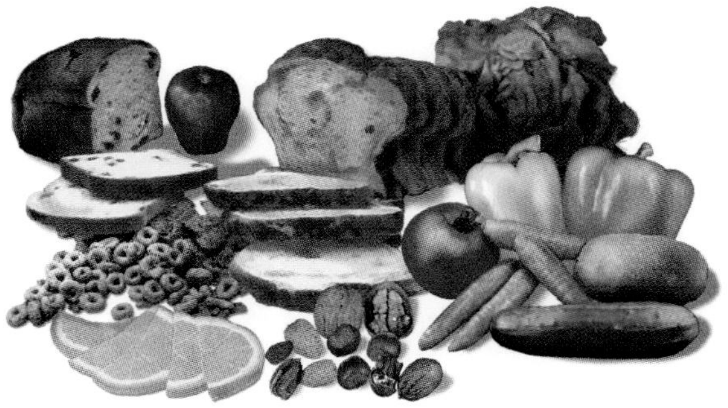

To reap the benefits of fiber, drink plenty of fluids to help pass the stool.

For constipated infants:

- Over 2 months old – try 2-4 ounces of fruit juice (grape, pear, apple, cherry, or prune) twice a day.
- Over 4 months old – if the baby has begun solid foods, try baby foods with high-fiber content (peas, beans, apricots, prunes, peaches, pears, plums, spinach) twice a day.

Regular exercise is also important in establishing regular bowel movements. If you are confined to a wheelchair or bed, change position frequently and perform abdominal contraction exercises and leg raises. A physical therapist can recommend exercises appropriate for your physical abilities.

Stool softeners (such as those containing docusate sodium) may help. Additionally, bulk laxatives such as Psyllium may help add fluid and bulk to the stool. Suppositories or gentle laxatives, such as mineral oil or milk of magnesia, may establish regular bowel movements. Enemas or laxatives should be reserved for severe cases only. In addition, laxatives should not be used over a long period because you can become dependent on them.

DO NOT give laxatives or enemas to children without instruction from a doctor.

When to contact a medical professional

Call your doctor if you have:

- Sudden constipation with abdominal cramps and an inability to pass gas or stool (DO NOT take any laxatives – call immediately!)
- Sharp or severe abdominal pain, especially if you're also bloated
- Blood in your stool
- Constipation alternating with diarrhea
- Thin, pencil-like stools
- Rectal pain
- Unexplained weight loss
- Been using laxatives for several weeks or self care is not working

Call if:

- An infant younger than 2 months is constipated.
- An infant (except those exclusively breastfed) goes 3 days without a stool. If vomiting or irritability is also present, call IMMEDIATELY.
- A child is holding back bowel movements in order to resist toilet training.

Corns and calluses

Corns and calluses are caused by pressure or friction on skin. A **corn** is thickened skin on the top or side of a toe, usually from shoes that do not fit properly. A **callus** is thickened skin on your hands or the soles of your feet.

The thickening of the skin is a protective reaction. For example, farmers and rowers get callused hands that prevent them from getting painful blisters. People with bunions often develop a callus over the bunion because it rubs against the shoe.

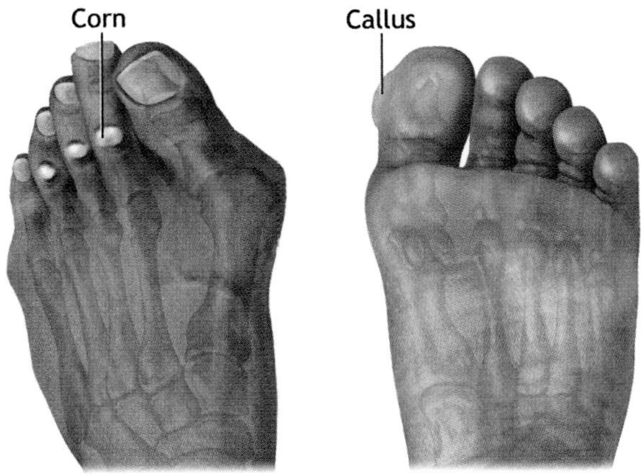

Home care

Usually, preventing friction is the only treatment needed. If a corn is the result of a poor-fitting shoe, changing to shoes that fit properly will usually eliminate the corn within a couple of weeks. Until then, protect the skin with donut-shaped corn pads, available in pharmacies. If desired, use a pumice stone to gently wear down the corn.

Calluses on the hands can be treated by wearing gloves during activities that cause friction, such as gardening and weight lifting.

When to contact a medical professional

People with diabetes who notice problems with their feet should contact their health care providers. Otherwise, simply changing to better-fitting shoes or wearing gloves should resolve most problems with corns and calluses.

If you suspect that your corn or callus is infected or is not getting better despite treatment, contact your health care provider.

Cough

Coughing is an important way to keep your throat and airways clear. However, excessive coughing may mean you have an underlying disease or disorder.

Some coughs are dry, while others are "productive." A productive cough is one that brings up phlegm (also called sputum or mucus). Coughs can be either acute or chronic:

- **Acute coughs** usually begin suddenly. They are often due to a cold, flu, or sinus infection. Typically, they do not last longer than 2-3 weeks.
- **Chronic coughs** last longer than 2-3 weeks.

Besides cold and flu, other common causes of coughs include:

- Allergies and asthma
- Lung infections like pneumonia or acute bronchitis (may start suddenly but then linger on)
- Chronic obstructive pulmonary disease (emphysema or chronic bronchitis)
- Sinusitis leading to postnasal drip
- Smoking cigarette smoke and pollutants
- Gastroesophageal reflux disease (GERD)

If a child has a barking cough, see *Croup*.

Home care

- Cough lozenges or hard candy can help dry, tickling coughs. These should never be given to a child under 3 years old because of the risk of choking.
- A vaporizer or steamy shower may help a dry cough by increasing the humidity in the air.
- Drink extra fluids to help thin the secretions in your throat and make them easier to cough up.

- Zinc lozenges can reduce cold symptoms, especially cough.

Medications available without a prescription include:

- Guaifenesin (like Robitussin) can help you bring up phlegm. Drink lots of fluids if taking this medication.
- Cough suppressants like dextromethor phan (Vicks 44, Robitussin DM) may lessen your cough. Although coughing can be a troubling symptom, it is usually your body's way of healing the underlying condition. Therefore, you may not want to suppress a cough unless it is interfering with sleep or other factors important for healing.
- Decongestants, like pseudoephedrine and phenylephrine, can be used to clear a runny nose and postnasal drip. These should NOT be used if you have high blood pressure or for a child under 6 years old unless prescribed by your doctor.

Don't expect a doctor to prescribe antibiotics for viral infections like colds or flu. Antibiotics have no effect on viruses. Antibiotics also will not help coughs from allergies.

When to contact a medical professional

Call 911 if you have:

- Shortness of breath or difficulty breathing
- Hives or swollen face or throat with difficulty swallowing

Call your doctor right away if you have:

- Violent cough that begins suddenly
- High-pitched sound (called stridor) when inhaling
- Cough that produces blood
- Fever (may indicate a bacterial infection requiring antibiotics)
- Thick, foul-smelling, yellowish-green phlegm (may indicate a bacterial infection)
- A history of heart disease, swelling in your legs, or a cough that worsens when you lie down (may indicate congestive heart failure)
- Exposure to someone with tuberculosis
- Unintentional weight loss or night sweats (may also indicate tuberculosis)
- Cough longer than 10-14 days
- Cough in an infant less than 3 months old

> **Tip**
>
> If a cough isn't improving over time, it is wise to look for a cause other than infection, such as asthma or GERD. Talk to your doctor about what else might be causing your lingering cough.

Prevention

- Don't smoke and stay away from secondhand smoke.
- If you have seasonal allergies like hay fever, stay indoors during days when airborne allergens are high. If possible, keep the windows closed and use an air conditioner. Avoid fans that draw in air from outdoors. Shower and change your clothes after being outside.

If you have allergies year round, cover your pillows and mattress with dust mite covers, use an air purifier, and avoid pets and other triggers.

Croup

Croup is breathing difficulty accompanied by a "barking" cough. Croup, which is swelling around the vocal cords, is common in infants and children and can have a variety of causes. Viral croup is the most common.

Other possible causes include bacteria, allergies, and inhaled irritants. Acid reflux from the stomach can trigger croup.

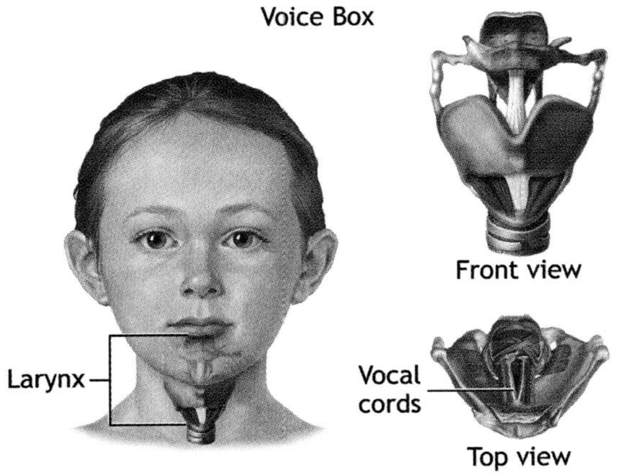

The name "croup" comes from an old German word meaning voice box, which is your larynx.

Before the era of immunizations and antibiotics, croup was a dreaded and deadly disease, usually caused by the diphtheria bacteria. Today, most cases of croup are mild. Nevertheless, it can still be dangerous.

Croup tends to appear in children between 3 months and 5 years old, but it can happen at any age. Some children are prone to croup and may get it several times.

In the Northern hemisphere, it is most common between October and March, but can occur at any time of the year.

Symptoms

Croup features a cough that sounds like a seal barking. Most children have what appears to be a mild cold for several days before the barking cough becomes evident. As the cough gets more frequent, the child may have labored breathing or stridor (a harsh, crowing noise made during inspiration).

Croup is typically much worse at night. It often lasts 5 or 6 nights, but the first night or two are usually the most severe. Rarely, croup can last for weeks. Croup that lasts longer than a week or recurs frequently should be discussed with your doctor to determine the cause.

Home care

Most cases of croup can be safely managed at home, but call your health care provider for guidance, even in the middle of the night.

Cool or moist air can bring relief. You might first try bringing the child into a steamy bathroom or outside into the cool night air. If you have a cool air vaporizer, set it up in the child's bedroom and use it for the next few nights.

Acetaminophen can make the child more comfortable and lower a fever, lessening his or her breathing needs. Avoid cough medicines unless you discuss them with your doctor first.

You may want your child to be seen. Steroid medicines can be very effective at promptly relieving the symptoms of croup. Medicated aerosol treatments, if necessary, are also powerful.

When to contact a medical professional

Most croup can be safely managed at home with telephone support from your health care provider. Call 911 if:

- The croup is possibly being caused by an insect sting or inhaled object
- The child has bluish lips or skin
- The child is drooling

Depending on the severity of the symptoms, call 911 or call your provider for any of the following:

- Stridor (noise when breathing in)
- Retractions (tugging-in between the ribs when breathing in)
- Struggling to breathe
- Agitatation or extreme irritability
- Not responding to home treatment

Prevention

Wash your hands frequently and avoid close contact with those who have a respiratory infection.

The diphtheria, Haemophilus influenzae (Hib), and measles vaccines protect children from some of the most dangerous forms of croup.

Dandruff and cradle cap

Dandruff in adults and cradle cap in infants are common yet harmless conditions that involve scaling and flaking of the scalp. The technical term is called seborrheic dermatitis, which is a type of rash that can occur in places other than the scalp. See the article entitled Rashes.

To get rid of your dandruff, use an over-the-counter anti-dandruff shampoo every day. Look for salicylic acid, selenium, sulfur, and tar as the active ingredients in the product. Work the shampoo into your hair as you actively massage your scalp. This is to make sure that the scales flake off. Rinse with lukewarm (not hot) water and avoid overuse of hair dryers and electric curlers.

If you have stubborn dandruff, try changing to another shampoo with a different active ingredient. Test different shampoos to see which gives you the best results. Meanwhile, light-colored clothing may make any dandruff that you still have less noticeable. If you don't find an over-the-counter solution, your doctor may consider a prescription shampoo.

For cradle cap:

- Massage your baby's scalp gently with your fingers or soft brush. This will loosen the scales and improve scalp circulation.
- Use a gentle, mild shampoo every day until the scales disappear. After that, use the same shampoo at least two times per week. Be sure to rinse off all of the soap.
- Brush your baby's hair with a clean, soft brush after each shampoo and several times during the day.
- If the scales do not loosen easily from massaging, shampooing, and brushing, try applying some mineral oil before shampooing.

These self-care measures almost always work for dandruff and cradle cap. If you or your baby has a severe case, however, and these steps do not work, there are prescription medications that your doctor would consider.

Depression

Depression may be described as feeling sad, blue, unhappy, miserable, or down in the dumps. Most of us feel this way at one time or another for short periods. But true clinical depression is a mood disorder in which feelings of sadness, loss, anger, or frustration interfere with everyday life for an extended time.

Depression is generally ranked in terms of severity – mild, moderate, or severe. The degree of your depression, which your doctor can determine, influences how you are treated. Symptoms of depression include:

- Trouble sleeping or excessive sleeping
- A dramatic change in appetite, often with weight gain or loss
- Fatigue and lack of energy
- Feelings of worthlessness, self-hate, and inappropriate guilt
- Extreme difficulty concentrating
- Agitation, restlessness, and irritability
- Inactivity and withdrawal from usual activities
- Feelings of hopelessness and helplessness
- Recurring thoughts of death or suicide

Low self esteem is common with depression. So are sudden bursts of anger and lack of pleasure from activities that normally make you happy, including sex.

Depressed children may not have the classic symptoms of adult depression. Watch especially for changes in school performance, sleep, and behavior. If you wonder whether your child might be depressed, it's worth bringing to a doctor's attention.

The main types of depression include:

- **Major depression** – five or more symptoms listed above must be present for at least 2 weeks, but major depression tends to continue for at least 6 months. (Depression is classified as minor depression if *less* than five depressive symptoms are present for at least 2 weeks.)
- **Dysthymia** – a chronic, generally milder form of depression but lasts longer – usually as long as two years.
- **Atypical depression** – depression accompanied by unusual symptoms, such as hallucinations (for example, hearing voices that are not really there) or delusions (irrational thoughts).

Other common forms of depression include:

- **Postpartum depression** – many women feel somewhat down after having a baby, but true postpartum depression is rare.
- **Premenstrual dysphoric disorder (PDD)** – depressive symptoms occur one week prior to menstruation and disappear after you menstruate.
- **Seasonal affective disorder (SAD)** – occurs during the fall-winter season and disappears during the spring-summer season. Likely to be due to lack of sunlight.

Depression may also occur with mania (known as manic-depression or bipolar disorder). In this condition, moods cycle between mania and depression.

Depression often runs in families. This may be from heredity, learned behavior, or both. Even with a genetic predisposition, it is usually a stressful or unhappy life event that triggers the onset of a depressive episode.

Depression may be brought on by:

- Disappointment at home, work, or school (in teens, this may be breaking up with a boyfriend or girlfriend, failing a class, or parents divorcing)
- Death of a friend or relative
- Prolonged pain or having a major illness
- Medical conditions such as hypothyroidism (underactive thyroid), cancer, or hepatitis
- Drugs such as sedatives and high blood pressure medications
- Alcohol or drug abuse
- Chronic stress
- Childhood events like abuse or neglect
- Social isolation (common in the elderly)
- Nutritional deficiencies (such as folate and omega-3 fatty acids)
- Sleeping problems

Home care

If you are depressed for 2 weeks or longer, you should contact your doctor, who can offer treatment options. Regardless of whether you have mild or major depression, the following self-care steps can help:

- Get enough sleep.
- Follow a healthy, nutritious diet.
- Exercise regularly.
- Avoid alcohol, marijuana, and other recreational drugs.
- Get involved in activities that make you happy, even if you don't feel like it.
- Spend time with family and friends.
- Try talking to clergy or spiritual advisors who may help give meaning to painful experiences.

- Consider prayer, meditation, tai chi, or biofeedback as ways to relax or draw on your inner strengths.
- Add omega-3 fatty acids to your diet, which you can get from cold-water fish like tuna, salmon, or mackerel.
- Take folate (vitamin B9) in the form of a multivitamin (400 to 800 micrograms).

If your depression occurs in the fall or winter months, try light therapy using a special lamp that mimics the sun.

Many people try a popular over-the-counter herb called St. John's Wort. Some studies do suggest that this herbal remedy may be helpful for mild depression, but not moderate or severe. Be aware that St. John's Wort has potential drug interactions and should NOT be taken with prescription antidepressants, birth control pills, protease inhibitors for HIV, theophylline, warfarin, digoxin, reserpine, cyclosporine, or loperamide. Talk to your doctor if you are thinking about trying this herb for mild depression.

If you have moderate to severe depression, the most effective treatment plan will likely be a combination of counseling and medication.

When to Contact a Medical Professional

Call 911, a suicide hotline, or get safely to a nearby emergency room if you have thoughts of suicide, a suicidal plan, or thoughts of harming yourself or others.

Call your doctor right away if:

- You hear voices that are not there.
- You have frequent crying spells with little or no provocation.
- You have had feelings of depression that disrupt work, school, or family life for longer than 2 weeks.
- You have 3 or more depressive symptoms.
- You think that one of your current medications may be making you feel depressed. DO NOT change or stop any medications without consulting your doctor.
- You believe that you should cut back on drinking, a family member or friend has asked you to cut back, you feel guilty about the amount of alcohol you drink, or you drink alcohol first thing in the morning.

Prevention

Healthy lifestyle habits can help prevent depression, or lessen the chances of it happening again. These habits include eating properly, sleeping adequately, exercising regularly, learning to relax, and not drinking alcohol or using drugs.

Counseling may help you through times of grief, stress, or low mood. Family therapy may be particularly important for teens who feel blue.

For elderly or others who feel socially isolated or lonely, try volunteering or getting involved in group activities.

> **Key Point**
>
> You may feel better if you add omega-3 fatty acids to your diet, which you can get from cold-water fish like tuna, salmon, or mackerel. Also, taking folate (vitamin B9) may be helpful. Appropriate amounts of folate (400 to 800 micrograms) are found in many multivitamins.

Diarrhea

Diarrhea is loose, watery, and frequent stools. Diarrhea is considered chronic (ongoing or prolonged) when you have had loose or frequent stools longer than 4 weeks.

Diarrhea in adults is usually mild and resolves quickly without complication. In infants and children (especially under age 3), diarrhea is more concerning. Children can become dehydrated fairly quickly.

The most common cause of diarrhea is a mild viral infection that resolves on its own within a few days. This is called viral gastroenteritis or "stomach flu." Viral gastroenteritis often appears in mini-epidemics in schools, neighborhoods, or families.

Food poisoning and traveler's diarrhea are two other common causes. They occur from eating food or drinking water contaminated with bacteria or parasites.

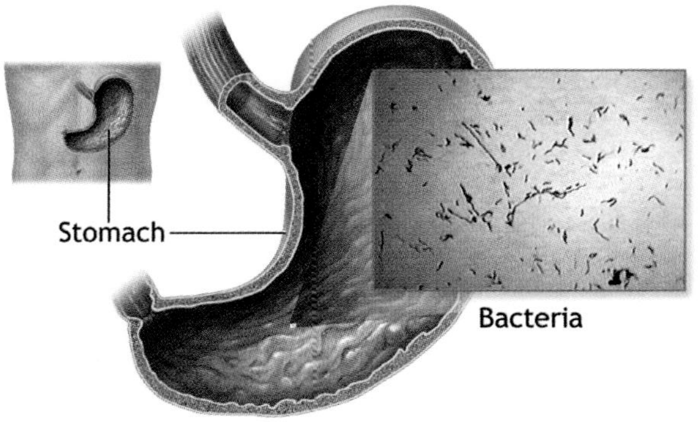

Certain medical conditions can also lead to diarrhea, such as:

- **Malabsorption syndromes** – you are unable to absorb or digest certain nutrients. Common examples include lactose intolerance, gluten malabsorption, and intolerance to specific foods like beans or fruit.
- **Inflammatory bowel diseases** – Crohn's disease and ulcerative colitis are two recurring types of diarrhea that are generally bloody and accompanied by abdominal pain.
- **Irritable bowel syndrome (IBS)** – a chronic form of stomach upset that gets worse from stress. You generally have alternating diarrhea and constipation.
- **Immune deficiency**.

Medications can also cause diarrhea, especially antibiotics, laxatives containing magnesium, and chemotherapy for cancer treatment.

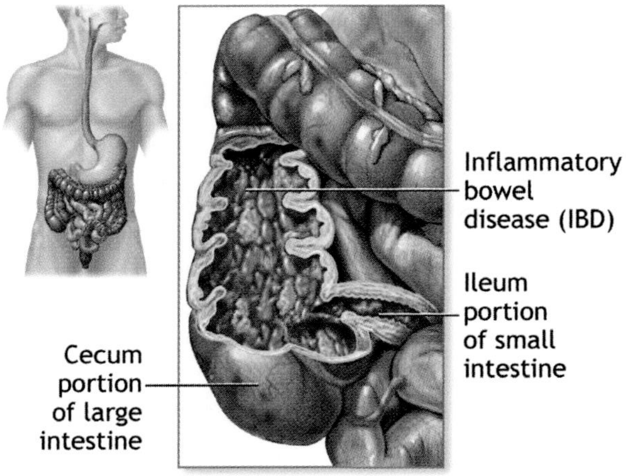

Inflammatory bowel disease causes inflammation and ulcers (open sores) along the inner lining of the intestinal wall.

Home care

- Drink plenty of fluid to avoid becoming dehydrated. Start with sips of any fluid other than caffeinated beverages. Milk may prolong loose stools, but also provides needed fluids and nourishment. Drinking milk may be fine for mild diarrhea. For moderate and severe diarrhea, electrolyte solutions available in drugstores are usually best.
- Active cultures of beneficial bacteria (probiotics) make diarrhea less severe and shorten its duration. Probiotics can be found in yogurt with live or active cultures and in supplements.
- Foods like rice, dry toast, and bananas may help some.
- Avoid over-the-counter diarrheal medications unless specifically instructed to use one by your doctor. Certain infections can be made worse by these drugs. When you have diarrhea, your body is trying to get rid of whatever food, virus, or other bug is causing it.
- Rest.

If you have a chronic form of diarrhea, like irritable bowel syndrome, try adding bulk to your diet to thicken the stool and regulate bowel movements. Such foods include rice, bananas, and fiber from whole-wheat grains and bran. Psyllium-containing products such as Metamucil or similar products can add bulk to stools.

When to contact a medical professional

Call your doctor if:

- You have blood or pus in your stools or if your stool is black.
- You have abdominal pain that is not relieved by a bowel movement.
- You have symptoms of dehydration – see article on dehydration.
- You have a fever above 101°F or your child has a fever above 100.4°F along with diarrhea.
- You have foul smelling or oily-looking stools.
- You have recently traveled to a foreign country.
- You have eaten with other people who also have diarrhea.
- You have started on a new medication.
- Your diarrhea does not get better in 5 days (2 days for an infant or child) or worsens before that.
- Your child has been vomiting for more than 12 hours. In a newborn (under 3 months), you should call as soon as vomiting or diarrhea begins.

Prevention

- Wash your hands often, especially after going to the bathroom and before eating.
- Teach children to not put objects in their mouth.
- When taking antibiotics, try using **Lactobacillus acidophilus**, a probiotic or healthy bacteria. This helps replenish the good bacteria that antibiotics can kill.

When traveling to underdeveloped areas, follow the steps below to avoid diarrhea:

- Drink only bottled water and DO NOT use ice.
- DO NOT eat uncooked vegetables or fruit without a peel.
- DO NOT eat raw shellfish or undercooked meat.
- DO NOT consume dairy products.

Dizziness / feeling faint

Dizziness may be experienced as lightheadedness, feeling like you might faint, being unsteady, loss of balance, or vertigo (a feeling that you or the room is spinning or moving).

Most causes of dizziness are not serious and either quickly resolve on their own or are easily treated.

Lightheadedness happens when there is not enough blood getting to the brain. This can happen if there is a sudden drop in your blood pressure or you are dehydrated from vomiting, diarrhea, fever, or other causes. Many people, especially as they get older, experience lightheadedness if they get up too quickly from a lying or seated position. Lightheadedness often accompanies the flu, common cold, or allergies.

More serious conditions that can lead to lightheadedness include heart problems (such as abnormal heart rhythm or heart attack), stroke, and severe drop in blood pressure (shock). If any of these serious disorders is present, you will usually have additional symptoms like chest pain, a feeling of a racing heart, loss of speech, change in vision, or other symptoms.

The most common causes of vertigo are benign positional vertigo and labyrinthitis. Benign positional vertigo is vertigo that happens when you change the position of your head. Labyrinthitis usually follows a cold or flu and is caused by a viral infection of the inner ear. Meniere's disease is another common inner ear problem. It causes vertigo, loss of balance, and ringing in the ears.

What is vertigo?

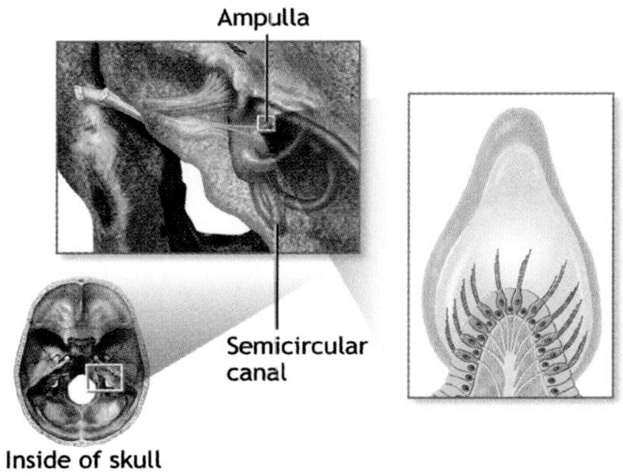

Deep inside the head is the inner ear, which contains 3 small, fluid-filled structures called the semicircular canals. Each canal has a swelling at the end called the ampulla, which contains tiny hair cells.

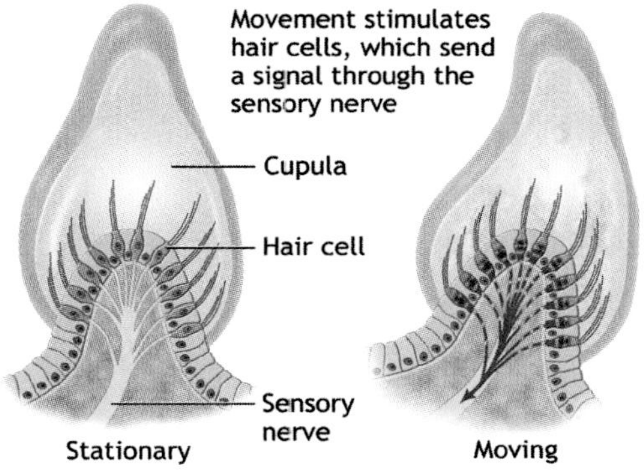

Head movements cause the fluid to bend the hair cells. The hair cells, in turn, send a signal to your brain that you are experiencing "motion".

Benign positional vertigo may be caused when small calcium particles are floating in the canals, disturbing the ampulla when you move. This causes your right and left ear to send different messages about your body's position, and your brain thinks you are spinning.

Home care

If you tend to get lightheaded when you stand up, avoid sudden changes in posture.

If you are thirsty or lightheaded, drink fluids. If you are unable to keep fluids down from nausea or vomiting, you may need intravenous fluids. These are delivered to you at the hospital.

Most times, benign positional vertigo and labyrinthitis go away on their own within a few weeks. During attacks of vertigo from any cause, try to rest and lie still. Avoid sudden changes in your position as well as bright lights. Be cautious about driving or using machinery.

Some vertigo can be reduced by working with a physical therapist. Medications from your doctor may help you feel better.

When to contact a medical professional

Call 911 or go to an emergency room if someone with dizziness also has:

- A head injury
- Fever over 101°F, headache, or very stiff neck
- Convulsions or ongoing vomiting
- Chest pain, heart palpitations, shortness of breath, weakness, inability to move an arm or leg, or change in vision or speech
- Fainting and losing consciousness for more than a few minutes

Call your doctor if:

- You have never had dizziness before.
- Symptoms you have had in the past are different (for example, last longer than usual, are worse than before, or are interfering with your daily activities).
- Medication is the suspected cause. Talk to your health care provider before making any changes to your medication.
- You have any hearing loss.

Prevention

Promptly treat ear infections, colds, flus, sinus congestion, and other respiratory infections. This may help prevent labyrinthitis and Meniere's disease.

If you have a cold, the flu, or other viral illness, drink plenty of fluids to prevent getting dehydrated.

Ear Infection

Ear infections are one of the most common reasons parents take their children to the doctor. While there are different types of ear infections, the most common is called otitis media, which means an inflammation and infection of the middle ear. The middle ear is located just behind the eardrum.

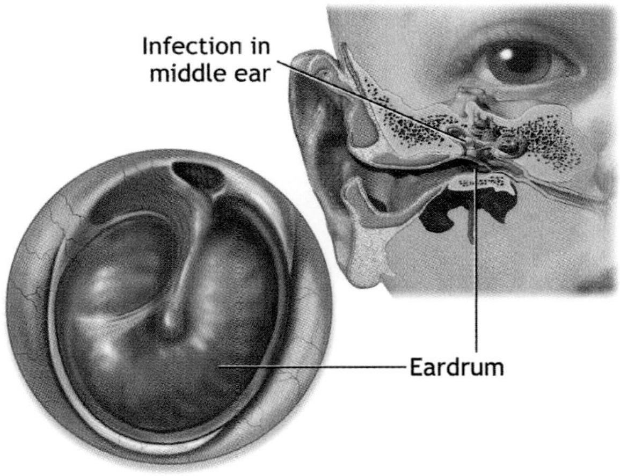

The term "acute" refers to a short and painful episode. An ear infection that lasts a long time or comes and goes is called "chronic" otitis media.

Ear infections are common in infants and children in part because their eustachian tubes become clogged easily. For each ear, a eustachian tube runs from the middle ear to the back of the throat. Its purpose is to drain fluid and bacteria that normally occurs in the middle ear. If the eustachian tube becomes blocked, fluid can build up and become infected.

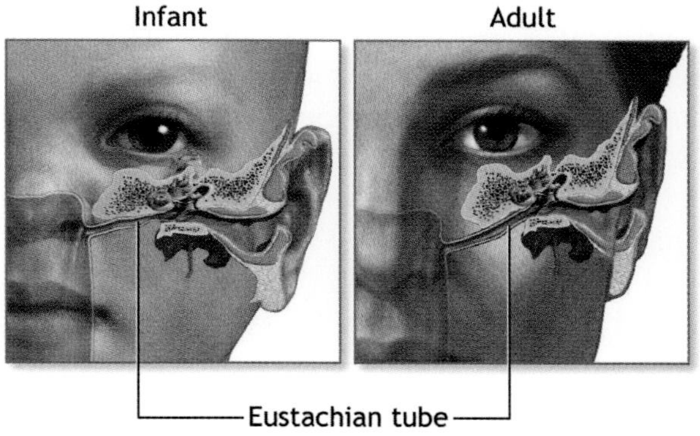

Children are more prone to ear infections than adults partly because of the more horizontal angle of their eustachian tube, making it less effective at draining fluids.

Anything that causes the eustachian tubes and upper airways to become inflamed or irritated, or cause more fluids to be produced, can lead to a blocked eustachian tube. These include:

- Colds and sinus infections
- Allergies
- Tobacco smoke or other irritants
- Infected or overgrown adenoids
- Excess mucus and saliva produced during teething

Ear infections are also more likely if a child spends a lot of time drinking from a sippy cup or bottle while lying on his or her back. Contrary to popular opinion, getting water in the ears will not cause an acute ear infection, unless the eardrum has a hole from a previous episode.

Ear infections occur most frequently in the winter. An ear infection is not itself contagious, but a cold may spread among children and cause some of them to get ear infections.

Symptoms

An acute ear infection causes pain (earache). In infants, the clearest sign is often irritability and inconsolable crying. Many infants and children develop a fever or have trouble sleeping. Parents often think that tugging on the ear is a symptom of an ear infection, but studies have shown that the same number of children going to the doctor tug on the ear whether or not the ear is infected.

Other possible symptoms include:

- Fullness in the ear
- Feeling of general illness
- Vomiting
- Diarrhea
- Hearing loss in the affected ear

The child may have symptoms of a cold, or the ear infection may start shortly after having a cold.

All acute ear infections include fluid behind the eardrum. You can use an electronic ear monitor, such as Earcheck, to detect this fluid at home. The device is available at pharmacies.

Home care

The goals for treating ear infections include relieving pain, curing the infection, preventing complications, and preventing recurrent ear infections. Most ear infections will safely clear up on their own without antibiotics.

Often, treating the pain and allowing the body time to heal itself is all that is needed:

- Apply a warm cloth or warm water bottle.
- Use over-the-counter pain relief drops for ears.
- Take over-the counter medications for pain or fever, like ibuprofen or acetaminophen. DO NOT give aspirin to children.
- Use prescription ear drops to relieve pain.

When to contact a medical professional

Call your child's doctor if:

- Pain, fever, or irritability do not improve within 24 to 48 hours
- At the start, the child seems sicker than just an ear infection
- Your child has a high fever or severe pain
- Severe pain suddenly stops hurting – this may indicate a ruptured eardrum
- Symptoms worsen
- New symptoms appear, especially severe headache, dizziness, swelling around the ear, or twitching of the face muscles

For a child under 6 months, let the doctor know right away if the child has a fever, even if no other symptoms are present.

Antibiotics – use with caution

Some ear infections require antibiotics to clear the infection and to prevent them from becoming worse. This is especially likely if your child is under age 2, has a fever, is acting sick (beyond just the ear), or is not improving over 24 to 48 hours. Most ear infections, however, heal well without antibiotics. Talk with your doctor about whether your child can be safely treated in other ways. Many times, a pain reliever is enough. Antibiotics do NOT make your child feel better faster. Antibiotics may cause unpleasant side effects and may make it more difficult to treat future ear infections.

You can also ask your doctor for a "SNAP." This stands for "Safety Net Antibiotic Prescription." This simply means you are given a prescription, but don't fill it unless the pain is getting worse or your child still has symptoms in 48 hours. In the meantime, use pain relief ear drops and/or a pain reliever like acetaminophen or ibuprofen.

Prevention

You can reduce your child's risk of ear infections with the following practices:

- Wash hands and toys frequently. Also, day care with 6 or fewer children can lessen your child's chances of getting a cold or similar infection. This leads to fewer ear infections.
- Avoid pacifiers, especially at daycare.
- Breastfeed – this makes a child much less prone to ear infections. But, if bottle feeding, hold your infant in an upright, seated position.
- Don't expose your child to secondhand smoke.
- The pneumococcal vaccine prevents infections from the organism that most commonly causes acute ear infections and many respiratory infections.
- Some evidence suggests that xylitol, a natural sweetener, may reduce ear infections.
- Avoid overusing antibiotics.

Ear wax

Contrary to popular belief, ear wax is actually good. In fact, our bodies are designed to dispose of it on their own.

A slow-flowing river of ear wax is created by our bodies to protect, lubricate, and clean our ear canals. Hairs within the ear canal move the wax out of the ear.

Once wax is visible at the opening of the ear, you can easily wipe it away with a cloth or cotton swab. If you seem to produce a lot of wax or your ear wax is especially thick, try ear drops that thin the wax.

DO NOT place cotton swabs down into the ear canal itself. This can cause infection in the ear canal, injury to the skin lining the ear canal, or perforation of the eardrum. In addition, a cotton swab in the canal stimulates the body to make more ear wax.

Ears - ringing

Tinnitus is the medical term for "hearing" noises in your ears when there is no outside source of the sounds.

The noises you hear can be soft or loud. They may sound like ringing, blowing, roaring, buzzing, hissing, humming, whistling, or sizzling. You may even think you are hearing air escaping, water running, the inside of a seashell, or musical notes.

Almost everyone experiences a mild form of tinnitus once in awhile that only lasts a few minutes. However, constant or recurring tinnitus is stressful and can interfere with your ability to concentrate or sleep.

It is not known exactly what causes a person to "hear" sounds with no outside source of the noise.

However, tinnitus can be a symptom of almost any ear problem, including ear infections, foreign objects or wax in the ear, and injury from loud noises. Alcohol, caffeine, antibiotics, aspirin, or other drugs can also cause ear noises.

Tinnitus may occur with hearing loss. Occasionally, it is a sign of high blood pressure, an allergy, or anemia. Rarely, tinnitus is a sign of a serious problem like a tumor or aneurysm.

Home care

- Tinnitus can be masked by competing sounds, such as low-level music, ticking clocks, or other noises. Tinnitus is often more noticeable when you go to bed at night because your surroundings are quieter. Any noise in the room, like a humidifier, white noise machine, or dishwasher, can help mask tinnitus and make it less irritating.

- Learn ways to relax. Feeling stressed or anxious can worsen tinnitus.
- Avoid caffeine, alcohol, and smoking.
- Get enough rest. Try sleeping with your head propped up in an elevated position. This lessens head congestion and noises may become less noticeable.

When to contact a medical professional

Call your doctor if:

- Ear noises start after a head injury.
- The noises are associated with other unexplained symptoms like dizziness, feeling off balance, nausea, or vomiting.
- You have unexplained ear noises that bother you even after self-help measures.

Prevention

Wear ear protection in any situations where ear damage is possible (such as loud concerts, or jackhammers). If you have hearing loss, avoid further damage to your hearing by avoiding excessive noise.

Make sure your blood pressure is normal by maintaining proper body weight, exercising regularly, and seeing your doctor for yearly check ups.

Elbow pain

Elbow pain can be caused by a variety of problems. A common cause in adults is tendinitis, an inflammation and injury to the tendons – soft tissues that attach muscle to bone.

People who play racquet sports are most likely to injure the tendons on the outside of the elbow. This condition is commonly called tennis elbow. Golfers are more likely to injure the tendons on the inside of the elbow.

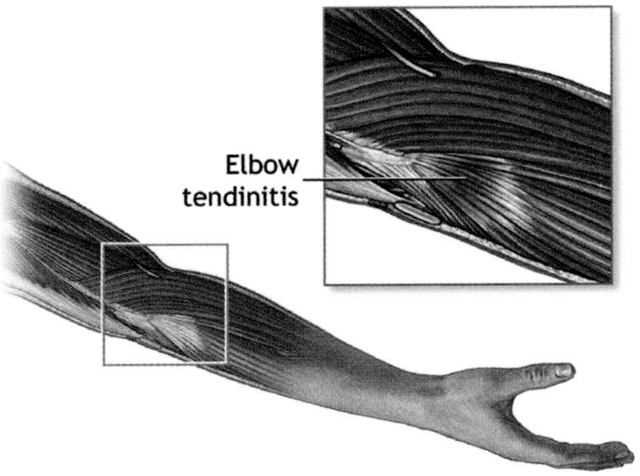

Other common causes of elbow tendinitis are gardening, playing baseball, using a screwdriver, or overusing your wrist.

Young children commonly develop "nursemaid's elbow," usually when someone is pulling on their straightened arm. The bones are stretched apart momentarily and a ligament slips in between, where it becomes trapped when the bones try to snap back into place. Children will usually quietly refuse to use the arm, but often cry out with any attempt to bend or straighten the elbow. This condition is also called an elbow subluxation (a partial dislocation).

Other common causes of elbow pain are:

- Bursitis – inflammation of a fluid-filled cushion beneath the skin
- Arthritis – narrowing of the joint space and loss of cartilage in the elbow
- Elbow strains
- Infection of the elbow

Home care

In adults, the following steps can help treat many cases of elbow pain:

- When you first notice the pain, apply ice up to 15 minutes every hour for the first day. Continue to apply ice every 3 to 4 hours for up to 3 days. Wrap the ice in a cloth – do not apply ice directly to the skin.

- Wrap the elbow with a bandage, such as an ACE bandage. You may need an air splint to keep the elbow immobilized.
- Keep the elbow elevated above your heart, if possible.
- Give the elbow joint complete rest for at least 2 days. DO NOT return to the activity that caused the problem for at least 3 weeks. Then, gradually strengthen the muscles around your elbow. A physical therapist can teach you how to do this.
- While you are resting the joint, take pain relievers such as acetaminophen or ibuprofen.
- After the initial rest period, you should begin to gradually strengthen the muscles around the elbow through gentle flexibility exercises.
- For nursemaid's elbow, call the child's doctor. This can be easily treated in a doctor's office.

When to contact a medical professional

Contact your doctor if:

- You have a prolonged case of tendinitis that doesn't improve with home care.
- The pain is due to a direct elbow injury.
- There is obvious deformity.
- You are unable to use the elbow.
- You have fever or swelling and redness of your elbow.
- A child has elbow pain.

Prevention

- Reduce how much time you spend doing the activity that causes the pain.
- Warm up slowly. Stretch the forearm before, during, and after exercise.
- Use an "elbow sleeve" to help keep your elbow warm while playing.
- Use ice or ibuprofen after the activity to prevent swelling and pain, if you have had an elbow injury in the past.
- Prevent tennis elbow by using the correct grip size, a two-handed backhand, and racquet strings that are not too tight.
- Wear an "elbow band" over an injured or rehabilitated area to prevent further injury and reduce pain.
- Perform regular stretching and strengthening exercises (given to you by your physical therapist or doctor).
- To prevent nursemaid's elbow in children, do not pull on a straightened arm. Avoid lifting or holding the child up by the hands or forearm. Children who get nursemaid's elbow once can easily get it again. Usually this is outgrown by age 4.

Erection problems

An erection problem is the inability to get or maintain an erection that is firm enough for a man to have intercourse. You may be unable to get an erection at all, or you may lose the erection during intercourse before you are ready. If the condition persists, the medical term is erectile dysfunction.

Erection problems are common in adult men. In fact, almost all men experience occasional difficulty getting or maintaining an erection. In many cases, it is a temporary condition that will go away with little or no treatment. In other cases, it can be an ongoing problem that can damage a man's self esteem and harm his relationship with his partner, and thus requires treatment.

In the past, erection problems were thought to be "all in the man's mind." Men often were given unhelpful advice such as "don't worry" or "just relax and it will take care of itself." Today, doctors believe that when the problem is not temporary or does not go away on its own, physical factors are often the cause.

One way to know if the cause is physical or psychologic is to determine if you are having nighttime erections. Normally, men have 3 to 5 erections per night, each lasting up to 30 minutes. Your doctor can explain a test to find out if you are having the normal number of nighttime erections.

An erection requires the interaction of your brain, nerves, hormones, and blood vessels. Anything that interferes with the normal process can become a problem. Common causes include:

- Diseases and conditions such as diabetes, high blood pressure, heart or thyroid conditions, poor circulation, low testosterone, depression, spinal cord injury, nerve damage (for example, from prostate surgery), or neurologic disorders (like multiple sclerosis or Parkinson's disease)
- Certain medications such as blood pressure medication (especially beta-blockers), heart medication (such as digoxin), some peptic ulcer medications, sleeping pills, and antidepressants
- Nicotine, alcohol, or cocaine
- Stress, fear, anxiety, or anger
- Unrealistic sexual expectations, which make sex a task rather than a pleasure.
- Poor communication with your partner
- A "vicious cycle" of doubt, failure, or negative communication that reinforces the erection problems

Home care

For many men, lifestyle changes can help:

- Cut down on smoking, alcohol, and illegal drugs.
- Get plenty of rest and take time to relax.
- Exercise and eat a healthy diet to maintain good circulation.
- Use safe sex practices, which reduces fear of HIV and STDs.
- Talk openly to your partner about sex and your relationship. If you are unable to do this, counseling can help.

If erection problems seem to be caused by a medication you are taking for an unrelated condition, consult your doctor. You may benefit from reducing the dose of the drug or changing to another drug that has the same result but not the same side effects. DO NOT adjust or discontinue medications without consulting your doctor first.

When to contact a medical professional

Call your doctor if:

- Self-care measures do not resolve the problem and you continue having difficulty with erections. Effective treatments are available.
- You suspect that a medication is causing the problem.
- The problems begin after an injury or prostate surgery.
- You have other symptoms like low back pain, abdominal pain, or change in urination.

Call your doctor immediately or go to an emergency room if medication for erection problems give you an unwanted erection that lasts more than an hour. Permanent impotence or other lasting damage to your penis may result from this condition.

Decision point

Although sildenafil (Viagra) and other medications have become very popular for impotence, taking a drug isn't always the best answer. First work with your doctor to figure out the underlying cause. For example, if you take a medication for high blood pressure that could be contributing to the problem, your doctor may be able to change or adjust your prescription. DO NOT alter or stop medications on your own. And, making some simple lifestyle changes may make a big difference.

Eye dryness

Dry eyes are caused by a lack of tears. Tears are necessary for the normal lubrication of your eyes and to wash away particles and foreign bodies.

If you have dry eyes, you will feel a burning, scratching, or stinging sensation. You may also have strained or tired eyes after reading, even for short periods of time. If you wear contacts, they will likely feel uncomfortable. Having dry eyes for a while can lead to tiny abrasions on the surface of your eyes.

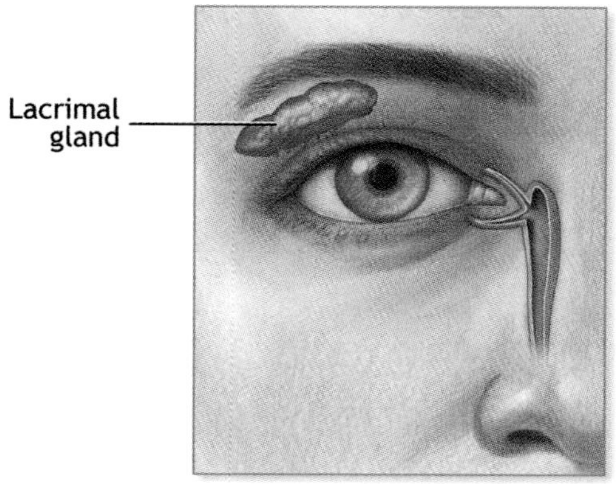

The lacrimal gland produces tears for the eye.

Home care

The following steps may help:

- Try artificial tears, available as either drops or ointment. Ointments last longer, but are thicker and can cause blurry vision.
- Don't smoke. Avoid second-hand smoke, direct wind, and air conditioning.
- Use a humidifier, especially in the winter.
- Purposefully blink more often. Rest your eyes.

When to contact a medical professional

Call your doctor if:

- Your have red or painful eyes.
- You have flaking, discharge, or a lesion on your eye or eyelid.
- You have had trauma to your eye, or you have a bulging eye or a drooping eyelid.
- You have joint pain, swelling, or stiffness.
- You also have a dry mouth.
- Your dry eyes do not respond to self-care measures within a few days.

Eye twitch

The most common things that make the muscle in your eyelid twitch are fatigue, stress, and caffeine. Once spasms begin, they may continue off and on for a few days. Then, they disappear. Most people experience this type of eyelid twitch on occasion and find it very annoying. In most cases, you won't even notice when the twitch has stopped.

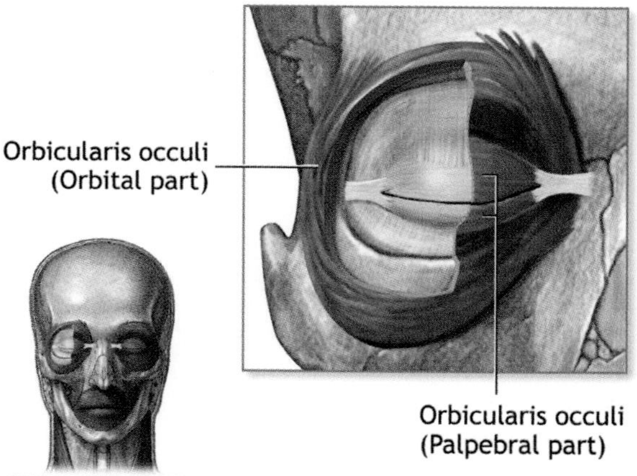

The muscles of your eyelid consist of the palpebral part of the orbicularis occuli muscle.

More severe contractions, where the eyelid completely closes, are possible. These can be caused by irritation of the surface of the eye (cornea) or the membranes lining the eyelids (conjunctiva).

Sometimes, the reason your eyelid is twitching cannot be identified. This form of eyelid twitching lasts much longer, is often very uncomfortable, and can also cause your eyelids to close completely.

Home care

Eyelid twitching usually disappears without treatment. In the meantime, the following steps may help:

- Get more sleep.
- Drink less caffeine.
- Lubricate your eyes with eye drops.

When to contact a medical professional

Call your primary care physician or eye doctor (ophthalmologist) if:

- Your eyelid twitching does not go away within one week.
- The twitching involves other parts of your face.
- You have redness, swelling, or a discharge from your eye.
- The twitching completely closes your eyelid.
- Your upper eyelid is drooping.

Eyelid bump

Most bumps on the eyelid are styes. A stye is an inflamed oil gland on the edge of your eyelid, where the lash meets the lid. It appears as a red, swollen bump that looks like a pimple. It is tender, especially to touch.

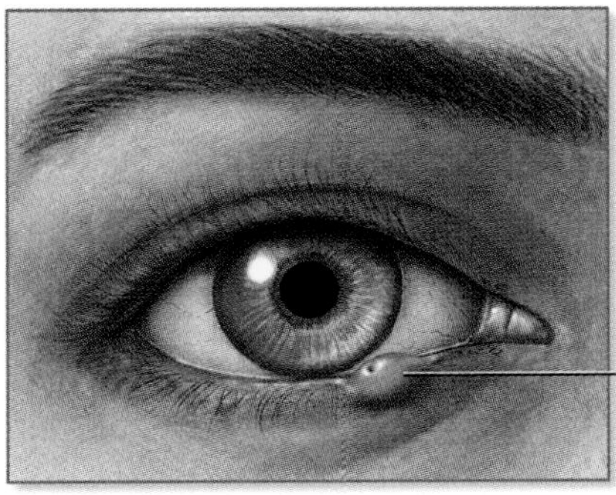

A stye is caused by bacteria from the skin that get into the hair follicle of the eyelash. Hair follicles contain oil glands that become inflamed from the bacteria. Styes are similar to common acne pimples that occur elsewhere on the skin. You may have more than one stye at the same time.

Styes usually develop over a few days and may drain and heal on their own. A stye can become a chalazion – this is when an inflamed oil gland becomes fully blocked. If a chalazion gets large enough, it can cause trouble with your vision.

If you have blepharitis (see *Eye Redness*), you are more likely to get styes.

Other possible eyelid bumps include:

- **Xanthelasma** – raised yellow patches on your eyelids that can happen with age. These are harmless, although they are occasionally a sign of high cholesterol.
- **Papillomas** – pink or skin colored bumps. They are harmless, but can slowly grow, affect your vision, or bother you for cosmetic reasons. If so, they can be surgically removed.
- **Cysts** – small fluid-filled sacs that can affect your vision.

Home care

- Styes and chalazions can be treated by applying warm compresses. Apply for 10 minutes. Do this 4 times a day.
- DO NOT attempt to squeeze a stye or any other type of eyelid bump. Let it drain on its own.
- Antibiotic creams may help recurrent or persistent styes. Some large styes need to be lanced to drain the infection.

When to contact a medical professional

Call your doctor if:

- Your have problems with your vision.

- The eyelid bump worsens or does not improve within a week or two of self-care.
- The eyelid bump or bumps become very large or painful.
- You have a blister on your eyelid.
- You have crusting or scaling of your eyelids.
- Your whole eyelid is red, or the eye itself is red.
- You are very sensitive to light or have excessive tears.
- A stye comes back soon after successful treatment of another one.
- Your eyelid bump bleeds.

Tip

You can usually cure a stye (the most common cause of an eyelid bump) on your own. Try the self-care measures outlined in this article before calling a nurse or doctor, unless you have trouble with your vision or other symptoms described.

Eye redness

There are many possible causes of a red eye or eyes. Some are quite concerning, even medical emergencies. Others are of no consequence or concern at all. The degree of redness or appearance of blood usually does not correlate to how serious it is. It is generally more important whether you also have eye pain or impaired vision.

Bloodshot eyes appear red because the vessels in the surface of the white portion of the eye (sclera) become enlarged and irritated. This may result from extremely dry air, sun exposure, dust, foreign body, an allergic reaction, infection, trauma, or other conditions.

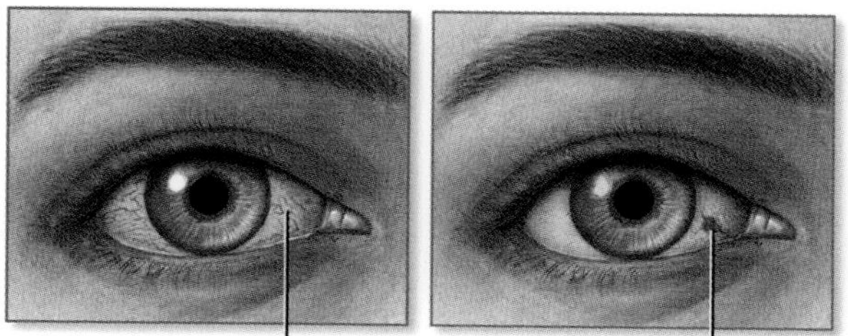

One common cause of a red eye is straining or coughing. This can lead to a bright red, uniformly dense bloody area on the sclera. This is called a subconjunctival hemorrhage. Although this bloody area may appear alarming, it is a fairly common occurrence and of little significance. If you notice a bloody blotch in one eye that doesn't hurt, but just looks bad, don't worry. It generally clears up on its own within a week or two.

Eye infections or inflammation can occur in different locations. They cause redness as well as possible itching, discharge, pain, or vision problems:

- **Blepharitis** – inflammation of the eyelash follicles along the eyelid. It is caused by skin bacteria. Itching is common and your eyelids may appear greasy or crusty.
- **Conjunctivitis** – inflammation or infection of the membrane that lines the eyelids and coats the surface of the eye (the conjunctiva). This condition is often referred to as "pink eye". It may be caused by a virus, bacteria, allergy, or irritation. If caused by an organism, this is highly contagious.
- **Corneal ulcers** – often caused by a bacterial or viral infection. (The cornea is the outer covering of the eye.)
- **Uveitis** – inflammation of the uvea, which includes the iris, ciliary body, and choroid. This is often related to an autoimmune disorder, infection, or exposure to toxins. Often, only the iris is inflamed, which is called iritis.

Home care

If you have conjunctivitis:

- Avoid touching the infected eye and then rubbing the other eye – the infection can spread from one eye to the other.
- Apply cool or warm compresses throughout the day.
- Over-the-counter homeopathic eye drops may provide relief.
- Do not use eye makeup or wear contact lenses until the infection has cleared. Throw away items like these that you used in your infected eye.
- Wash your hands frequently.

If you have blepharitis:

- Apply warm compresses to your eyes for 5 minutes. Do this at least 2 times per day.
- Using a cotton swab, gently rub a solution of warm water and no-tears baby shampoo along your eyelid, where the lash meets the lid. Do this in the morning and before you go to bed.

When to contact a medical professional

Go to the hospital or call 911 if:

- Your eye is red after a penetrating injury.
- You have a headache along with blurred vision or confusion.
- You are seeing halos around lights.
- You have nausea and vomiting.

Call your doctor if:

- Your eyes are red longer than 1-2 days.
- You have eye pain or vision changes.
- You take blood thinning medication, like warfarin.
- You may have an object in your eye.
- You are very sensitive to light.
- You have a yellow or greenish discharge from one or both eyes.

Tip

Drops that only clear redness don't treat the cause of your eye trouble. In fact, redness-reliever ingredients may even mask the underlying problem. Instead, look for drops that lubricate dry and irritated eyes. Be sure to call your doctor if you have pain or any change in vision.

Prevention

To prevent conjunctivitis:

- DO NOT share anything that has touched the eye of someone with this contagious condition – like pillowcases, sheets, towels, or eyeliner.
- Wash your hands right away if you have come in contact with someone with conjunctivitis.
- Wash out any chemicals or objects from your eye immediately.

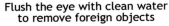

Flush the eye with clean water to remove foreign objects

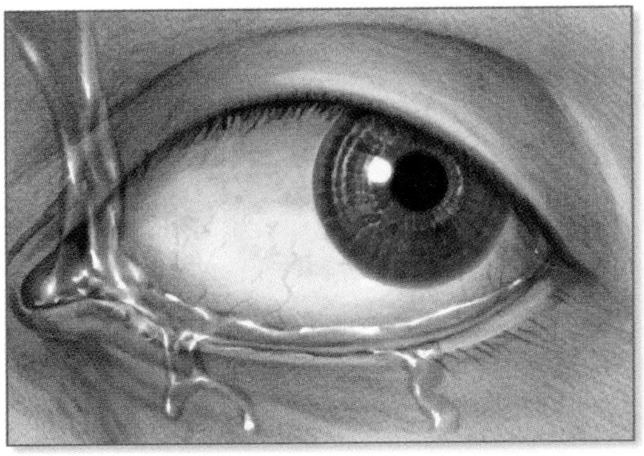

Fever

Normal body temperature varies by person, age, activity, and time of day. The average normal body temperature is 98.6°F (37°C).

Your body temperature is usually highest in the evening. It can be raised by physical activity, strong emotion, eating, heavy clothing, medications, high room temperature, and high humidity. This is especially true in children.

A rectal temperature up to 100.4°F (38°C) may be entirely normal. A rectal temperature of 100.5°F or above should always be considered a fever. Lower values might be a fever, depending on the person.

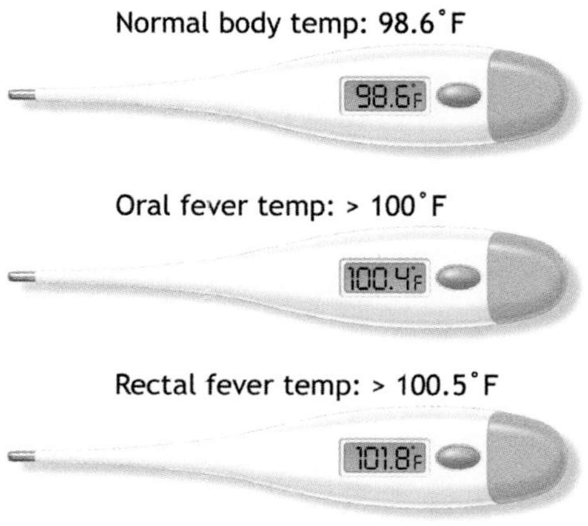

Fever is not an illness. Far from being an enemy, it is an important part of the body's defense against infection. Many infants and children develop high fevers with minor viral illnesses. While a fever signals to us that a battle might be going on in the body, the fever is fighting **for** the person, not against.

Most bacteria and viruses that cause infections in people thrive best at 98.6°F. Raising the temperature a few degrees can give your body the winning edge. In addition, a fever activates the body's immune system to make more white blood cells, antibodies, and other infection-fighting agents.

Many parents fear that fevers will cause brain damage. Brain damage from a fever generally will not occur unless the fever is over 107.6°F (42°C). Many parents also fear that untreated fevers will keep going higher and higher. Untreated fevers caused by infection will seldom go over 105°F unless the child is overdressed, or trapped in a hot place. The brain's thermostat will stop the fever from climbing above 106°F.

Some parents fear that fevers will cause seizures. For the great majority of children, this is not the case. However, febrile seizures do occur in some children. Once a child is already known to have a high fever, a febrile seizure is unlikely with the current illness. In any event, simple febrile seizures are over in moments with no lasting consequences.

Although infections are the most common causes of elevated body temperature, fevers have a long list of other causes, including toxins, cancers, and autoimmune diseases.

Heatstroke is a particularly dangerous type of high temperature, because the body is not able to stop the temperature from continuing to rise. It can happen when a child is left in a hot car or when you exercise too strenuously without enough to drink.

Home care

If the fever is mild and no other problems are present, no medical treatment is required. Drink fluids and rest. If a child is playful and comfortable, drinking plenty of fluids, and able to sleep, fever treatment is not likely to help.

Take steps to lower a fever if you or your child is uncomfortable, vomiting, dehydrated, or having difficulty sleeping. The goal is to lower, not eliminate, the fever.

When trying to reduce a fever:

- DO NOT bundle up someone who has the chills.
- Remove excess clothing or blankets. The environment should be comfortably cool. For example, one layer of lightweight clothing, and one lightweight blanket to sleep. If the room is hot or stuffy, a fan may help.
- A lukewarm bath or sponge bath may help cool someone with a fever. This is especially effective after medication is given – otherwise the temperature might bounce right back up.
- DO NOT use cold baths or alcohol rubs.

These cool the skin, but often make the situation worse by causing shivering, which raises the core body temperature.

- Drink cool liquids, as tolerated.

Here are some guidelines for taking medicine:

- Acetaminophen and ibuprofen help reduce fever in children and adults.
- Take acetaminophen every 4-6 hours. It works by turning down the brain's thermostat. Take ibuprofen every 6-8 hours. Like aspirin, it helps fight inflammation at the source of the fever. Sometimes doctors advise you to use both types of medicine. Ibuprofen is not approved for use under 6 months of age.
- Aspirin is very effective for treating fever in adults. DO NOT give aspirin to children.
- Fever medicines come in different concentrations, so always check the instructions on the package.
- DO NOT use any medicine to reduce fever in children under three months of age without first contacting a doctor.

When to contact a medical professional

- A baby less than 90 days old has a rectal temperature of 100.2°F (37.9°C) or higher.
- A baby 3 to 6 months old has a fever of 101°F (38.3°C) or higher.
- A baby 6 to 12 months old has a fever of 103°F (39.4°C) or higher.
- A child under age two years has a fever that lasts longer than 24 to 48 hours.
- A fever lasts longer than 48 to 72 hours in older children and adults.
- Anyone has a fever over 105°F (40.5°C), unless it comes down readily with treatment and the person is comfortable.
- There are other worrisome symptoms. For example, irritability, confusion, difficulty breathing, stiff neck, inability to move an arm or leg, or first-time seizure.
- There are other symptoms that suggest an illness may need to be treated, such as a sore throat, earache, or cough.
- You think you may have incorrectly dosed acetaminophen or ibuprofen.

Don't forget

Fever is your friend! In most cases, it is a sign your body is helping itself.

Fever convulsions

A febrile seizure is a convulsion in a child triggered by a fever. Such convulsions occur without any underlying brain or spinal cord infection or other neurologic cause.

About 3-5% of otherwise healthy children between the ages of 9 months and 5 years will have a seizure caused by a fever. Toddlers are most commonly affected. There is a tendency for febrile seizures to run in families. Most febrile seizures are triggered by a rapid rise of body temperature over 102.2°F. Most occur well within the first 24 hours of an illness, not necessarily when the fever is highest. The seizure is often the first sign of a fever.

The first febrile seizure is one of life's most frightening moments for parents. Most parents are afraid that their child will die or have brain damage. Thankfully, simple febrile seizures are harmless. There is no evidence that simple febrile seizures cause death, brain damage, epilepsy, mental retardation, a decrease in IQ, or learning difficulties.

Most febrile seizures are triggered by fevers from viral upper respiratory infections, ear infections, or roseola. Meningitis causes less than 0.1% of febrile seizures but should ALWAYS be considered, especially in children less than one year old or those who still look ill when the fever comes down.

A simple febrile seizure stops by itself within a few seconds to 10 minutes, usually followed by a brief period of drowsiness or confusion. Anticonvulsant medicines are generally not needed.

A complex febrile seizure is one that lasts longer than 15 minutes, occurs in an isolated part of the body, or recurs during the same illness.

About a third of children who have had a febrile seizure will have another one with a subsequent fever. Of those who do, about half will have a third seizure. Few children have more than three febrile seizures in their lifetime.

Symptoms

A febrile seizure may be as mild as the child's eyes rolling or limbs stiffening. Quite often a fever triggers a full-blown convulsion that involves the whole body.

Febrile seizures may begin with the sudden sustained contraction of muscles on both sides of a child's body – usually the muscles of the face, trunk, arms, and legs. A haunting, involuntary cry or moan often emerges from the child, from the force of the muscle contraction. The contraction continues for seemingly endless seconds, or tens of seconds. The child will fall, if standing, and may pass urine. He may vomit. He may bite his tongue. The child will not be breathing, and may begin to turn blue. Finally, the sustained contraction is broken by repeated brief moments of relaxation – the child's body begins to jerk rhythmically. The child is unresponsive to the parent's screams.

Home care

During the seizure, leave your child on the floor. You may want to slide a blanket under him if the floor is hard. Move him only if he is in a dangerous location. Remove objects that may injure him. Loosen any tight clothing, especially around the neck. If possible, open or remove clothes from the waist up. If he vomits, or if saliva and mucus build up in the mouth, turn him on his side or stomach. This is also important if it looks like the tongue is getting in the way of breathing.

DO NOT try to force anything into his mouth to prevent him from biting the tongue, as this increases the risk of injury. DO NOT try to restrain your child or try to stop the seizure movements.

Focus your attention on bringing the fever down. Inserting rectal acetaminophen is a great first step – if you happen to have some. DO NOT try to give anything by mouth. Apply cool washcloths to the forehead and neck. Sponge the rest of the body with lukewarm (not cold) water. Cold water or alcohol may make the fever worse. After the seizure is over and your child is awake, give the normal dose of ibuprofen or acetaminophen.

After the seizure, the most important step is to identify the cause of the fever.

When to contact a medical professional

- Children should see a doctor as soon as possible after their first febrile seizure.
- If the seizure is lasting several minutes, call 911 to have an ambulance bring your child to the hospital.
- If the seizure ends quickly, drive the child to an emergency room when it is over.
- A child should also see a doctor if repeated seizures occur during the same illness, or if this looks like a new type of seizure for your child.
- Call or go in if any other symptoms occur before or after the seizure, such as nausea, vomiting, rash, tremors, abnormal movements, problems with coordination, drowsiness, restlessness, confusion, or sedation. It is normal for children to sleep or be briefly drowsy or confused immediately following a seizure.

Prevention

To prevent future febrile seizures, give acetaminophen or ibuprofen at the first sign of a fever. (You may want to keep acetaminophen suppositories on hand). Then sponge your child with lukewarm water. Give him cool liquids to drink – both to lower the temperature and keep him well hydrated.

Because febrile seizures can occur as the first sign of illness, prevention is often not possible. Neither an initial nor recurrent febrile seizure suggests that your child is not being properly cared for.

Occasionally, a doctor will prescribe diazepam to prevent or treat recurrent febrile seizures.

FLU

The flu is a contagious infection of the nose, throat, and lungs caused by the influenza virus.

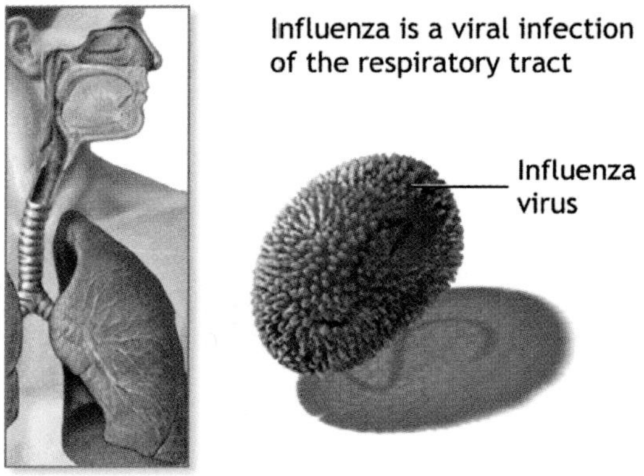
Influenza is a viral infection of the respiratory tract
Influenza virus

The flu usually begins abruptly, with a fever between 102 to 106°F (with adults on the lower end of the spectrum). Other common symptoms include a flushed face, body aches, and lack of energy. Some people have dizziness or vomiting. The fever usually lasts for a day or two, but can last 5 days.

Somewhere between day 2 and day 4 of the illness, the "whole body" symptoms begin to subside, and respiratory symptoms begin to increase. The virus can settle anywhere in the respiratory tract, producing symptoms of a cold, croup, sore throat, bronchiolitis, ear infection, or pneumonia.

The most prominent of the respiratory symptoms is usually a dry, hacking cough. Most people also develop a sore (red) throat and a headache. Nasal discharge and sneezing are common. These symptoms (except the cough) usually disappear within 4-7 days. Sometimes there's a second wave of fever at this time. Cough and tiredness usually last for weeks after the rest of the illness is over.

The most common way to catch the flu is by inhaling droplets from coughs or sneezes. Less often, it is spread when you touch a surface such as a faucet handle or phone that has the virus on it, and then touch your own mouth, nose, or eyes.

Anyone at any age can have serious complications from the flu, but those at highest risk include:

- People over 50 years of age
- Children 6-23 months
- Women more than 3 months pregnant during the flu season
- Anyone living in a long-term care facility
- Anyone with chronic heart, lung, or kidney conditions, diabetes, or weakened immune system

Sometimes people confuse cold and flu, which share some of the same symptoms and occur at the same time of the year (cold and flu season). However, the two diseases are very different. Most people get a cold several times each year, and the flu only once every several years.

HOME CARE

If you have mild illness and are not at high-risk, take these steps:

- Rest
- Take medicines that relieve symptoms and help you rest
- Drink plenty of liquids
- Avoid aspirin (especially teens and children)

- Avoid alcohol and tobacco
- Avoid antibiotics (unless necessary for another illness)

When to contact a medical professional

Call your health care provider if someone in a high-risk category develops symptoms of the flu. For healthy, non-pregnant people between 2 and 49 years old, see the articles on fever, cough, vomiting, and other specific symptoms about when it is important to call a health care provider.

Prevention

A yearly flu vaccine is recommended for those people in high-risk categories. The vaccine is also recommended for people who work with (or live with) others at high risk.

Anyone can get the flu shot if they want to lower their chances of getting the flu, as long as they:

- Are over 6 months old
- Don't have a serious allergy to eggs
- Haven't had a serious reaction to flu shots in the past

The FluMist nasal spray is an alternative. Unlike the regular vaccine, it is a live virus. Therefore, it is best if the person receiving it does not have close contact with people with a weakened immune system.

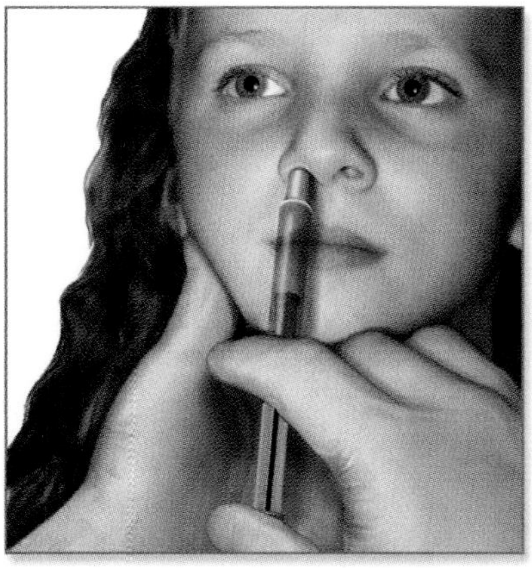

FluMist is a liquid product sprayed into the nose.

Remember!

The flu is a viral illness, and is NOT helped by antibiotics.

Food poisoning

Food poisoning is the result of eating organisms or toxins in contaminated food. Most cases of food poisoning are from common bacteria like *Staphylococcus* or *E. coli*.

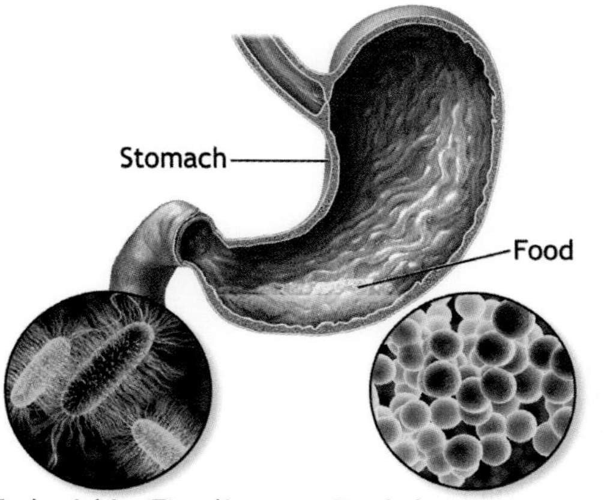

Food poisoning may occur if bacteria are growing in the food you eat.

Food poisoning tends to occur at picnics, school cafeterias, and large social functions. These are situations where food may be left unrefrigerated too long or food preparation techniques are not clean. Food poisoning often occurs from undercooked meats or dairy products (like mayonnaise mixed in coleslaw or potato salad) that have sat out too long.

Infants and elderly people have the greatest risk for food poisoning. You are also at higher risk if you have a serious medical condition, like kidney disease or diabetes, a weakened immune system, or you travel outside of the U.S. to areas where there is more exposure to organisms that cause food poisoning. Pregnant and breastfeeding women have to be especially careful.

Symptoms

The symptoms from the most common types of food poisoning generally start within 2 to 6 hours of eating the food responsible. That time may be longer (even a number of days) or shorter, depending on the toxin or organism responsible for the food poisoning. The possible symptoms include:

- Nausea and vomiting
- Abdominal cramps
- Diarrhea (may be bloody)
- Fever and chills
- Weakness (may be serious and lead to respiratory arrest as in the case of botulism)
- Headache

Botulism is a very serious form of food poisoning that can be fatal. It can come from improper home canning

Home care

You will usually recover from the most common types of food poisoning within a couple of days. The goal is to make you feel better and avoid dehydration. Drink any fluid (except milk or caffeinated beverages) to replace fluids lost by diarrhea and vomiting. Children should be given an electrolyte sold in drugstores. Don't eat solid foods until the diarrhea has passed, and avoid dairy, which can worsen diarrhea.

For the most common causes of food poisoning, your doctor would NOT prescribe antibiotics. Antibiotics can actually prolong diarrhea and keep the organism in your body longer.

When to contact a medical professional

Call your doctor if:

- You have diarrhea and are unable to drink fluids due to nausea or vomiting.
- You are on diuretics and have diarrhea, nausea, or vomiting.
- Diarrhea lasts for more than 2 to 3 days.
- There is blood in your stools.
- You have a fever over 101°F.

Call 911 if:

- You have signs of dehydration (thirsty, dizzy, lightheaded, faint).
- Bleeding is excessive or your stools are maroon or black.
- You are short of breath or having trouble breathing.
- Your heart is racing, pounding, or skipping.
- You may have poisoning from mushrooms, fish, or botulism.
- You have any nervous system symptoms like weakness, double vision, difficulty speaking, or paralysis.
- You have trouble swallowing.

Prevention

To prevent food poisoning, take the following steps when preparing food:

- Carefully wash your hands and clean dishes and utensils.
- Use a thermometer when cooking. Cook beef to at least 160°F, poultry to at least 180°F, and fish to at least 140°F.
- DO NOT place cooked meat or fish back onto the same plate or container that held the raw meat, unless the container has been thoroughly washed.
- Promptly refrigerate any food you will not be eating right away. Keep the refrigerator set to around 40°F and your freezer at or below 0°F. DO NOT eat meat, poultry, or fish that has been refrigerated uncooked for longer than 1 to 2 days.
- DO NOT use outdated foods, packaged food with a broken seal, or cans that are bulging or have a dent.
- DO NOT use foods that have an unusual odor or a spoiled taste.

Other steps to take:

- If you take care of young children, wash your hands often and dispose of diapers carefully so that bacteria can't spread to other surfaces or people.
- If you make canned food at home, be sure to follow proper canning techniques to prevent botulism.
- DO NOT feed honey to children under 1 year of age.
- DO NOT eat wild mushrooms.
- When traveling where contamination is more likely, eat only hot, freshly cooked food. Drink water only if it's been boiled. DO NOT eat raw vegetables or unpeeled fruit.
- DO NOT eat shellfish exposed to red tides.
- If you are pregnant or have a weakened immune system, DO NOT eat soft cheeses, especially imported from countries outside the U.S.

If other people may have eaten the food that made you sick, let them know. If you think the food was contaminated when you bought it from a store or restaurant, tell the store and your local health department.

Foot pain

Pain or discomfort can be felt anywhere in the foot, including the heel, toes, arch, instep, sole, or ankles. See also *Ankle Pain* and *Heel Pain*.

Foot pain can be caused by:

- **Bunions** – a protrusion at the base of the big toe, which can become inflamed. Bunions often develop over time from wearing narrow-toed shoes.
- **Hammer toes** – toes that curl downward into a claw-like position.
- **Calluses and corns** – thickened skin from friction or pressure. Calluses are on the balls of the feet or heels. Corns appear on your toes.
- **Plantar warts** – from pressure on the soles of your feet.
- **Fallen arches** – also called flat feet.

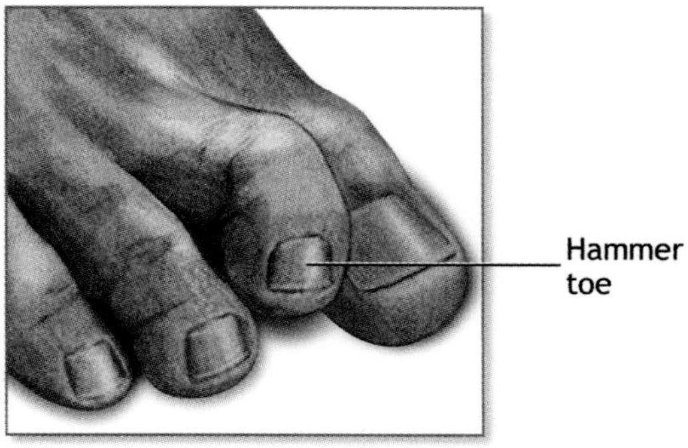

Ill-fitting shoes often cause these problems. Aging and being overweight also increase your chances of having foot problems.

Other common causes of foot pain include:

- Broken bones
- Stress fracture
- Arthritis
- Gout – common in the big toe, which becomes red, swollen, and very tender
- Plantar fasciitis – see *Heel Pain*
- Bone spur – see *Heel Pain*
- Sprains – see *Ankle Pain*
- Bursitis of the heel – see *Heel Pain*
- Tendinitis – see *Heel Pain*

Home care

- Apply ice to reduce pain and swelling. Do this just after an activity that aggravates your pain.
- Elevate your painful foot as much as possible.
- Reduce activity until the problem improves.

- Wear foot pads in areas of friction or pressure. This will prevent rubbing and irritation.
- Take over-the-counter pain medicine, like ibuprofen or acetaminophen. Try this for 2 to 3 weeks (unless you have a history of an ulcer, liver disease, or other condition that does not allow you to take one of these drugs).

For plantar warts, try an over-the-counter wart removal preparation.

For calluses, soak in warm water and then rub them down with a pumice stone. DO NOT cut or burn corns or calluses.

For foot pain caused by a stress fracture, an extended rest period is often necessary. Crutches may be used for a week or so to take the pressure off, if your foot is particularly painful.

For foot pain due to plantar fasciitis, shoe inserts may help.

When to contact a medical professional

Call your doctor if:

- You have sudden, severe pain.
- Your pain began following an injury – especially if there is bleeding, bruising, deformity, or you cannot bear weight.
- You have redness or swelling of the joint, an open sore or ulcer on your foot, or a fever.
- You have diabetes or peripheral vascular disease – a condition characterized by poor circulation.
- You do not respond to self-care within 1 to 2 weeks.

Prevention

The following steps can prevent foot problems and foot pain:

- Wear comfortable, properly fitting shoes. They should have good arch support and cushioning.
- Wear shoes with adequate room around the ball of your foot and toe.
- Wear sneakers as often as possible, especially when walking.
- Avoid narrow-toed shoes and high heels.
- Replace running shoes frequently.
- Warm up before exercise, cool down after exercise, and stretch adequately.
- Increase your amount of exercise SLOWLY over time to avoid putting excessive strain on your feet.
- Lose weight if you need to.
- Learn exercises to strengthen your feet and avoid pain. This can help flat feet and other potential foot problems.
- Keep feet dry to avoid friction. This may help prevent corns and calluses.
- Avoid alcohol to prevent attacks of gout.

Foot, leg, ankle swelling

Painless swelling of the feet and ankles is a common problem, particularly in older people.

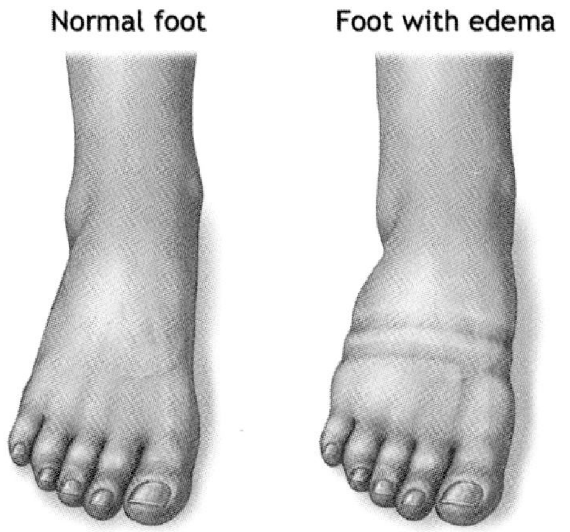

The clinical name for swelling caused by abnormal fluid buildup is "edema".

It may affect both legs and may include the calves or even the thighs. Because of the effect of gravity, swelling is particularly noticeable in these locations.

Foot, leg, and ankle swelling is common with the following situations:

- Prolonged standing
- Long airplane flights or automobile rides
- Menstrual periods (for some women)
- Pregnancy – excessive swelling may be a sign of pre-eclampsia (a serious condition that includes high blood pressure and swelling; sometimes called toxemia)
- Being overweight
- Increased age
- Injury or trauma to your ankle or foot

Swollen legs may be a sign of heart failure, kidney failure, or liver failure. In these conditions, there is too much fluid in your body.

Other conditions that can cause swelling to one or both legs include:

- Blood clot
- Leg infection
- Venous insufficiency (when the veins in your legs are unable to adequately pump blood back to the heart)
- Varicose veins
- Burns including sunburn
- Insect bite or sting
- Starvation or malnutrition
- Surgery to your leg or foot

Certain medications may also cause your legs to swell:

- Hormones like estrogen (in birth control pills or hormone replacement therapy) and testosterone
- A group of blood pressure lowering drugs called calcium channel blockers (such as nifedipine, amlodipine, diltiazem, felodipine, and verapamil)
- Steroids
- Antidepressants, including MAO inhibitors (such as phenelzine and tranylcypromine) and tricyclics (such as nortriptyline, desipramine, and amitriptyline)

Home care

- Elevate your legs above your heart while lying down.
- Exercise your legs. This helps pump fluid from your legs back to your heart.
- Wear support stockings (sold at most drug and medical supply stores).
- Try to follow a low-salt diet, which may reduce fluid retention and swelling.

When to contact a medical professional

Call 911 if:

- You feel short of breath.
- You have chest pain, especially if it feels like pressure or tightness.

Call your doctor right away if:

- You have decreased urine output.
- You have a history of liver disease and now have swelling in your legs or abdomen.
- Your swollen foot or leg is red or warm to the touch.
- You have a fever.
- You are pregnant and have more than just mild swelling or have a sudden increase in swelling.

Also call your doctor if self care measures do not help or swelling worsens.

Prevention

Avoid sitting or standing without moving for prolonged periods of time. When flying, stretch your legs often and get up to walk when possible. When driving, stop to stretch and walk every hour or so. Avoid wearing restrictive clothing or garters around your thighs. Exercise regularly. Lose weight if you need to.

GAS (FLATULENCE)

Gas is formed in the intestines as food is being digested. Gas can make you feel bloated, which may cause crampy or colicky abdominal pain.

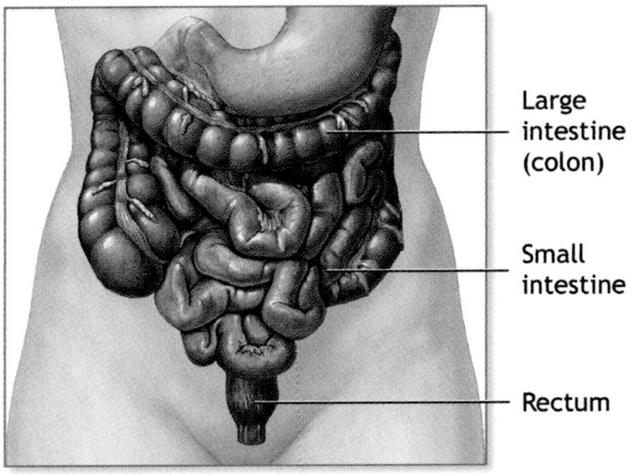

Gas (flatulence) is formed in the intestines.

Gas can be caused by any of the following:

- Swallowing air while eating.
- Eating foods that are difficult to digest, such as fiber. If you recently introduced fiber into your diet, having gas may be temporary. Give it a little time. Your body may adjust and stop producing gas.
- Eating foods that you cannot tolerate – for example, if you have lactose intolerance and eat dairy products.
- Irritable bowel syndrome – a chronic form of stomach upset that gets worse from stress.
- Malabsorption (when your body cannot absorb or digest a particular nutrient properly, often accompanied by diarrhea).
- Antibiotics.

HOME CARE

- Eat more slowly.
- Chew your food thoroughly.
- Avoid gum chewing.
- Relax while you eat.
- Avoid beans, cabbage, and carbonated beverages.
- Try Beano, a product sold over-the-counter at most drugstores, if you eat a lot of beans, fruits, vegetables, and other high-fiber foods.
- Walk for 10 to 15 minutes after eating.
- Drink peppermint or chamomile tea after a meal.

GASTROINTESTINAL DIAGNOSTIC TESTS

Your doctor may order diagnostic tests to further evaluate your gastrointestinal tract, such as:

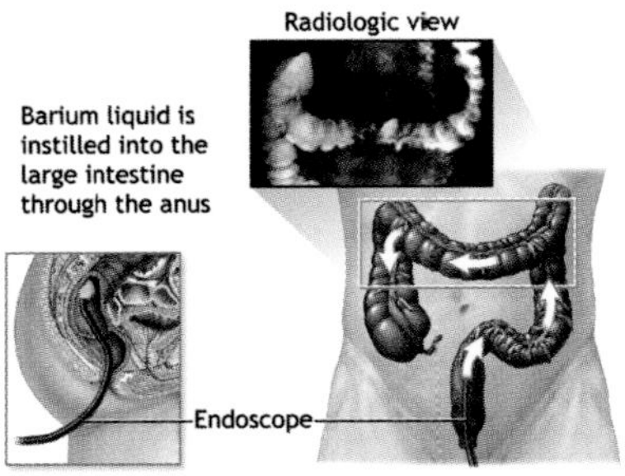

Barium enema x-ray

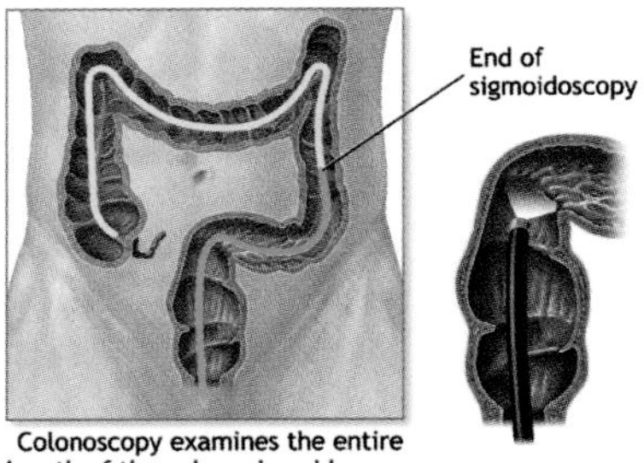

Colonoscopy examines the entire length of the colon; sigmoidoscopy examines only the lower third

Sigmoidoscopy or colonoscopy

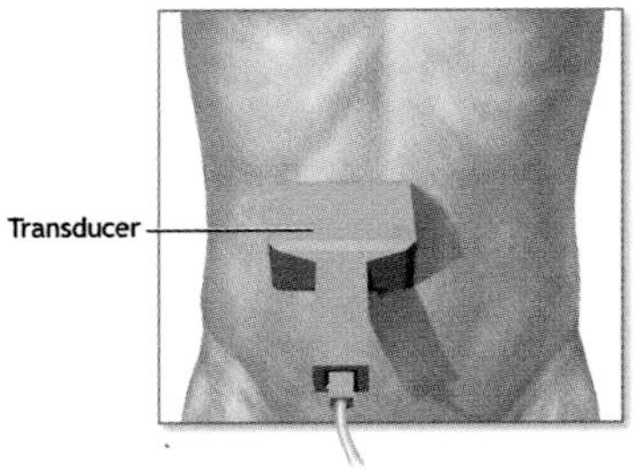

Abdominal ultrasound

When to contact a medical professional

Call your doctor if:

- Your have other symptoms in addition to gas, like abdominal or rectal pain, heartburn, nausea, vomiting, diarrhea, constipation, or weight loss.
- You have oily, foul-smelling, or bloody stools.

Genital sores

Sores or lesions on your genitals have many possible causes. Most are caused by sexually transmitted diseases (STDs). These include:

- **Genital warts** – see the article on genital warts.
- **Herpes** – small, painful blisters that commonly recur in the same area. Before the skin lesions appear, you feel tingling, burning, itching, or pain at the site.
- **Syphilis** – initially, one or more painless lesions on your genitals, rectum, or mouth. Then a rash may develop that can involve your palms and soles. Lymph nodes swell.
- **Chancroid** – appears as a small bump or bumps that turn into ulcers. This STD is more common in developing countries, uncircumcised men, and those with HIV. It may be mistaken for the initial syphilis lesion.
- **Molluscum contagiosum** – appears as small, flesh-colored, raised lesions that spread in crops if you scratch them. It can occur anywhere on the skin, including the genitals, except for your palms and soles. It is not always an STD, especially in children. In adults, however, it is usually transmitted sexually and is a common problem in those with AIDS.

Other STDs, such as gonorrhea and chlamydia, cause discharge, itching, and pain with intercourse but don't tend to cause visible lesions on the genitalia. When you see your doctor for a genital lesion, however, you will likely be tested for these infections as well.

Less commonly, genital lesions may be from pre-cancerous changes of the vulva (outer part of the vagina), or an allergic reaction to soap, lotion, detergent, or other substance.

Prevention

You can greatly reduce your chances of getting an STD by wearing latex condoms and following other safe-sex practices. However, condoms are not a guarantee. Some lesions may not be covered by the condom, and could still be spread from person to person.

Treatment

Antibiotics and other prescription medications are needed to clear most STDs. In people with a normal immune system, molluscum contagiosum usually clears on its own within 2 to 3 months, while those with a compromised immune system may need to have them frozen off or removed through another method.

All of your sexual partners should be notified and, if infected, treated. Certain STDs, like syphilis, must be reported to the Department of Public Health.

Also, if left untreated, many STDs may be passed on to an unborn fetus or baby during pregnancy or delivery.

Hair - unwanted

The normal amount of body hair varies widely among women. When coarse, dark hairs grow where women typically do not grow dark hair, such as the lip, chin, chest, abdomen, or back, the condition is called hirsutism.

Excessive hair growth in women is usually from too much male hormone (androgen). A common cause is polycystic ovarian syndrome (PCOS). In most cases, however, the specific cause is never identified. It tends to run in families. In general, hirsutism is a harmless condition. But many women find it bothersome, even embarrassing.

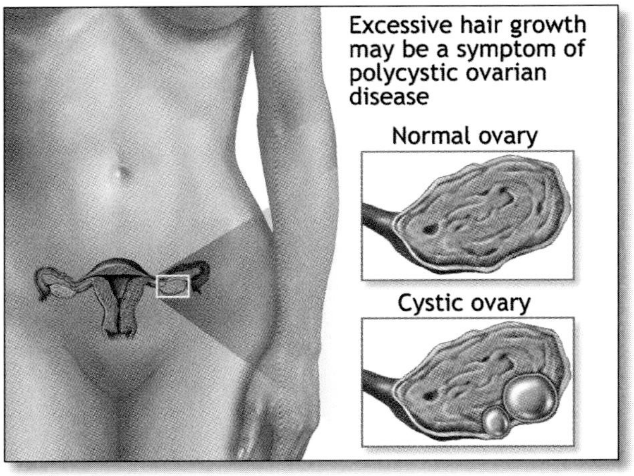
Excessive hair growth may be a symptom of polycystic ovarian disease
Normal ovary
Cystic ovary

Home care

There are a variety of ways to remove unwanted hair:

- **Bleaching** – lightening hair to make it less noticeable.
- **Hair removal** – shaving, plucking, waxing, or chemical depilation.
- **Electrolysis** – using electrical current to damage individual hair follicles so they do not grow back. This is expensive and requires multiple treatments.
- **Laser hair removal** – using laser to damage individual hair follicles so they do not grow back. This is expensive and requires multiple treatments.
- **Weight loss** – in overweight women, weight loss can decrease male hormone levels and reduce hair growth.

Birth control pills and anti-androgen medications can also help reduce hair growth. A doctor must prescribe these medications.

When to contact a medical professional

Call your doctor if:

- The hair grows rapidly.
- The hair growth is associated with male features such as acne, deepening voice, increased muscle mass, and decreased breast size.
- You are concerned that medication may be worsening unwanted hair growth.

Hair loss

Each hair sits in a cavity in the skin called a follicle. Baldness in men occurs when the follicle shrinks over time, resulting in shorter and finer hair. The end result is a very small follicle with no hair inside. Ordinarily, hair should grow back. However, in men who are balding, the follicle fails to grow a new hair.

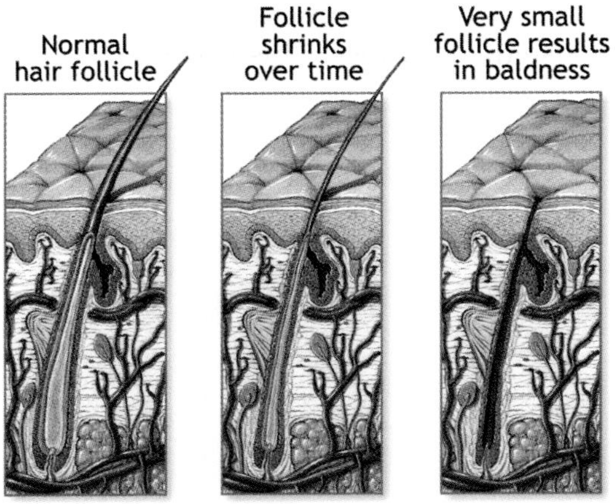
Normal hair follicle
Follicle shrinks over time
Very small follicle results in baldness

Why this occurs is not well understood, but it is related to your genes and male sex hormones. Even though the follicles are small, they remain alive, suggesting the possibility of new growth.

Symptoms

The typical pattern of male baldness begins at the hairline. The hairline gradually recedes to form an "M" shape. The existing hair may become finer and shorter. The hair at the crown also begins to thin. Eventually the top of the hairline meets the thinned crown, leaving a horseshoe pattern of hair around the sides of the head.

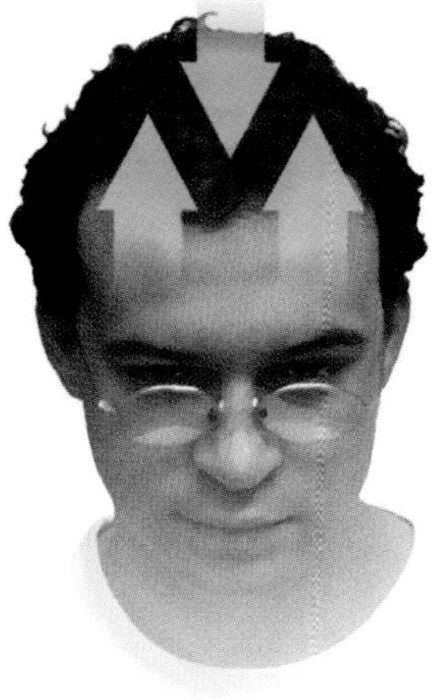
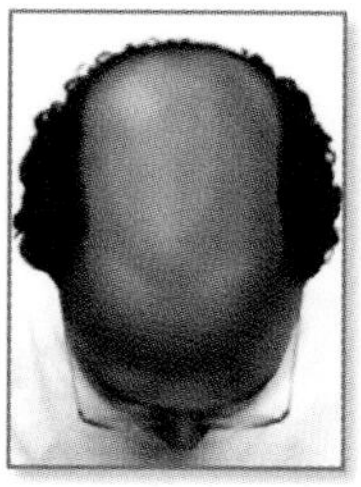

In male pattern baldness, hair recedes in an "m" shape. The crown bald patch eventually meets the top points to form a horseshoe shape.

Home care

Treatment is not necessary if you are comfortable with your appearance. Hair weaving, hairpieces, or change of hairstyle may disguise the hair loss. This is usually the least expensive and safest approach for male baldness.

There are two main drugs used to treat male pattern baldness:

- **Minoxidil** (Rogaine) – a solution that you apply directly to the scalp to stimulate the hair follicles. It slows hair loss for many men, and some men grow new hair. The previous degree of hair loss returns when you stop applying the solution.
- **Finasteride** (Propecia, Proscar) – a prescription pill that inhibits the production of the male hormone dihydrotestosterone. Like minoxidil, you are more likely to have slower hair loss than actual new hair growth. In general, it is somewhat more effective than minoxidil. The previous degree of hair loss returns when you stop taking the drug.

Hair transplants consist of removing tiny plugs of hair from areas where the hair is continuing to grow and placing them in areas that are balding. This can cause minor scarring in the donor areas and carries a modest risk for skin infection. The procedure usually requires multiple transplantation sessions and may be expensive. Results, however, are often excellent and permanent.

When to contact a medical professional

Call your doctor if:

- Your hair loss occurs in an atypical pattern – rapid hair loss, diffuse shedding, hair loss in patches, or breaking of hair shafts.
- Your hair loss is accompanied by itching, skin irritation, redness, scaling, pain, or other symptoms.
- Your hair loss begins after starting a medication.
- You want to attempt to treat your hair loss.

Hair loss in women

In female pattern baldness, the hair typically thins all over the head, but the frontal hairline is maintained. There may be a moderate loss of hair on the crown, but this rarely progresses to total or near baldness as it may in men. The treatment options for women are quite similar to men, except that finasteride is not prescribed to women.

Other reasons for hair loss

Hair loss can occur for reasons other than pattern baldness. These may include temporary shedding of hair, breaking of hair (from such things as styling treatments and twisting or pulling of hair), patchy areas of total hair loss (alopecia areata – an immune disorder causing temporary hair loss), stress, some medications, thyroid disease, and ringworm or other skin diseases. Hair loss from menopause or childbirth often returns to normal 6 months to 2 years later.

Headache

A headache is pain or discomfort in the head, scalp, or neck. Serious causes of headaches are extremely rare. Most people with headaches can feel much better by making lifestyle changes, learning ways to relax, and occasionally by taking medications.

Tension headaches are due to tight, contracted muscles in your shoulders, neck, scalp, and jaw.

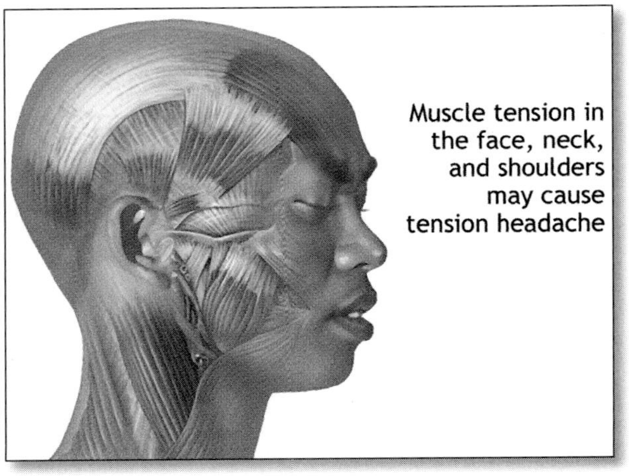
Muscle tension in the face, neck, and shoulders may cause tension headache

They are often related to stress, depression, or anxiety. Overworking, not getting enough sleep, missing meals, and using alcohol or street drugs can make you more susceptible to them. Headaches can be triggered by chocolate, cheese, and monosodium glutamate (MSG). People who drink caffeine can have headaches when they don't get their usual daily amount.

Other common causes include:

- Holding your head in one position for a long time, like at a computer, microscope, or typewriter
- Poor sleep position
- Overexerting yourself
- Clenching or grinding your teeth

Tension headaches tend to be on both sides of your head. They often start at the back of your head and spread forward. The pain may feel dull or squeezing, like a tight band or vice. Your shoulders, neck, or jaw may feel tight and sore.

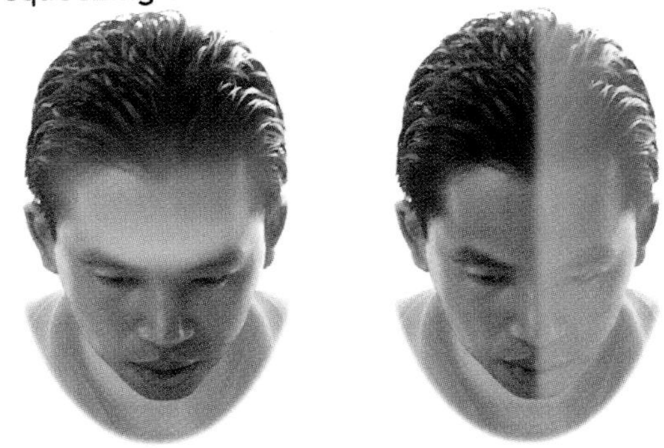
Tension headache: pain is like a band squeezing the head
Migraine headache: pain, nausea, and visual changes are typical of the classic form

Most headaches are due to tension, migraine, or a combination of both.

For information on migraine, see *Migraine Headache*.

Other types of headaches:

- **Cluster headaches** are sharp, extremely painful headaches that tend to occur several times per day for months and then go away for a similar period. They are far less common.
- **Sinus headaches** cause pain in the front of your head and face. They are due to inflammation in the sinus passages that lie behind the cheeks, nose, and eyes. The pain tends to be worse when you bend forward and when you first wake up in the morning. Postnasal drip, sore throat, and nasal discharge usually occur with these headaches.

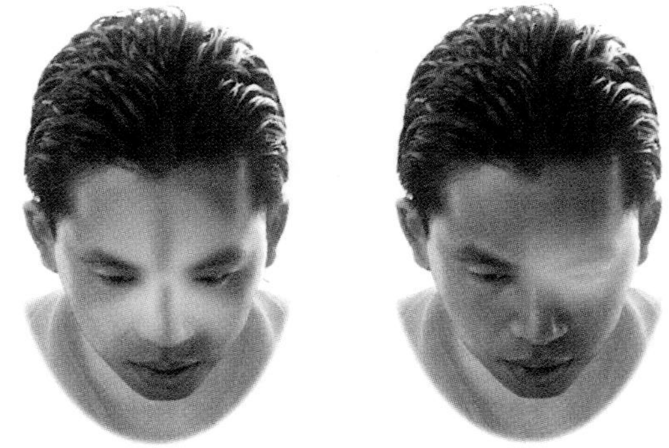
Sinus headache: pain is behind browbone and/or cheekbone
Cluster headache: pain is in and around one eye

Headaches may occur if you have a cold, the flu, fever, or premenstrual syndrome.

Home care

Keep a headache diary to help identify the source or trigger of your symptoms. Then modify your environment or habits to avoid future headaches. When a headache occurs, write down the date and time the headache began, what you ate for the past 24 hours, how long you slept the night before, what you were doing and thinking about just before the headache started, any stress in your life, how long the headache lasts, and what you did to make it stop. After a period of time, you may begin to see a pattern.

A headache may be relieved by resting with your eyes closed and head supported. Relaxation techniques can help. A massage or heat applied to the back of the upper neck can be effective in relieving tension headaches.

Try acetaminophen, aspirin, or ibuprofen for tension headaches. DO NOT give aspirin to children because of the risk of Reye's syndrome.

Migraine headaches may respond to aspirin, naproxen, or combination migraine medications.

If over-the-counter remedies do not control your pain, talk to your doctor about possible prescription medications.

When to contact a medical professional

Take the following symptoms seriously. If you cannot see your health care provider immediately, go to the emergency room or call 911:

- Your headache comes on suddenly and is explosive or violent.
- You would describe your headache as "your worst ever", even if you are prone to headaches.
- Your headache is associated with slurred speech, change in vision, problems moving your arms or legs, loss of balance, confusion, or memory loss.
- Your headache gets progressively worse over a 24-hour period.
- Your headache is accompanied by fever, stiff neck, nausea, and vomiting.
- Your headache occurs with a head injury.
- Your headache is severe and localized to one eye with redness in that eye.
- You are over age 50 and your headaches just began, especially with impaired vision and pain while chewing.

See your provider soon if:

- Your headaches wake you up from sleep.
- A headache lasts more than a few days.
- Headaches are worse in the morning.
- You have a history of headaches but they have changed in pattern or intensity.
- You have headaches frequently, and there is no known cause.

Prevention

The following healthy habits can lessen stress and reduce your chance of getting headaches:

- Getting adequate sleep
- Eating a healthy diet
- Exercising regularly
- Stretching your neck and upper body, especially if your work involves typing or using a computer
- Learning proper posture
- Quitting smoking
- Learning to relax using meditation, deep breathing, yoga, or other techniques

Headache - Migraine

Migraine headaches are a type of headache that some people get repeatedly over time. Migraines are different from other headaches because they occur with symptoms such as nausea, vomiting, or sensitivity to light.

Some people who get migraines have warning symptoms, called an aura, before the actual headache begins. Most people, however, do not have such warning symptoms.

The exact cause of migraine is not known. Migraine headaches are related to problems with blood flow through parts of the brain. At the start of a migraine, blood vessels in certain areas of the brain constrict (narrow), leading to symptoms like visual disturbances, difficulty speaking, weakness, or numbness. Minutes to hours later, the blood vessels dilate (enlarge), leading to increased blood flow in the brain and a bad headache.

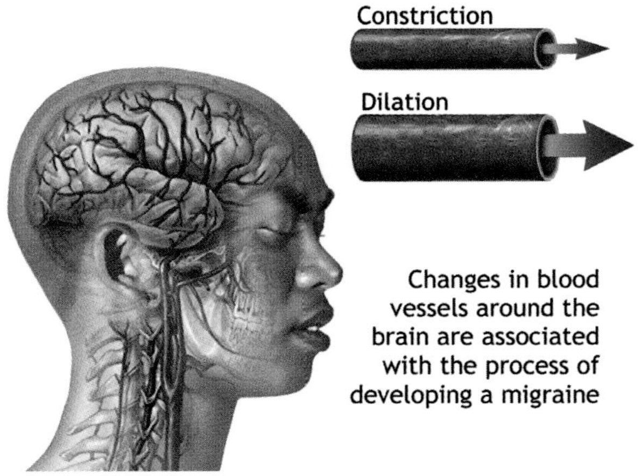

Changes in blood vessels around the brain are associated with the process of developing a migraine

Why these changes in blood vessels and blood flow occur in the brain is not understood. Certain triggers, however, make it more likely for you to get migraines:

- Allergic reactions
- Bright lights, loud noises, and certain odors or perfumes
- Physical or emotional stress
- Changes in sleep patterns
- Smoking or exposure to smoke
- Skipping meals
- Alcohol or caffeine
- Menstrual cycle fluctuations, birth control pills
- Tension headaches
- Foods containing tyramine (red wine, aged cheese, smoked fish, chicken livers, figs, and some beans), monosodium glutamate (MSG), or nitrates (like bacon, hot dogs, and salami)
- Other foods such as chocolate, nuts, peanut butter, avocado, banana, citrus, onions, dairy products, and fermented or pickled foods

Keep a headache diary

Keep a headache diary to identify things that trigger your migraines, like certain foods, stress, or allergies. You can reduce your migraines without medication by avoiding these triggers and making lifestyle changes. (See Prevention section.)

Symptoms

Migraine headaches, which can be dull or severe, usually:

- Feel throbbing, pounding, or pulsating
- Are worse on one side of the head
- Last 6 to 48 hours

Symptoms accompanying migraines include:

- Nausea and vomiting
- Sensitivity to light or sound
- Loss of appetite
- Fatigue
- Numbness, tingling, or weakness

Warning signs that a migraine is coming include seeing stars or zigzag lines, having tunnel vision, or temporary blind spot.

Home care

There is no specific cure for migraine headaches. The goal is to prevent symptoms by avoiding or altering triggers. When you do get migraine symptoms, try to treat them right away. The headache may be less severe.

A good way to identify triggers is to keep a headache diary. See *Headache*.

When migraine symptoms begin:

- Rest in a quiet, darkened room.
- Drink fluids to avoid dehydration (especially if you have vomited).
- Try placing a cool cloth on your head.

Over-the-counter pain medications like acetaminophen, ibuprofen, or aspirin are often helpful, especially when your migraine is mild. If these don't help, ask your doctor about prescription medications.

Many of the prescription medications for migraines narrow your blood vessels. Therefore, these drugs should not be used if you have heart disease, unless specifically instructed by your doctor.

If you wish to consider an alternative, feverfew is a popular herb for migraines. Several studies, but not all, support using feverfew for treating migraines. If you are interested in trying feverfew, make sure your doctor approves. Also, know that herbal remedies sold in drugstores and health food stores are not regulated. Work with a trained herbalist when selecting herbs.

When to contact a medical professional

Call 911 if:

- You have unusual symptoms not experienced with a migraine before, like speech or vision problems, loss of balance, or difficulty moving a limb.
- You are experiencing "the worst headache of your life."

Call your doctor immediately if:

- Your headache pattern or intensity is different.
- Your headache gets worse when you lie down.

Also, call your doctor if:

- Previously effective treatments no longer help.
- Side effects from medication occurs (irregular heartbeat, pale or blue skin, extreme sleepiness, persistent cough, depression, fatigue, nausea, vomiting, diarrhea, constipation, stomach pain, cramps, dry mouth, extreme thirst, or others).
- You are likely to become pregnant. (Some medications should not be taken when pregnant.)

Prevention

- Avoid smoking, caffeine, and alcohol.
- Exercise regularly.
- Get enough sleep each night.
- Learn to relax and reduce stress. Try progressive muscle relaxation (contracting and releasing muscles throughout your body), meditation, biofeedback, or joining a support group.

If you get at least three headaches per month, your doctor may prescribe medication for you to prevent recurrent migraines.

Heart palpitations

Palpitations are heartbeat sensations that feel like pounding or racing. You may simply have an unpleasant awareness of your own heartbeat. You may feel skipped or stopped beats. The heart's rhythm may be normal or abnormal. Palpitations can be felt in your chest, throat, or neck.

Normally the heart beats between 60-100 times per minute. In people who exercise routinely or take medications that slow the heart, the rate may drop below 55 beats per minute.

If your heart rate is very fast (over 100 beats per minute), this is called tachycardia. An unusually slow heart rate is called bradycardia, and an occasional extra heart beat is known as extrasystole.

Palpitations are often not serious. However, it depends on whether or not the sensations represent an abnormal heart rhythm (called an arrhythmia). You are more likely to have an abnormal heart rhythm if you have:

- Known heart disease at the time the palpitations begin
- Significant risk factors for heart disease
- An abnormal heart valve
- An electrolyte abnormality – for example, low potassium

Heart palpitations can be caused by:

- Exercise
- Anxiety, stress, fear
- Fever
- Caffeine, nicotine, cocaine, diet pills
- Overactive thyroid
- Anemia
- Hyperventilation
- Low levels of oxygen in your blood
- Medications such as thyroid pills, asthma drugs, beta blockers for high blood pressure or heart disease, or anti-arrhythmics (medications to treat an irregular heart rhythm can sometimes cause a different irregular rhythm)
- Mitral valve prolapse – the valve that separates the left upper chamber (atrium) from the left lower chamber (ventricle) of the heart does not close properly
- Heart disease

Heartbeat and Electrocardiogram (ECG)

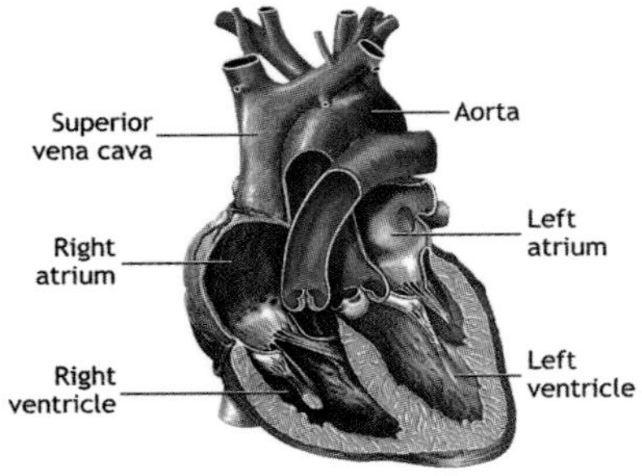

The heart contains 4 chambers – right and left atria and ventricles. The ventricles contract to pump blood to the body's organs and tissues.

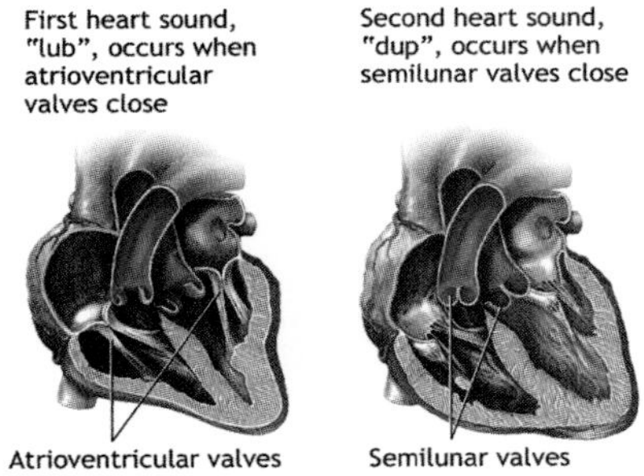

A heartbeat can be describe by "lub" and "dup" sounds, made by the closing of heart valves.

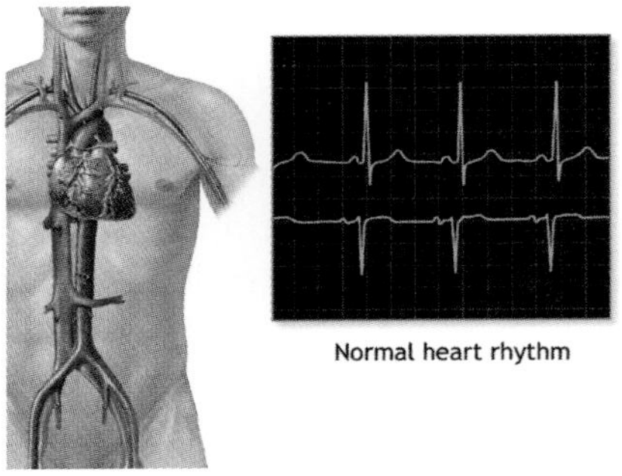

A normal heartbeat rhythm has a very distinctive pattern, as seen in the above ECG tracing.

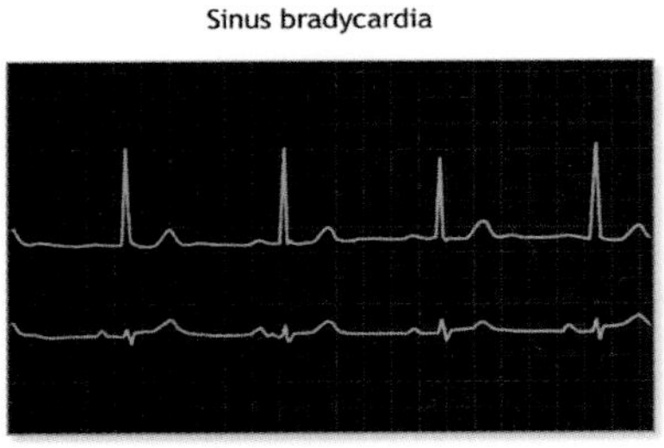

ECG testing can detect abnormal heartbeat rhythms. Sinus bradycardia, or abnormally slow heart rate, is pictured above.

Home care

Reducing stress and anxiety can help lessen your heart palpitations. Try breathing exercises or deep relaxation (a step-by-step process of tensing and then relaxing every muscle group in your body) at the time of your heartbeat sensations. Also, consider practicing yoga or tai chi on a regular basis to reduce the frequency of your palpitations.

Keep a record of how often you have palpitations, when they happen, how long they last, your heart rate at the time of the palpitations, and what you are feeling at the time. This information may help your doctor figure out both their seriousness and the cause.

Once a serious cause has been ruled out by your doctor, try NOT to pay attention to heart palpitations, unless you notice a sudden increase or a change in them.

If you have never had heart palpitations before, bring them to the attention of your doctor. He or she will do a work up to determine the cause and whether they are treatable or not.

How to check your pulse

With light pressure, press down as shown below until you feel your pulse. Count the number of beats for a full minute.

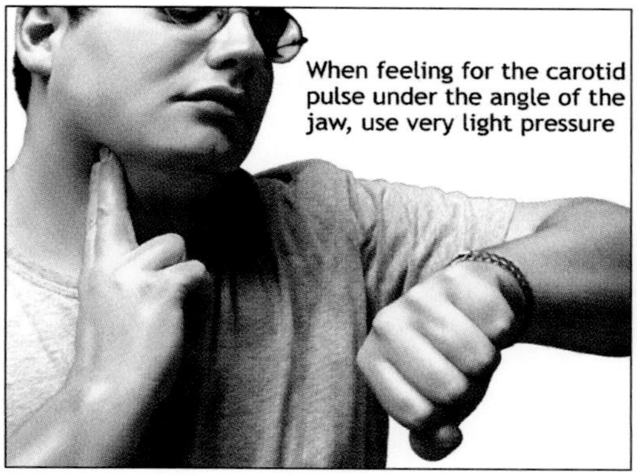
When feeling for the carotid pulse under the angle of the jaw, use very light pressure

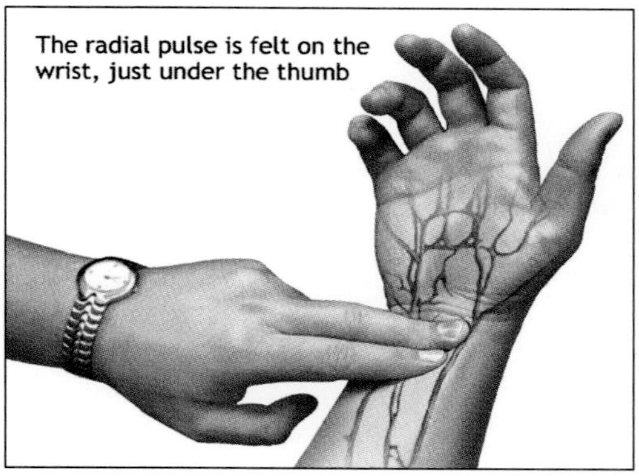
The radial pulse is felt on the wrist, just under the thumb

When to contact a medical professional

Call 911 if:

- You have fainted or someone you are with loses consciousness.
- You have shortness of breath, chest pain, unusual sweating, dizziness, or lightheadedness.

Call your doctor right away if:

- You feel frequent extra heartbeats (more than 6 per minute or coming in runs of 3 or more).
- You have risk factors for heart disease like high cholesterol, diabetes, or high blood pressure.
- You have new or different heart palpitations.
- Your pulse is more than 100 beats per minute (without exercise, anxiety, or fever).

Prevention

Try to reduce stress and risk factors for heart disease:

- Don't smoke.
- Eat a well-balanced, low-fat diet.
- Exercise regularly.
- Try stress management techniques like yoga, tai chi, or meditation.
- Make sure that your blood pressure and cholesterol are under control.

Heartburn

Heartburn is a painful burning sensation in the esophagus, just below the breastbone. The pain often rises in your chest and may radiate to your neck or throat.

Almost everyone has occasional heartburn. If you have frequent, ongoing heartburn, you may have gastroesophageal reflux disease (GERD).

Normally, when food or liquid enters your stomach, a band of muscle at the end of your esophagus (called the lower esophageal sphincter or LES) closes off the esophagus. If this muscle fails to close tightly enough, stomach contents can back up (reflux) into the esophagus. This partially digested material is usually acidic and can irritate the esophagus, causing heartburn and other symptoms.

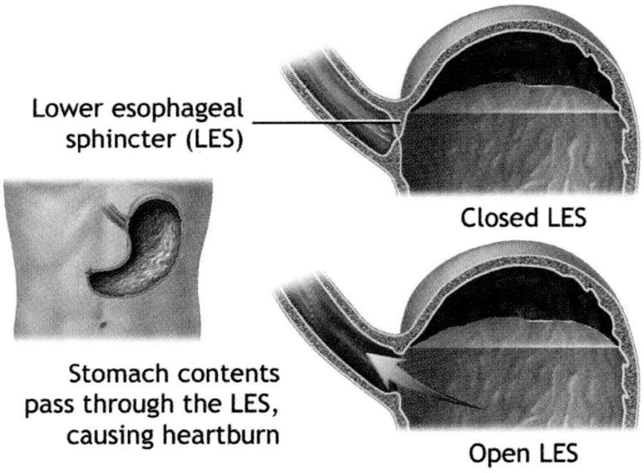

Sometimes GERD is related to a hiatal hernia. This is when part of the stomach protrudes upward through a hole in the diaphragm, putting pressure on the LES. Heartburn can also be a side effect of many different medications.

If you suspect that one of your medications may be causing heartburn, talk to your doctor. NEVER change or stop medication you take regularly without talking to your doctor. If you take an occasional aspirin or ibuprofen for headache or mild pain, try acetaminophen instead.

Home care

Pay attention to heartburn and treat it, especially if you feel symptoms often. Over time, ongoing reflux can damage the lining of your esophagus and cause serious problems. The good news is that making changes to certain habits can go a long way to preventing heartburn and other symptoms of GERD.

The following tips will help you avoid heartburn and other GERD symptoms. If these measures are not working, talk to your doctor.

First, avoid foods and beverages that can trigger reflux, such as:

- Alcohol
- Caffeine, carbonated beverages
- Chocolate
- Citrus fruits and juices
- Tomatoes and tomato sauces
- Spicy or fatty foods, full-fat dairy products
- Peppermint and spearmint

Lifestyle changes go a long way

For some people, medication is necessary to treat GERD. However, not everyone benefits from the most expensive new drug. Many people can avoid a lifetime of medication costs and side effects by simply making lifestyle changes. If you have ever wanted to lose weight, quit smoking, or cut down on alcohol, now you have even more motivation to do it – you can solve your heartburn problem at the same time!

Next, try changing your eating habits:

- Eat smaller meals. A full stomach puts extra pressure on the lower esophageal sphincter (LES), increasing the chance that food will reflux.
- Avoid eating or lying down within 2-3 hours of bedtime. Lying down with a full stomach results in stomach contents pressing harder against the LES.
- Avoid bending over or exercising just after eating.
- Drink plenty of fluids, especially when taking medications.

Make other lifestyle changes as needed:

- Lose weight if you are overweight. Obesity increases abdominal pressure, which can push stomach contents up into the esophagus. In some cases, GERD symptoms disappear completely after an overweight person loses 10-15 pounds.
- Stop smoking. Chemicals in cigarette smoke weaken the LES.
- Sleep with your head raised about 6 inches. Sleeping with the head higher than the stomach reduces the likelihood that partially digested food will reflux into the esophagus. Place books, bricks, or blocks securely under the legs at the head of your bed. Or use a wedge-shaped pillow under your mattress. Sleeping on extra pillows does NOT work well for relieving heartburn.
- Avoid tight-fitting belts or garments around the waist. They squeeze the stomach, and may force food to reflux.
- Reduce stress. Try yoga, tai chi, or meditation.

If you still do not have full relief, try over-the-counter medications:

- Antacids, like Maalox or Mylanta, work by neutralizing stomach acid.
- H2 blockers, like Pepcid AC, Tagamet, and Zantac, reduce stomach acid production.
- Proton pump inhibitors, like Prilosec OTC, nearly stop all stomach acid production.

When to contact a medical professional

Call 911 if:

- You vomit material that is bloody or black like coffee grounds.
- Your stools are black (like tar) or maroon.
- The burning sensation is accompanied by chest squeezing, crushing, or pressure. Sometimes a heart attack is mistaken for heartburn.

Call your doctor if:

- The problem becomes frequent or doesn't go away with a few weeks of self-care.
- You start losing weight unintentionally.
- You have difficulty swallowing (food feels stuck as it goes down).
- You have a persistent, unexplained cough or wheezing.
- Your symptoms get worse with antacids or H2 blockers.
- You think that one of your medications may be causing heartburn. DO NOT change or stop your medication on your own, without discussing with your doctor.

Heel pain

The most frequent causes of heel pain are not single injuries, such as a fall or twist, but repetitive or excessive heel pounding.

Plantar fasciitis is inflammation of the thick connective tissue on the sole of your foot that attaches to your heel. The pain is usually felt at the bottom of your heel and is often worse in the morning because of stiffness that occurs overnight.

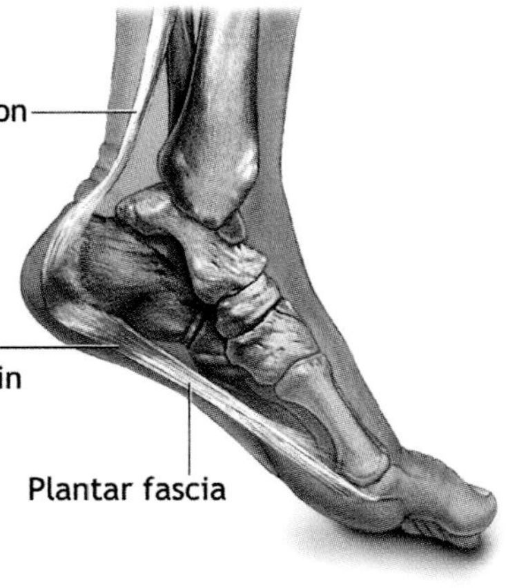

The following increase your risk of developing this painful problem:

- Shoes with poor arch support or stiff soles.
- Quick turns that put stress on your foot.
- Tight calf muscles.
- Repetitive pounding on your feet from long-distance running, especially running downhill or on uneven surfaces.
- Pronation – when you tend to land on the outside of your foot and roll inward when walking or running. To know if you pronate, check the soles of your shoes to see if they are worn along the outer edge.

Bone spurs in the heel can accompany plantar fasciitis, but are generally not the source of the pain. If you treat the plantar fasciitis appropriately, the bone spur is likely to no longer bother you.

Heel bursitis (inflammation of the back of the heel) can be caused by landing hard or awkwardly on the heel, or by pressure from shoes.

Achilles tendinitis is inflammation of the large tendon that connects your calf muscle to your heel. This can be caused by:

- Running, especially on hard surfaces like concrete.
- Tightness and lack of flexibility in your calf muscles.
- Shoes with inadequate stability or shock absorption.
- Sudden inward or outward turning of your heel when hitting the ground.

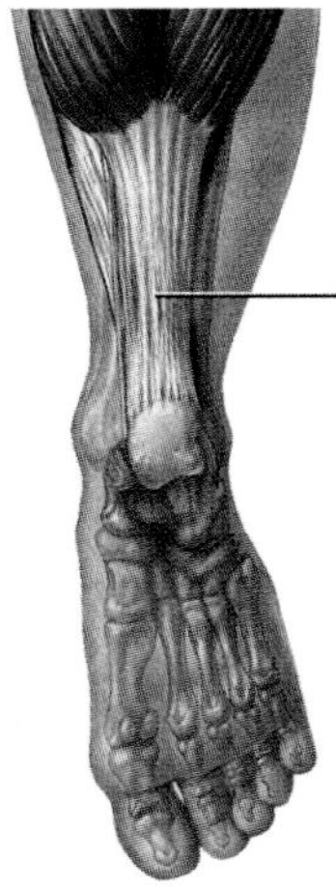

Home care

- Rest as much as possible for at least a week.
- Apply ice to the painful area. Do this at least twice a day for 10 to 15 minutes, more often in the first couple of days.
- Take acetaminophen for pain or ibuprofen for pain and inflammation.
- Wear proper-fitting shoes.
- A heel cup, felt pads in the heel area, or an orthotic device may help.
- Night splints can help some types of heel pain.

Additional steps:

- Apply moleskin to avoid pressure if you have bursitis.
- See a physical therapist to learn stretching and strengthening exercises. These help prevent plantar fasciitis or Achilles tendinitis from returning.

When to contact a medical professional

Call your doctor if:

- Your pain is getting worse despite home treatment.
- There is little progress after 2 to 3 weeks of home treatment.

- Your pain is sudden and severe.
- You have redness or swelling of your heel or you cannot bear weight.

Prevention

To prevent plantar fasciitis and Achilles tendinitis, maintain flexible and strong muscles in your calves, ankles, and feet.

Wear comfortable, properly fitting shoes with good arch support and cushioning. If you pronate, look for athletic shoes with an anti-pronation device. If orthotics are prescribed by your provider, wear them in all of your shoes, not just while exercising.

Hemorrhoids

Hemorrhoids are painful, swollen veins in the lower portion of the rectum or anus.

This condition is very common, especially during pregnancy and after childbirth. Hemorrhoids result from increased pressure in the veins of the anus. The pressure causes the veins to bulge and expand, making them painful, particularly when you are sitting.

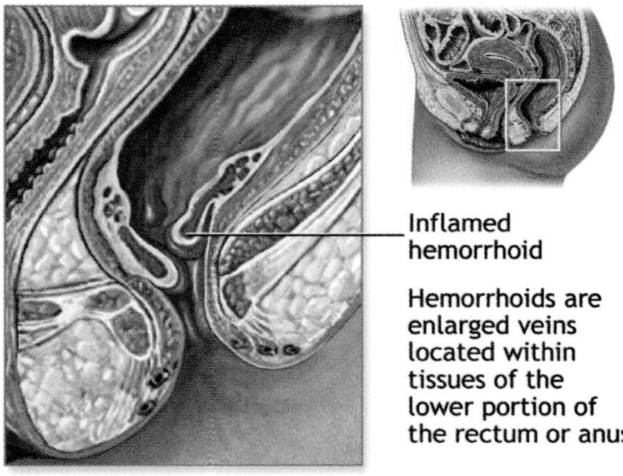

Hemorrhoids are enlarged veins located within tissues of the lower portion of the rectum or anus

The most common cause is straining during bowel movements. Hemorrhoids may result from constipation, sitting for long periods of time, and anal infections. In some cases they may be caused by other diseases, such as liver cirrhosis.

Internal hemorrhoids occur just inside the anus, at the beginning of the rectum. External hemorrhoids occur at the anal opening and may hang outside the anus.

Symptoms

Symptoms of hemorrhoids include:

- Anal itching
- Anal ache or pain, especially while sitting
- Bright red blood on toilet tissue, stool, or in the toilet bowl
- Pain during bowel movements
- One or more hard tender lumps near the anus

Home care

Over-the-counter corticosteroid creams can reduce pain and swelling. Hemorrhoid creams with lidocaine can reduce pain. Witch hazel (applied with cotton swabs) can reduce itching. Other steps for anal itching include:

- Wear cotton undergarments.
- Avoid toilet tissue with perfumes or colors.
- Try not to scratch the area.

Sitz baths can help you to feel better. Sit in warm water for 10 to 15 minutes. Stool softeners help reduce straining and constipation.

When to contact a medical professional

Call for an appointment with your health care provider if hemorrhoid symptoms do not improve with home treatment. You should also be seen if you have rectal bleeding. Your provider may want to check for other, more serious causes of the bleeding, especially if you have never bled from hemorrhoids before.

Call 911 if blood loss is significant or if you feel dizzy, lightheaded, or faint.

Prevention

Avoid straining during bowel movements. You can help prevent hemorrhoids by preventing constipation. Drink plenty of fluids, at least eight glasses per day. Eat a high-fiber diet of fruits, vegetables, whole grains. Consider fiber supplements.

Hepatitis

Hepatitis is inflammation of the liver.

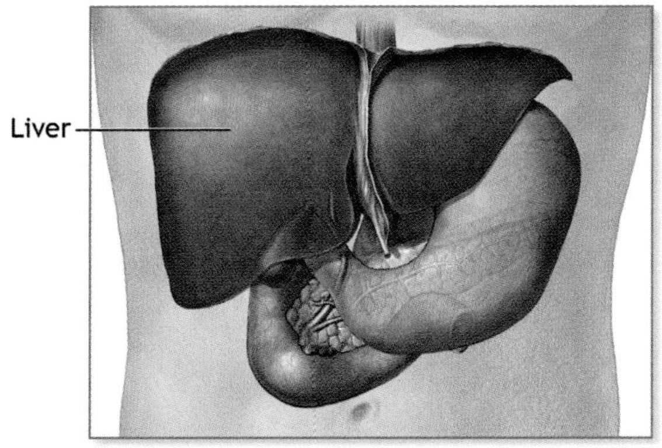

The disease can be caused by:

- Infections from parasites, bacteria, or viruses (such as Hepatitis A, B, or C)
- Liver damage from alcohol, drugs, or poisonous mushrooms
- An overdose of acetaminophen, which is rare but deadly
- Immune cells in the body attacking the liver and causing autoimmune hepatitis

Hepatitis may start and resolve quickly (acute hepatitis), or cause long-term disease (chronic hepatitis). In some instances, progressive liver damage, liver failure, or even liver cancer may result.

The severity of hepatitis depends on many factors, including the cause of the liver damage and any underlying illnesses you have. Hepatitis A, for example, is generally short-lived, not leading to chronic liver problems.

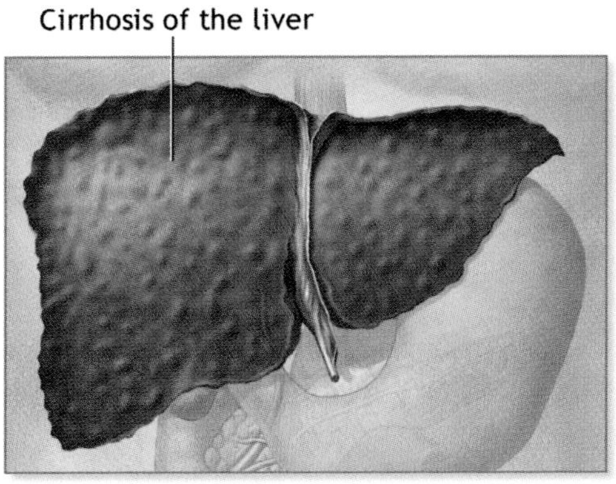

50% of people with Hepatitis C go on to have chronic liver disease, and possibly liver cirrhosis.

Symptoms

The symptoms of hepatitis include:

- Dark urine and pale or clay colored stools
- Loss of appetite
- Fatigue
- Abdominal pain or distention
- General itching
- Jaundice (yellowing of the skin or whites of the eyes)
- Nausea and vomiting
- Low grade fever
- Weight loss
- Breast development in males

Many people with hepatitis B or C do not have symptoms when first infected and can still develop liver failure later. If you have any risk factors for either type of hepatitis, you should be tested periodically.

Home care

Your doctor will discuss possible treatments with you, depending on the cause of your liver disease. Your doctor may recommend a high-calorie diet if you are losing weight. You can take these steps yourself:

- Eat the bulk of your calories early in the day.

- Rest, especially when you feel symptoms.

When to contact a medical professional

Call 911 if you:

- Have symptoms related to acetaminophen or other medicines; you may need stomach pumping
- Vomit blood
- Are confused or delirious

Call your doctor if:

- You have any symptoms of hepatitis or believe that you have been exposed to hepatitis A, B, or C.
- You cannot keep food down due to excessive vomiting. You may need to receive nutrition intravenously (through a vein).
- You have been traveling to an endemic area like Asia, Africa, South or Central America.

Prevention

The following hepatitis vaccines are available:

- Hepatitis A vaccine is available for people in high-risk groups, like day care and nursing home workers, laboratory workers, and those traveling to endemic parts of the world.
- Hepatitis B vaccine is now given to all infants and unvaccinated children under 18. The vaccine is available for adults at high risk, such as health care professionals, IV drug users, and those with risky sexual behavior.

A shot of immunoglobulin may also prevent infection. This is true even after you have been exposed:

- It may be given soon after you have had close contact (like kissing or sharing utensils) with someone who was diagnosed with hepatitis A within the last two weeks.
- It should be given right away, along with the hepatitis B vaccine, to an infant born to a woman with hepatitis B.

Other steps to take:

- Avoid contact with blood or blood products. Take precautions if this is part of your work.
- Avoid sexual contact with a person infected with hepatitis or unknown health history. Practice safe sex at all times.
- Wash your hands after going to the bathroom and before handling food.
- Avoid sharing plates, utensils, or bathrooms with someone who has hepatitis A.
- Do not share razors, needles, or toothbrushes.
- When traveling to endemic areas, do not eat uncooked or partially cooked foods. Drink bottled water.
- Do not use recreational IV drugs. If you are already an IV drug user, never share needles and seek help from a needle exchange or drug treatment program.
- Be cautious when receiving tattoos or piercings.
- DO NOT drink alcohol at the same time that you take acetaminophen. If you already have hepatitis, do not use either (to avoid further liver damage).

Take-home point

Hepatitis A and B vaccines are available to help keep you and your children safe. Read the Prevention section of this article to find out if you qualify for a vaccine and to learn methods to prevent many types of hepatitis.

When to get tested for hepatitis:

- Get tested for hepatitis B or C if you had sexual contact or shared needles with someone who may have had one of these viruses.
- Do this even if you have no symptoms.

Hernia

A hernia occurs when part of an organ (usually the intestines) protrudes through a weak point or tear in the thin muscular wall that holds the abdominal organs in place.

There are several types of hernias, based on where it occurs:

- **Inguinal hernia** – appears as a bulge in the groin or scrotum. This type is more common in men than women.
- **Femoral hernia** – appears as a bulge in the upper thigh. This type is more common in women than in men.
- **Incisional hernia** – can occur through a scar if you had abdominal surgery.
- **Umbilical hernia** – a bulge around the belly button. Happens if the muscle around the navel doesn't close completely.

Usually, there is no obvious cause of a hernia, although they are sometimes associated with heavy lifting.

Hernias can be seen in infants and children. This can happen when the lining around the abdominal organs does not close properly before birth. About 5 out of 100 children have inguinal hernias (more boys than girls). Some may not have symptoms until adulthood.

If you have any of the following, you are more likely to develop a hernia:

- Family history of hernias
- Cystic fibrosis
- Undescended testicles
- Extra weight
- Chronic cough
- Chronic constipation from straining to have bowel movements
- Straining to urinate from an enlarged prostate

Various types of hernias

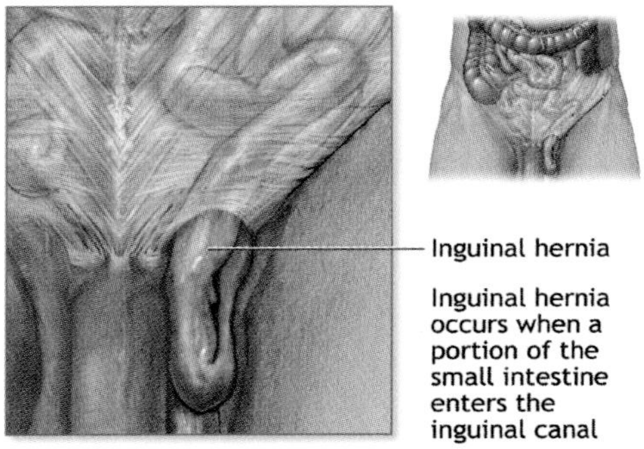

Inguinal hernia
Inguinal hernia occurs when a portion of the small intestine enters the inguinal canal

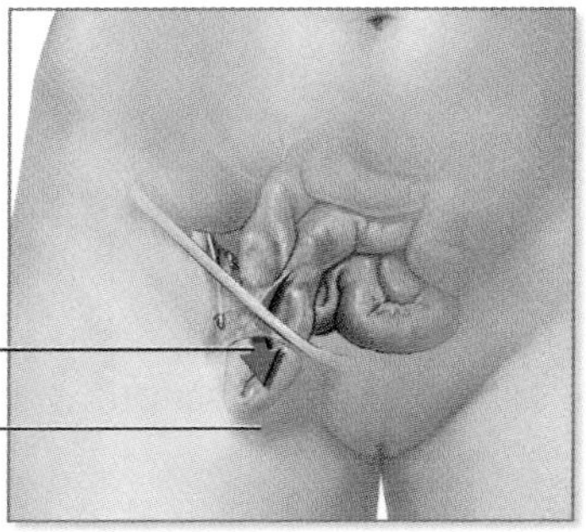

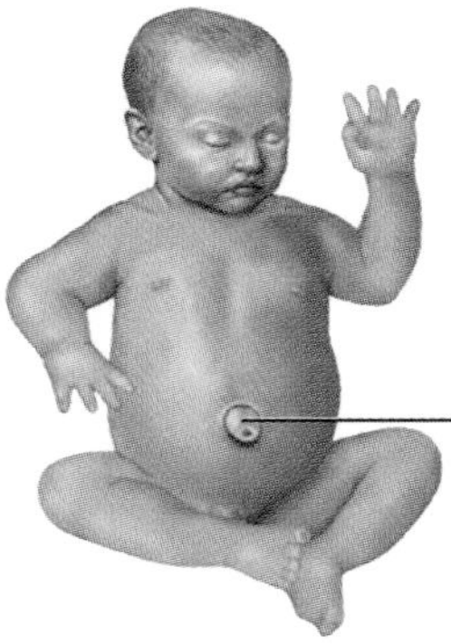

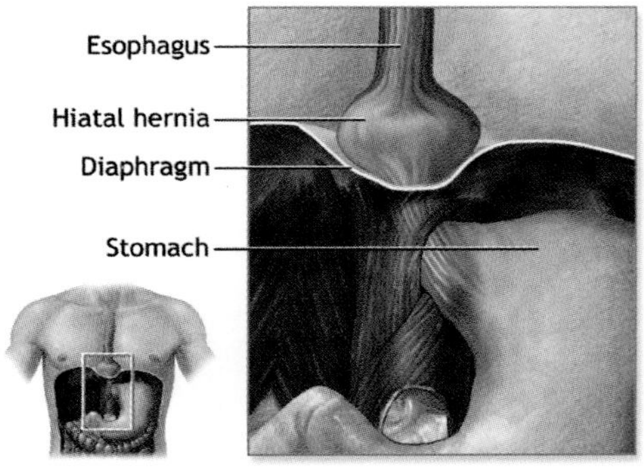

Symptoms

- Groin discomfort or groin pain aggravated by bending or lifting
- A tender groin lump or scrotum lump
- A non-tender bulge or lump in children

Home care

Most hernias can be pushed back into the abdominal cavity. However, if it cannot be pushed back through the abdominal wall, this can lead to a strangulated loop of intestine. If left untreated, this dies because of loss of blood supply.

Almost all hernias require surgery, preferably before complications occur, to reposition the herniated loop of intestine and secure the weakened muscles in the abdomen.

When to contact a medical professional

Call your doctor right away if:

- You have a hernia and the contents cannot be pushed back into the abdomen using gentle pressure.
- You develop nausea, vomiting, or a fever with your hernia.
- The hernia becomes red, purple, dark, or discolored.

Call your doctor if:

- You have groin pain, swelling, or a bulge.
- An umbilical hernia fails to heal on its own by the time your child is 5 years old.

Prevention

- Use proper lifting techniques.
- Lose weight if you are overweight.
- Relieve or avoid constipation by eating plenty of fiber, drinking lots of fluid, going to the bathroom as soon as you have the urge, and exercising regularly.

Hip pain

Two common and concerning causes of hip pain are fractures and insufficient blood flow to the hip (aseptic necrosis).

A hip fracture can change the quality of your life significantly. Fewer than 50% of those with a hip fracture return to their former level of activity. In addition, while recovering from a hip fracture, several possible complications can be life-threatening. These include pneumonia and a blood clot in the leg, which can dislodge and cause a clot in the lungs. Both are due to immobility following a hip fracture and hip surgery.

Hip fractures become more common as people age because falls are more likely and bones become less dense. People with osteoporosis can get a fracture from simple, everyday activities, not just a dramatic fall or injury.

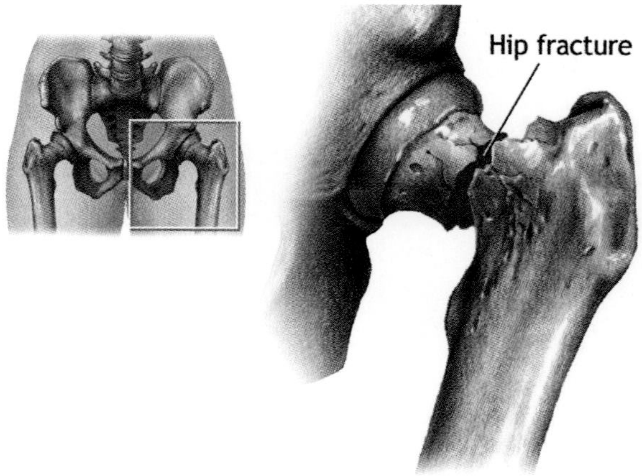

Aseptic necrosis can happen if you have been on steroids for a long time or you have sickle cell anemia. Regular use of alcohol and injury also increase your risk.

Other possible causes of hip pain include:

- Arthritis – often felt in the front part of your thigh.
- Trochanteric bursitis – inflammation of the bursa that sits on the outside of your hip joint. This hurts when you get up from a chair, walk, climb stairs, and drive.

- Tendinitis from repetitive or strenuous activity.
- Strain or sprain.
- Low back pain such as sciatica.
- Infection.

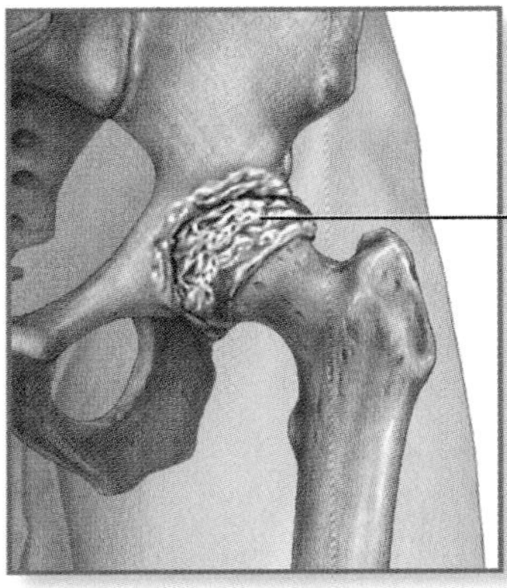

Arthritis, such as osteoarthritis, is a common cause of hip pain. Osteoarthritis is caused by loss of cartilage in the joint. Cartilage normally protects the joint and absorbs the shock of movement.

Home care

- Try to avoid activities that aggravate the pain.
- Take over-the-counter pain medication, like ibuprofen or acetaminophen.
- Sleep on your non-painful side with a pillow between your legs.

A hip fracture is considered a medical emergency. Therefore, if suspected, you should be seen right away.

As the pain improves, gradually begin to exercise. It is best to work with a physical therapist to learn proper exercises and how to advance your activity. Swimming may be a good option because it stretches the muscles and builds good muscle tone without straining your hip joint. However, swimming does not build bone mass. When you are ready (a physical therapist can help determine that), slowly and carefully resume walking or another activity against the resistance of gravity.

When to contact a medical professional

Go to a hospital or call 911 if:

- Your hip pain is caused by a fall or other injury.
- Your hip is misshapen, badly bruised, or bleeding.
- You are unable to move your hip or bear any weight.

Call your doctor if:

- Your hip is still painful after 1 week of home treatment.
- You also have a fever or rash.
- You have sudden hip pain, plus sickle cell anemia or long-term steroid use.
- You have pain in both hips or other joints.

Prevention

- Avoid activities that raise one of your hips above the other for extended periods of time, like running on an uneven surface. Running on a treadmill can keep your hips level.
- Warm up before exercising and cool down afterward. Stretch your hips, low back, and thighs.
- Avoid falls.
- Wear hip pads for contact sports like football and hockey. For those at high risk for a hip fracture, pads with a streamline design can be worn in undergarments.
- Learn how to prevent osteoporosis.

Hives

Hives are raised, often itchy red welts on the surface of the skin. They are usually an allergic reaction to food or medicine.

When you have an allergic reaction to a substance, histamine and other chemicals are released into your bloodstream, causing itching, swelling, and other symptoms. Hives are a common reaction, especially in people with other allergies like hay fever.

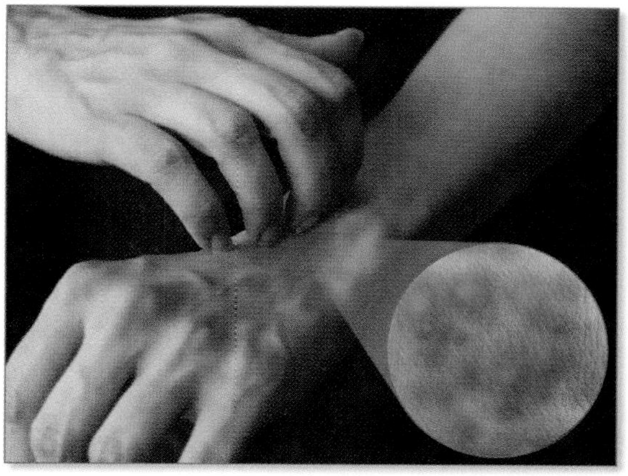

Hives

Many substances can trigger hives:

- Medications
- Shellfish, fish, nuts, eggs, milk, and other foods

Shellfish

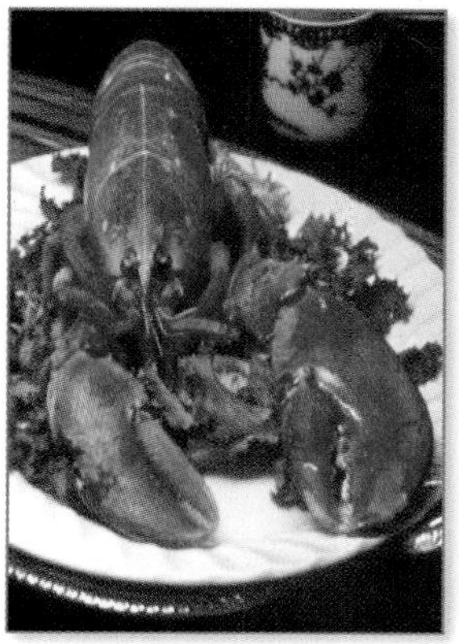

Peanuts and nuts

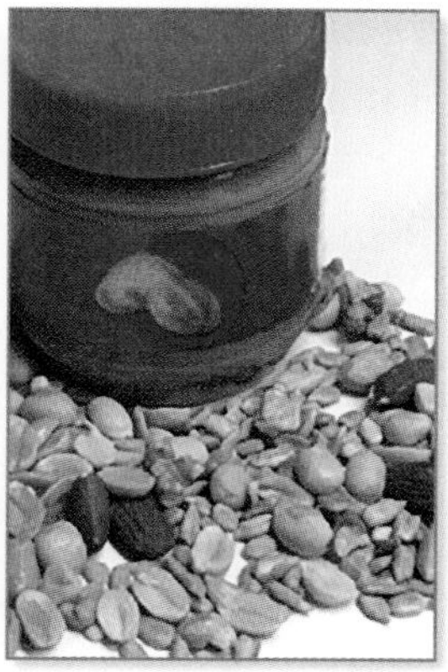

- Pollen
- Animal dander (especially cats)
- Insect bites

Hives may also develop from:

- Infections like mononucleosis or illness (including lupus, other autoimmune diseases, and leukemia)
- Emotional stress
- Extreme cold or sun exposure
- Excessive perspiration

Symptoms

The welts may enlarge, spread, and join together to form larger areas of flat, raised skin. They can also change shape, disappear, and reappear within minutes or hours. The welts tend to start suddenly and resolve quickly. When you press the center of a red welt, it blanches (turns white).

Home care

Treatment may not be needed if the hives are mild. They may disappear on their own. To reduce itching and swelling:

- Apply cool compresses to the welts. This may reduce swelling and pain. If a large part of your body is affected, soak in a cool bath. Avoid hot baths or showers.
- Avoid irritating the area with tight-fitting clothing.
- Apply Calamine lotion.
- Take antihistamines.

If your reaction is severe, especially if the swelling involves your throat, you may require an emergency shot of epinephrine (adrenaline) or steroids. Hives in the throat can obstruct your airway, making it difficult to breathe.

When to contact a medical professional

Call 911 if you experience:

- Tightness in your throat
- Shortness of breath
- Tongue or face swelling
- Fainting
- Wheezing

Call your health care provider if the hives are severe, uncomfortable, and do not respond to self-care.

Hyperactivity and ADHD

ADHD is a problem with inattentiveness, over-activity, impulsivity, or a combination. For these problems to be diagnosed as ADHD, they must be out of the normal range for the child's age and development.

ADHD affects school performance and relationships with others. Parents of children with ADHD are often exhausted and frustrated.

ADHD is often genetic. Whatever the specific cause may be, it seems to be set in motion early in life as the brain is developing.

Depression, sleep deprivation, learning disabilities, tic disorders, and behavior problems may be confused with, or appear along with, ADHD. Every child suspected of having ADHD deserves a careful evaluation to sort out exactly what is contributing to the concerning behaviors.

Most children with ADHD also have at least one other developmental or behavioral problem.

Symptoms

To be diagnosed with ADHD, children should have at least 6 attention symptoms or 6 activity / impulsivity symptoms – to a degree beyond what would be expected for children their age.

The symptoms must be present for at least 6 months, observable in 2 or more settings, and not caused by another problem. The symptoms must be severe enough to cause significant difficulties. Some symptoms must be present before age 7.

Inattention symptoms:

1. Fails to give close attention to details or makes careless mistakes in schoolwork
2. Difficulty sustaining attention in tasks or play
3. Does not seem to listen when spoken to directly
4. Does not follow through on instructions and fails to finish schoolwork, chores, or duties in the workplace
5. Difficulty organizing tasks and activities
6. Avoids or dislikes tasks that require sustained mental effort (such as schoolwork)
7. Often loses toys, assignments, pencils, books, or tools needed for tasks or activities
8. Easily distracted
9. Often forgetful in daily activities

Hyperactivity symptoms:

1. Fidgets with hands or feet or squirms in seat
2. Leaves seat when remaining seated is expected
3. Runs about or climbs in inappropriate situations
4. Difficulty playing quietly
5. Often "on the go", acts as if "driven by a motor", talks excessively

Impulsivity symptoms:

1. Blurts out answers before questions have been completed
2. Difficulty awaiting turn
3. Interrupts or intrudes on others (butts into conversations or games)

Home care

The American Academy of Pediatrics has guidelines for treating ADHD:

- Set specific, appropriate target goals to guide therapy.
- Medication and / or behavior therapy should be started.
- When treatment has not met the target goals, evaluate the original diagnosis, the possible presence of other conditions,

and how well the treatment plan has been implemented.

- Systematic follow-up is important to regularly reassess target goals, results, and any side effects of medications. Information should be gathered from parents, teachers, and the child.

ADHD is a frustrating problem. Alternative remedies have become quite popular, including herbs, supplements, and chiropractic manipulation. However, there is little or no solid evidence for many remedies marketed to parents.

Key point

If you suspect your child has ADHD, don't just guess. Review the criteria in this article for a doctor to make a diagnosis. Also, work with your doctor to make sure nothing else might be responsible for your child's symptoms.

Children who receive both behavioral treatment and medication often do the best. Medications should not be used just to make life easier for the parents or the school. There are now several different classes of ADHD medications that may be used alone or in combination. The following may also help:

- Limit distractions in the child's environment.
- Provide one-on-one instruction with teacher.
- Make sure the child gets enough sleep.
- Make sure the child gets a healthy, varied diet, with plenty of fiber and basic nutrients.

Ingrown toenails

An ingrown toenail is when the edge of the nail grows into the skin of the toe. There may be pain, redness, and swelling around the nail.

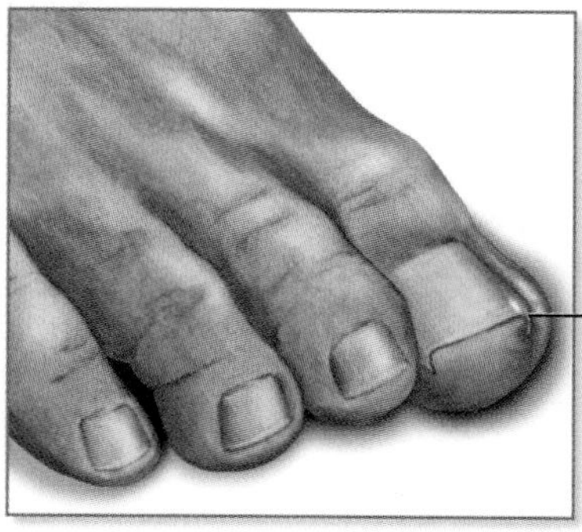

An ingrown toenail can result from curved toenails, poorly fitting shoes, toenails that are trimmed improperly, or a toe injury. The skin around the toenail may become red and infected. The great toe is usually affected, but any toenail can become ingrown.

The condition may become serious in people with diabetes.

Home care

To treat an ingrown nail at home:

1. Soak the foot in warm water.
2. Use a nail file to separate the nail from the inflamed skin.
3. Place a small piece of cotton under the nail. Wet the cotton with water or antiseptic.

Repeat those steps, several times a day if necessary, until the nail begins to grow out and the pain goes away. Also trim the toenail and apply over-the-counter antibiotics. If this does not work and the ingrown nail gets worse, see a foot specialist (podiatrist) or skin specialist (dermatologist).

When to contact a medical professional

Call your health care provider if you are unable to trim an ingrown toenail or have severe pain, redness, swelling, or fever.

If you have diabetes, your risk for complications is higher. See your provider.

Prevention

To prevent an ingrown toenail:

- Wear shoes that fit properly.
- Trim toenails straight across the top and not too short.
- Keep the feet clean and dry.
- People with diabetes should have routine foot exams and nail care.

Intercourse - painful

For both men and women, pain can occur in the pelvic area during or soon after sexual intercourse. It can happen at any time during sex – for example, at the time of penetration, erection, or ejaculation. Eventually, if pain from intercourse is ongoing, you could lose interest in any sexual activity.

Home care

For painful intercourse in women after pregnancy:

- Wait at least 6 weeks after childbirth before resuming sexual relations.
- Be gentle and patient.

For vaginal dryness/inadequate lubrication:

- Try water-based lubricants.
- If you are going through menopause and lubricants don't work, talk to your doctor about estrogen creams or other prescription medications.

For painful intercourse caused by prostatitis:

- Soak in a warm bath.
- Drink plenty of fluids, but avoid alcohol and caffeine.
- Take acetaminophen or ibuprofen.
- Take antibiotics as prescribed.

For hemorrhoids, try stool softeners. Antibiotics may be required for urinary tract infections, sexually transmitted diseases, or vaginal infections.

Other causes of painful intercourse may require prescription medications or, rarely, surgery.

Sex therapy may be helpful, especially if no underlying medical cause is identified. Guilt, inner conflict, or unresolved feelings about past abuse may be involved which need to be worked through in therapy. It may be best for your partner to see the therapist with you.

When to contact a medical professional

Call your doctor if:

- Home remedies are not working.
- You have other symptoms with painful intercourse, like bleeding, genital lesions, irregular periods, discharge from penis or vagina, or involuntary vaginal muscle contraction.

Jock itch

Jock itch, also called tinea cruris or ringworm of the groin, is an infection of the groin area caused by fungi.

The body normally hosts a variety of bacteria and fungi. Some of these are useful to the body. Others can multiply rapidly and form infections. Jock itch occurs when a particular type of fungus grows and multiplies in the groin area.

Jock itch occurs almost exclusively in adult men. It can sometimes accompany athlete's foot and ringworm. The fungus that causes jock itch thrives in warm, moist areas. Jock itch can be triggered by friction from clothes and prolonged wetness in the groin area (such as from sweating).

Jock itch may be contagious. It can be passed from one person to the next by direct skin-to-skin contact or contact with unwashed clothing. Jock itch usually stays around the creases in the upper thigh and does not involve the scrotum or penis. It is often less severe than other tinea infections, but may last a long time. Jock itch may spread to the anus, causing anal itching and discomfort.

Symptoms

- Itching in groin, thigh skin folds, or anus.
- Red, raised, scaly patches that may blister and ooze. The patches often have sharply-defined edges. They are often redder around the outside with normal skin tone in the center. This may create the appearance of a ring.
- Abnormally dark or light skin.

Home care

Jock itch usually responds to self-care within a couple of weeks:

- Keep the skin clean and dry.
- Don't wear clothing that rubs and irritates the area.
- Apply topical over-the-counter antifungal or drying powders, such as those that contain miconazole, clotrimazole, or tolnaftate.

When to contact a medical professional

Call your doctor if jock itch does not respond to home care after two weeks, or you have other symptoms.

Knee pain

Knee pain usually results from overuse, poor form during physical activity, not warming up or cooling down, or inadequate stretching. Simple causes of knee pain often clear up on their own with self care. Being overweight can put you at greater risk for knee problems.

Knee pain can be caused by:

- Arthritis – including rheumatoid, osteoarthritis, and gout, or other connective tissue disorders like lupus.

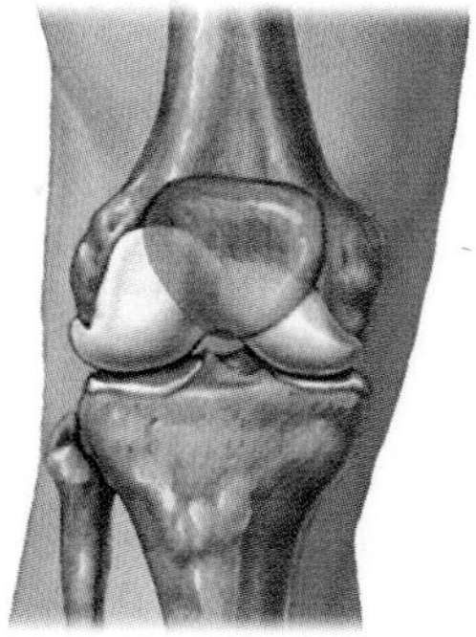

Healthy knee joint

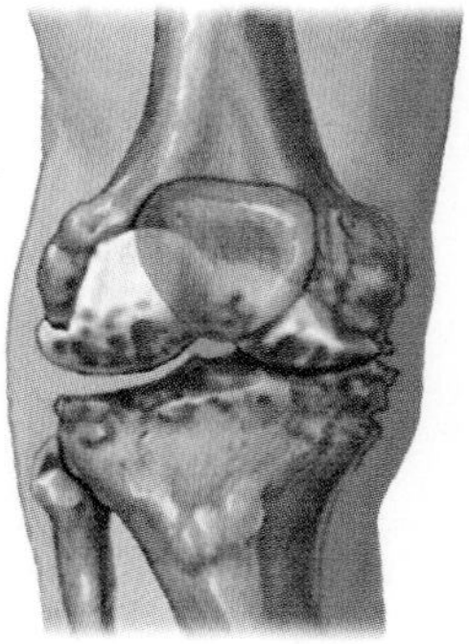

Osteoarthritis

- Bursitis – inflammation from repeated pressure on the knee (like kneeling for long periods of time, overuse, or injury).

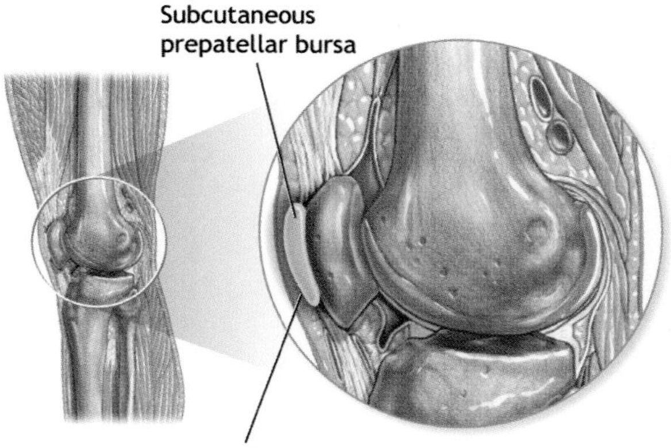

- Tendinitis – a pain in the front of your knee that gets worse when going up and down stairs or inclines. Happens to runners, skiers, and cyclists.

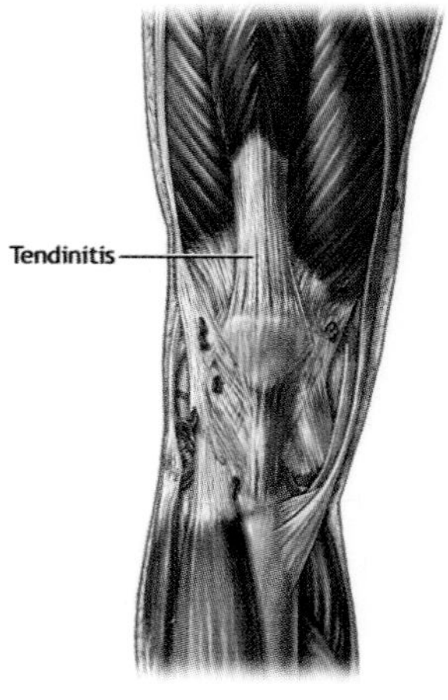

- Baker's cyst – a fluid-filled swelling behind the knee that may accompany inflammation from other causes, like arthritis. If the cyst ruptures, pain in the back of your knee can travel down your calf.

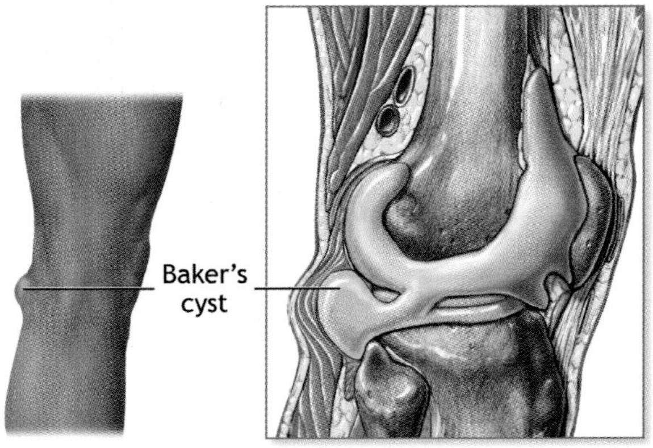

- Torn or ruptured ligaments or torn cartilage (a meniscus tear) – can cause severe pain and instability of the knee joint.
- Strain or sprain – minor injuries to the ligaments caused by sudden or unnatural twisting.
- Dislocation of the kneecap.
- Infection in the joint.
- Knee injuries – can cause bleeding into your knee, which worsens the pain.
- Hip disorders – may cause pain that is felt in the knee. For example, iliotibial band syndrome is injury to the thick band that runs from your hip to the outside of your knee.

Home care

Many causes of knee pain, especially those related to overuse or physical activity, respond well to self-care:

- Rest and avoid activities that aggravate the pain, especially weight bearing activities.
- Apply ice. First, apply it every hour for up to 15 minutes. After the first day, apply it at least 4 times per day.
- Keep your knee elevated as much as possible to bring any swelling down.
- Gently compress the knee by wearing an ace bandage or elastic sleeve. Either can be purchased at most pharmacies. This may reduce swelling and provide support.
- Take acetaminophen for pain or ibuprofen for pain and swelling.
- Sleep with a pillow underneath or between your knees.

When to contact a medical professional

Call your doctor if:

- You cannot bear weight on your knee.
- You have severe pain, even when not bearing weight.
- Your knee buckles, clicks, or locks.
- Your knee is deformed or misshapen.
- You have a fever, redness or warmth around the knee, or significant swelling.
- You have pain, swelling, numbness, tingling, or bluish discoloration in the calf below the sore knee.
- You still have pain after 3 days of home treatment.

Prevention

- Increase your activity level slowly over time. For example, when you begin exercising again, walk rather than run.
- Always warm up before exercising and cool down afterward. Stretch your quadriceps and hamstrings.
- Replace your sports shoes often. Get good advice about proper footwear for your foot shape and mechanics. For example, if you pronate (land on the outside of your heel and turn your foot inward), consider anti-pronation footwear.

Leg pain

Leg pain can be due to a muscle cramp (also called a charley horse).

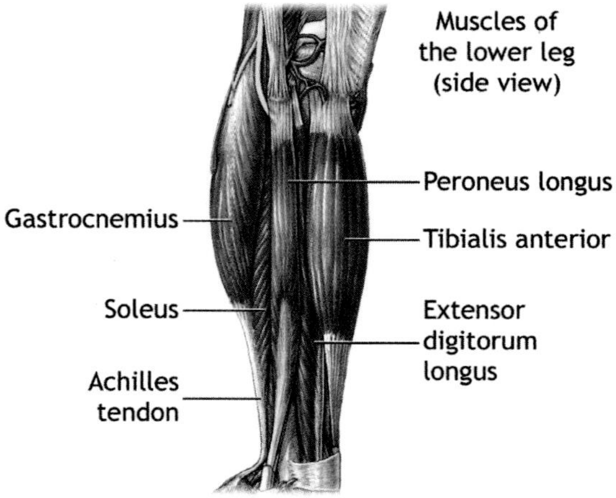

"Charley horse" may describe a leg cramp in the big muscle of the calf, called the gastrocnemius muscle.

Common causes of cramps include:

- Muscle fatigue or strain from overuse, excessive exercise, or holding a muscle in the same position for a long time.
- Dehydration or depletion of potassium, sodium, calcium, or magnesium.
- Medications like diuretics, which can cause you to lose too much fluid or minerals, and cholesterol-lowering drugs called statins.

An injury can also cause leg pain from:

- Shin splints – pain in the front of your leg related to overuse or repetitive pounding

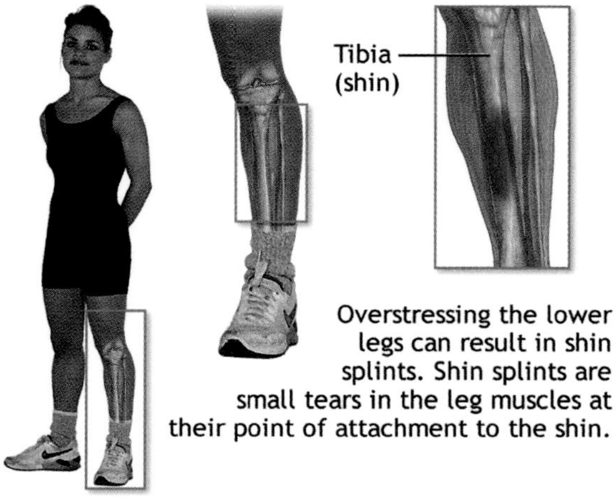

Overstressing the lower legs can result in shin splints. Shin splints are small tears in the leg muscles at their point of attachment to the shin.

- Hairline crack in the bone (stress fracture)
- A torn or overstretched muscle (strain)
- Inflamed tendon (tendinitis)

Other common causes of leg pain include:

- Blood clot (deep vein thrombosis) from prolonged bed rest.
- Atherosclerosis (plaque buildup) that blocks blood flow in the arteries. This type of pain, called claudication, is generally felt when exercising or walking and relieved by rest.
- Inflammation of the leg joints by arthritis or gout.
- Nerve damage – common in diabetics, smokers, and alcoholics. You may feel numbness, tingling, or a sensation of pins-and-needles.
- Infection of the bone (osteomyelitis) or skin and soft tissue (cellulitis).
- Varicose veins.

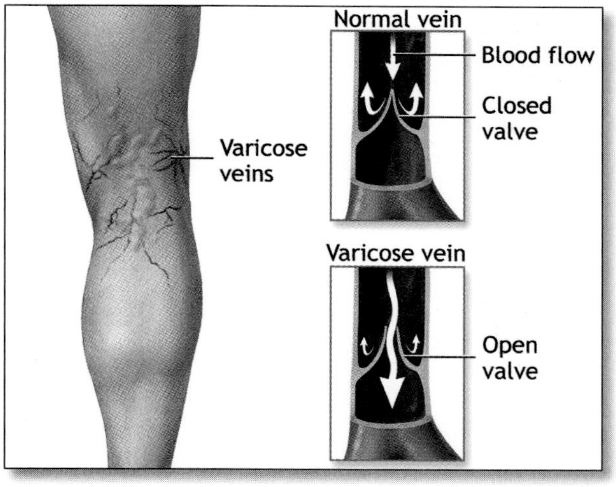

Home care

If you have leg pain from cramps or overuse, take these steps first:

- Rest as much as possible.
- Elevate your leg.
- Apply ice for 15 minutes. Do this 4 times per day, more often for the first few days.
- Gently stretch and massage cramping muscles.

Take over-the-counter pain medications like acetaminophen or ibuprofen.

For leg pain caused by varicose veins, leg elevation and compression with elastic bandages or support hose can help.

For leg pain caused by nerve disorders or claudication, control diabetes, eliminate alcohol and tobacco, and avoid ill-fitting shoes.

When to contact a medical professional

Call your doctor if:

- The painful leg is swollen or red.
- You have a fever.
- Your pain worsens when walking or exercising and improves with rest.
- The leg is black and blue.
- The leg is cold and pale.
- You are on medications that may be causing leg pain. DO NOT stop or change any of your usual medications without talking to your doctor.
- Self-care steps do not help.

Prevention

To prevent claudication and nerve damage:

- Don't smoke or use tobacco.
- Limit how much alcohol you drink.
- Keep your blood sugars under good control if you have diabetes.
- Reduce other heart disease risk factors, including high cholesterol and high blood pressure.

To prevent overuse injuries, like shin splints, muscle cramps, and other causes of leg pain:

- Warm up before physical activity and cool down afterward. Be sure to stretch.
- Drink plenty of fluids throughout the day, especially before, during, and after exercise.

Lice

There are three common types of lice: head lice, body lice, and pubic lice (also called crabs). Head lice infect the scalp hair and are easiest to see at the nape of the neck and over the ears. Tiny eggs can be seen on the hair, appearing much like flakes of dandruff, but stuck firmly to the hair shaft instead of flaking off the scalp.

Lice can also live on clothing, carpets, or bedding.

Head lice are spread easily and cause intense itching, but they do not lead to a serious medical problem. Lice are more common in close, overcrowded living conditions. Lice spread readily among school children.

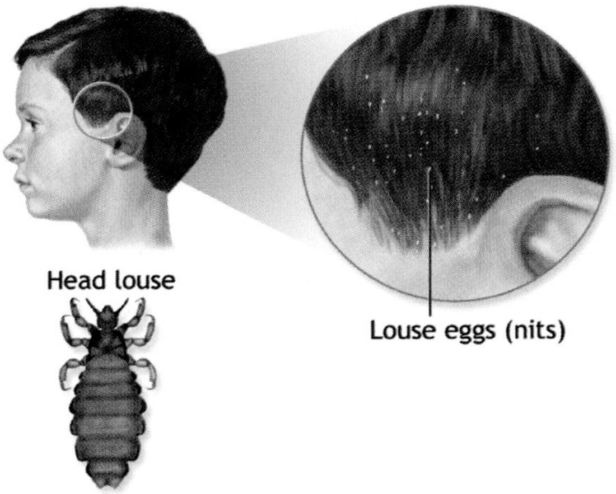

Home care

Lotions and shampoos containing permethrin are usually effective. They are available over-the-counter. If these do not work, other products are available by prescription. The medications used for lice are insecticides. Therefore, they should be used exactly as directed and no more frequently than recommended.

Certain products loosen the bond between the egg sack (nit) and hair shaft so that eggs can be easily removed. Remove the eggs with a nit comb. Removing eggs may prevent reinfection if the medication fails to kill all of them.

Treat children and adults with lice promptly and thoroughly. Wash all clothes and bed linens. This also helps prevent head lice from spreading to others.

When to contact a medical professional

First, apply home treatment. Call your health-care provider if symptoms continue after home treatment, or if you develop an irritation from the medicine.

Prevention

- Check policies at schools, daycares, preschools, and nurseries. Many do not allow infected children to be at school until the lice have been completely treated. Sometimes, however, the insects get into carpets or other areas at the school. It is helpful if the school has policies to ensure the environment is cleared of lice.
- DO NOT share hair brushes, combs, hair pieces, hats, bedding, towels, or clothing with someone who has lice.

Menopause symptoms

Menopause is the transition period in a woman's life when her ovaries stop producing eggs, her body produces less estrogen and progesterone, and menstruation becomes less frequent, eventually stopping altogether.

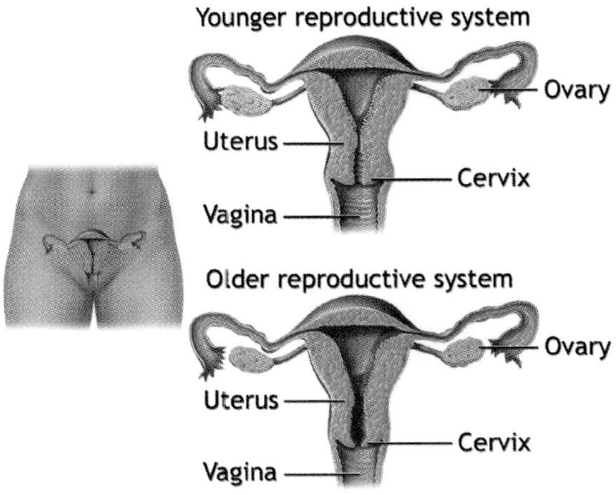

During menopause, the ovaries stop producing eggs and reduce slightly in size.

Menopause is a natural event that normally occurs between the ages of 45 and 55.

In some women, menstrual flow comes to a sudden halt. More commonly, it tapers off. During this time, your menstrual periods generally become either more closely or more widely spaced. This irregularity may last for 1 to 3 years before menstruation finally ends completely.

Symptoms

The potential symptoms include:

- Hot flashes and skin flushing
- Night sweats
- Insomnia
- Mood swings including irritability, depression, and anxiety
- Irregular menstrual periods
- Spotting of blood in between periods
- Vaginal dryness and painful sexual intercourse
- Decreased sex drive
- Vaginal infections
- Urinary tract infections

In addition, the long-term effects of menopause include:

- Bone loss and eventual osteoporosis
- Changes in cholesterol levels and greater risk of heart disease

Home care

Menopause is a natural process. It does not require treatment unless the symptoms, such as hot flashes or vaginal dryness, are particularly bothersome.

One big decision you may face is whether or not to take hormones to relieve your symptoms. Discuss this thoroughly with your doctor, weighing your risks against any possible benefits. Pay careful attention to the many options currently available to you that do not involve taking hormones.

HORMONE REPLACEMENT THERAPY

For years, hormone replacement therapy (HRT) was the main treatment for menopause symptoms. Many doctors believed that HRT was not only good for reducing menopausal symptoms, but also reduced the risk of heart disease and bone fractures from osteoporosis. However, the results of a major study – called the Women's Health Initiative – has led doctors to revise their recommendations.

In fact, this important study was stopped early because the health risks outweighed the health benefits. Women taking the hormones did see some benefits for their bones. But they greatly increased their risk for breast cancer, heart attacks, strokes, and blood clots.

If your symptoms are severe, you may still want to consider HRT for short-term use (two to four years) to reduce vaginal dryness, hot flashes, and other symptoms.

ALTERNATIVES TO HRT

The good news is that you can take many steps to reduce your symptoms without taking hormones:

- Dress lightly and in layers.
- Avoid caffeine, alcohol, and spicy foods.
- Practice slow, deep breathing whenever a hot flash starts to come on. (Try taking 6 breaths per minute.)
- See an acupuncturist.
- Use relaxation techniques like yoga, tai chi, or meditation.
- Eat soy foods.
- Remain sexually active to preserve elasticity of your vagina.
- Perform Kegel exercises daily to strengthen the muscles of your vagina and pelvis.
- Use water-based lubricants during sexual intercourse.

When to contact a medical professional

Call your health care provider if:

- You are spotting blood between periods.
- You have had 12 consecutive months with no period and suddenly vaginal bleeding begins again.

Prevention

Menopause is a natural and expected part of a woman's development and does not need to be prevented. However, there are ways to reduce or eliminate some of the symptoms that accompany menopause. You can also reduce your risk of long-term problems like osteoporosis and heart disease.

- DO NOT smoke – cigarette use can cause early menopause.
- Exercise regularly to strengthen your bones. Include activity against the resistance of gravity.
- Take calcium and vitamin D.
- Eat a low-fat diet.
- If you show early signs of bone loss, talk to your doctor about medications that can help stop further weakening.
- Control your blood pressure, cholesterol, and other risk factors for heart disease.

Know your options

Now that taking estrogen has come into such strong question, it is more important than ever to learn lifestyle steps to lessen your menopause symptoms and go through this time of transition more smoothly.

Menstruation - Heavy or Irregular

The menstrual cycle is not the same for every woman. On average, menstrual flow occurs every 28 days and lasts about 4 days. However, there is wide variation in timing and duration that is still considered normal, especially if your periods began within the last two years.

If you soak through a sanitary pad or tampon every hour for 6 consecutive hours, this is considered a very heavy period. A prolonged period is one that lasts longer than 7 days. Irregular periods happen more often than every 21 days or less often than every 35 days.

These variations may be normal and are less concerning than bleeding, pain, or discharge between periods.

Bleeding may be something to worry about if you are over age 50, especially if you have already gone through menopause. The risk of cancer increases with age.

Often, if you are bleeding from the rectum or in your urine, you think it is coming from the vagina. To know for certain, insert a tampon into the vagina to confirm that it's the source of your bleeding.

Home care

Keep a record of your menstrual cycles, including when menstruation begins and ends, how much flow you have (count numbers of pads and tampons used, noting whether they are soaked), and any other symptoms you experience. Tampons should be changed at least twice a day to avoid infection.

Bed rest may be recommended if bleeding is heavy.

Because aspirin may prolong bleeding, it should be avoided. Ibuprofen is usually more effective than aspirin for relieving menstrual cramps.

When to contact a medical professional

Call your doctor if:

- You have soaked through a pad or tampon every hour for 6 hours.

Female reproductive system

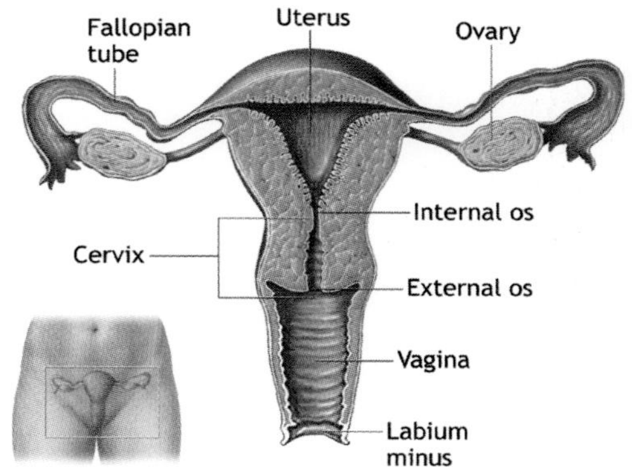

Common causes of heavy menstrual periods

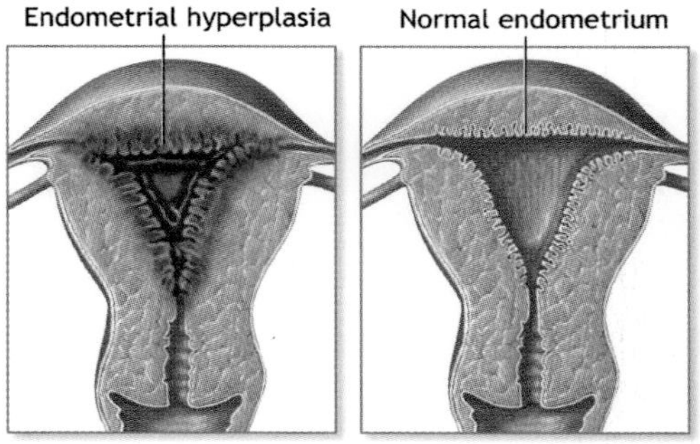

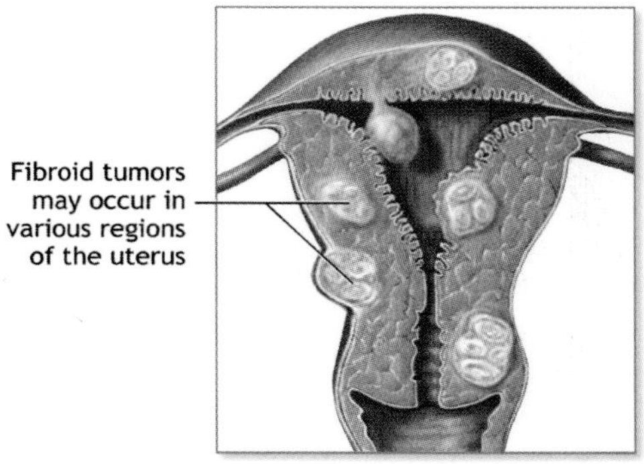

- Your bleeding has lasted longer than one week.
- You are pregnant.
- You have severe pain, especially if you also have pain when not menstruating.
- Your periods have been heavy or prolonged for 3 or more cycles, compared to what is normal for you.
- You have a fever or abnormal vaginal discharge, especially if it has an odor.
- You have bleeding after menopause.
- You have bleeding or spotting between periods.
- You have nipple discharge, excessive hair growth, deepening voice, unintentional weight loss or gain, or new acne.

Prevention

- Follow a healthy diet, avoiding fat.
- If you are trying to lose weight, do so gradually.
- Change exercise routine slowly. Work your way up over time to more strenuous activities.
- Practice relaxation techniques.

Menstruation - painful

Painful menstruation is when menstrual periods are accompanied by either sharp, intermittent pain or dull, aching pain, usually in the pelvis or lower abdomen.

Painful menstruation affects many women. For a small number of women, such discomfort makes it next to impossible to perform normal household, job, or school-related activities for a few days during each menstrual cycle. Painful menstruation is the leading cause of lost time from school and work among women in their teens and 20's.

The pain may begin several days before or just at the start of your period. It generally subsides as menstrual bleeding tapers off.

Home care

The following steps may allow you to avoid prescription medications:

- Apply a heating pad to your lower abdomen (below your navel). Be careful NOT to fall asleep with it on.
- Take warm showers or baths.
- Drink warm beverages.
- Do light circular massage with your fingertips around your lower abdomen.
- Walk or exercise regularly, including pelvic rocking exercises.
- Follow a diet rich in complex carbohydrates, like whole grains, fruits, and vegetables, but low in salt, sugar, alcohol, and caffeine.
- Eat light but frequent meals.
- Try over-the-counter anti-inflammatory medicine, such as ibuprofen.
- Practice relaxation techniques like meditation or yoga.
- Try vitamin B6, calcium, and magnesium supplements, especially if your pain is from PMS.
- Keep your legs elevated while lying down. Or lie on your side with knees bent.

When to contact a medical professional

Call your doctor right away if:

- You have a fever.
- Vaginal discharge is increased in amount or foul-smelling.
- Your pain is significant, your period is over one week late, and you have been sexually active.

Also call your doctor if:

- Your pain is severe or sudden.

- Self-care measures don't relieve your pain after 3 months.
- You pass blood clots or have other symptoms with the pain.
- Your pain occurs at times other than menstruation, begins more than 5 days prior to your period, or continues after your period is over.
- You have an IUD that was placed more than 3 months ago.

Mononucleosis

Mononucleosis is a viral infection causing fevers, sore throat, and swollen lymph glands, especially in the neck. It is typically caused by the Epstein-Barr virus (EBV), but can also be caused by other organisms such as cytomegalovirus (CMV). Both viruses are members of the herpesvirus family.

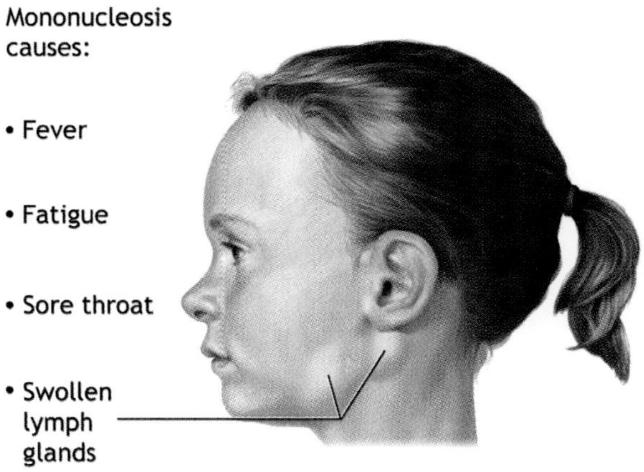
Mononucleosis causes:
• Fever
• Fatigue
• Sore throat
• Swollen lymph glands

Mononucleosis is often transmitted by saliva. While it is known as "the kissing disease," occurring most often in 15- to 17-year-olds, the infection may occur at any age.

Mono may begin slowly with fatigue, malaise, headache, and sore throat. The sore throat becomes progressively worse, often with enlarged tonsils covered with a whitish-yellow covering. The lymph nodes in the neck are frequently enlarged and painful.

A pink, measles-like rash can occur and is more likely if the patient is given ampicillin or amoxicillin for a throat infection. (Antibiotics should NOT be given without a positive strep test.) The symptoms of mono gradually subside on their own over a period of weeks to months.

Home care

Most patients recover within 2-4 weeks without medication. Younger children often don't have symptoms, while some older patients may have fatigue for up to 6 weeks.

There is no specific treatment available. Antiviral medications do not help. Steroid medication may be considered for patients with severe symptoms.

To relieve typical symptoms:

- Take acetaminophen or ibuprofen for pain and fever.
- Gargle with warm salt water for sore throat.
- Get plenty of rest. Drink plenty of fluids.
- Avoid contact sports while the spleen is enlarged (to prevent it from rupturing).

When to contact a medical professional

The initial symptoms of mono feel very much like a typical viral illness. It is not necessary to contact a health care provider unless symptoms last longer than 10 days or you develop the following:

- Severe sore throat or swollen tonsils
- Difficulty breathing
- Abdominal pain
- Severe headache
- Persistent high fevers (more than 101.5°F)
- Yellow discoloration of your eyes or skin
- Weakness in the arm or legs

Call 911 or go to an emergency room if you develop:

- Sharp, sudden, severe abdominal pain

- Significant difficulty swallowing or breathing
- A stiff neck or severe weakness

Prevention

The infection is probably spread by saliva and close contact. People may be contagious while they have symptoms and for up to a few months afterwards. The virus can live for several hours outside the body. Avoid kissing or sharing utensils if you or someone close to you has mono. The exact period that people are contagious varies.

Morning sickness

Morning sickness is very common. Most pregnant women have at least some nausea, and about a third have vomiting. Morning sickness usually begins during the first month of pregnancy and continues until the 14th to 16th week. Some women have nausea and vomiting through their entire pregnancy.

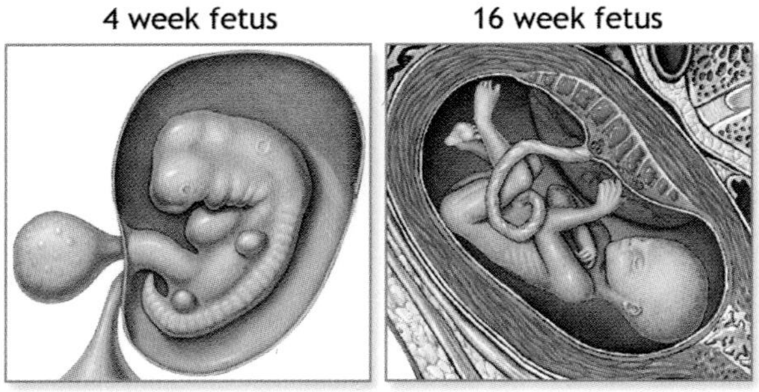
4 week fetus
16 week fetus

Morning sickness typically continues from the 4th week of pregnancy through the 16th week

Morning sickness does not hurt the baby in any way. The degree of morning sickness during one pregnancy does not predict how you will feel in future pregnancies.

The exact cause of morning sickness is unknown. It may be caused by hormonal changes or lower blood sugar during early pregnancy. Emotional stress, traveling, or some foods can aggravate the problem.

Home care

Try to maintain a positive attitude. Remember that morning sickness usually stops after the first 3 or 4 months of pregnancy. To minimize nausea, try:

- A few soda crackers or dry toast when you first wake up, even before you get out of bed in the morning.
- A small snack at bedtime and when getting up to go to the bathroom at night.
- Avoiding large meals. Instead, snack as often as every 1 to 2 hours during the day and drink plenty of fluids.
- Eating food high in protein and complex carbohydrates, like peanut butter on apple slices or celery; nuts; cheese and crackers; milk; cottage cheese; or yogurt. Avoid foods high in fat and salt but low in nutrition.

Here are some more tips:

- When you feel nauseated, bland foods like gelatin, broth, ginger ale, and saltine crackers can soothe your stomach.
- Take your prenatal vitamins at night. Increase vitamin B6 in your diet by eating whole grains, nuts, seeds, and legumes. Talk to your doctor about possibly taking vitamin B6 supplements.

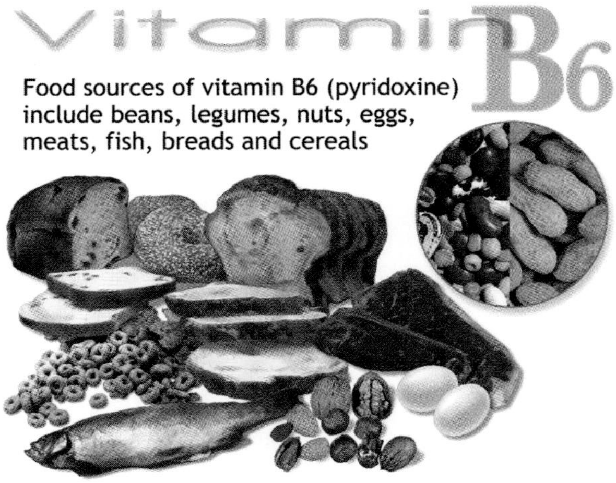
Vitamin B6
Food sources of vitamin B6 (pyridoxine) include beans, legumes, nuts, eggs, meats, fish, breads and cereals

- Keep rooms well-ventilated to reduce odors.
- Avoid smoking and secondhand smoke.

- Avoid taking medications for morning sickness. If you do, consult a doctor first.
- Acupressure wrist bands or acupuncture may help. You can find these bands in drug, health food, and travel stores. If considering acupuncture, talk to your doctor and seek an acupuncturist trained to work with pregnant women.

When to contact a medical professional

Call your doctor if:

- Morning sickness does not improve, despite trying home remedies.
- You vomit blood or material that looks like coffee grounds. (Call IMMEDIATELY.)
- You lose more than 2 pounds.
- You vomit more than 3 times per day or you cannot keep food or liquid down.
- Nausea and vomiting continue beyond your 4th month of pregnancy. This happens to some women and is usually normal, but have it checked out.

Mouth sores

Mouth sores are most often mechanical irritations, cold sores (also called fever blisters), or canker sores.

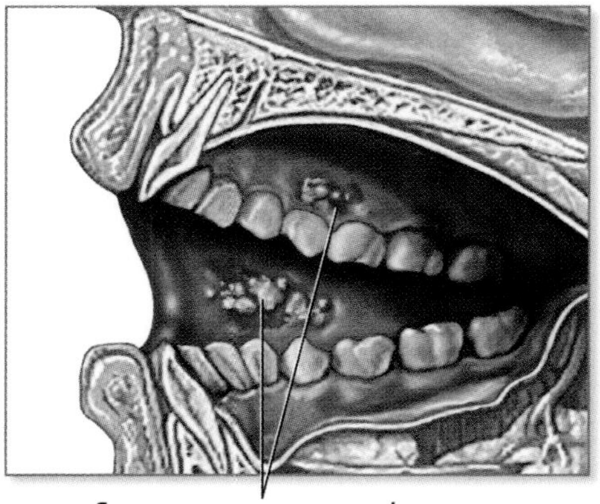

Irritation can happen from:

- Biting your cheek, tongue, or lip
- Chewing tobacco
- Braces
- A sharp or broken tooth or poorly fitting dentures
- Burning your mouth from hot food or drinks

Cold sores are caused by herpes simplex virus and are very contagious. Usually, you have tenderness, tingling, or burning before the actual lesion appears. Herpes lesions begin as blisters and then crust over.

The herpes virus can reside in your body for years, appearing as a mouth sore only when something provokes it. Such circumstances may include another illness, especially if there is a fever, stress, hormonal changes (like menstruation), and sun exposure.

Canker sores are NOT contagious and can appear as a single pale or yellow ulcer with a red outer ring, or as a cluster of such lesions.

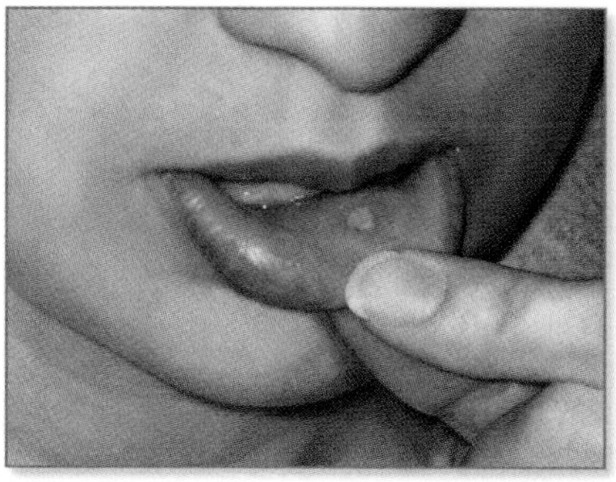

Canker sore

The cause of canker sores is not entirely clear, but may be related to:

- A virus
- A temporary weakness in your immune system (for example, from cold or flu)
- Hormonal changes
- Mechanical irritation
- Stress
- Low levels of vitamin B12 or folate

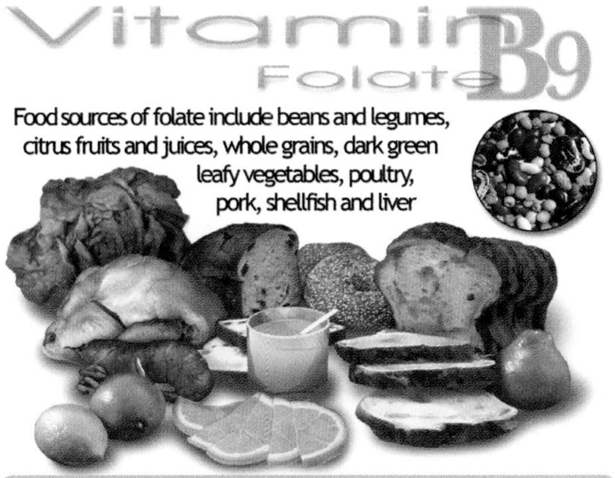
Vitamin B9
Folate
Food sources of folate include beans and legumes, citrus fruits and juices, whole grains, dark green leafy vegetables, poultry, pork, shellfish and liver

Canker sores may be related to low levels of folate.

Home care

Mouth sores generally last 7 to 10 days, even if you don't do anything. They sometimes last up to 2 weeks. The following steps can make you feel better:

- Gargle with cool water or eat popsicles. This is particularly helpful if you have a mouth burn.
- Avoid hot beverages and foods, spicy and salty foods, and citrus.
- Take pain relievers like acetaminophen.

For canker sores:

- Rinse with salt water.
- Apply a thin paste of baking soda and water.
- Mix 1 part hydrogen peroxide with 1 part water and apply this mixture to the lesions using a cotton swab.

Nonprescription preparations, like Orabase, can protect a sore inside the lip and on the gums. Blistex or Campho-Phenique may provide some relief of canker sores and fever blisters, especially if applied when the sore initially appears.

Additional steps that may help cold sores or fever blisters:

- Apply ice to the lesion.
- Take L-lysine tablets.

When to contact a medical professional

Call your doctor if:

- The sore begins soon after you start a new medication
- You have large white patches on the roof of your mouth or your tongue (this may be thrush or another type of lesion)
- Your mouth sore lasts longer than 2 weeks
- You are immunocompromised (for example, from HIV or cancer)
- You have other symptoms like fever, skin rash, drooling, or difficulty swallowing

Prevention

You can reduce your chance of getting common mouth sores by:

- Reducing stress. Practice relaxation techniques like yoga or meditation.
- Avoiding very hot foods or beverages.

To avoid mechanical irritation, also:

- See your dentist promptly for a sharp or broken tooth or misfitting dentures.
- Chew slowly.
- Use a soft-bristle toothbrush.

If you seem to get canker sores often, talk to your doctor about taking folate and vitamin B12 to prevent outbreaks.

If you get cold sores often, taking L-lysine tablets or increasing lysine in your diet (found in fish, chicken, eggs, and potatoes) may reduce outbreaks. However, if you have high cholesterol, heart disease, or high triglycerides, DO NOT use L-lysine.

To prevent the spread of herpes lesions, do not kiss or have oral sex with someone with a cold sore or fever blister. Do not participate in these activities when you have an active cold sore. Do not share razors, lip balm, toothbrushes, or lipsticks.

To prevent cancerous mouth lesions:

- Do not smoke or use tobacco.
- Limit alcohol to 2 drinks per day.
- Wear a wide-brimmed hat to shade your lips. Wear a lip balm with SPF 15 at all times.

Muscle aches and pains

Muscle aches and pains are common and can involve more than one muscle. Muscle pain can also involve ligaments, tendons, and fascia, the soft tissues that connect muscles, bones, and organs together.

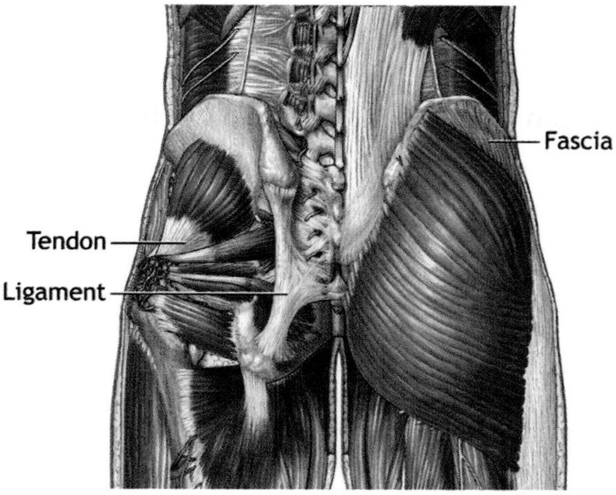

Muscle pain is most frequently related to tension, overuse, or muscle injury from exercise or physically demanding work. In these situations, the pain tends to involve specific muscles and starts during or just after the activity. It is usually obvious which activity is causing the pain.

Muscle pain also can be a sign of conditions affecting your whole body, like some infections (including the flu) and disorders that affect connective tissues throughout the body (such as lupus).

One common cause of muscle aches and pains is fibromyalgia, a condition that includes tenderness in your muscles and surrounding soft tissue, sleep difficulties, fatigue, and headaches.

Home care

For muscle pain from overuse or injury, rest that body part and take acetaminophen or ibuprofen. Apply ice for the first 24 to 72 hours of an injury to reduce pain and inflammation. After that, heat often feels more soothing.

Muscle aches from overuse and fibromyalgia often respond well to massage. Gentle stretching exercises after a long rest period are also helpful.

Regular exercise can help restore proper muscle tone. Walking, cycling, and swimming are good aerobic activities to try. A physical therapist can teach you stretching, toning, and aerobic exercises to feel better and stay pain free. Begin slowly and increase workouts gradually. Avoid high-impact aerobic activities and weight lifting when injured or while in pain.

Be sure to get plenty of sleep and try to reduce stress. Yoga and meditation are excellent ways to help you sleep and relax.

When to contact a medical professional

Call your doctor if:

- Your muscle pain persists beyond 3 days.
- You have severe, unexplained pain.
- You have any sign of infection, like swelling or redness around the tender muscle.
- You have poor circulation in the area where you have muscles aches (for example, in your legs).
- You have a tick bite or a rash.

Call 911 if:

- You have sudden weight gain, water retention, or you are urinating less than usual.
- You are short of breath or have difficulty swallowing.

- You have muscle weakness or inability to move any part of your body.
- You have vomiting, a very stiff neck, or high fever.

Prevention

- Warm up before exercising and cool down afterward.
- Stretch before and after exercising.
- Drink lots of fluids before, during, and after exercise.
- If you work in the same position most of the day (like sitting at a computer), stretch at least every hour.

> **Remember...**
>
> Stretching exercises, gentle massages, getting enough sleep, and reducing your stress can go a long way for treating and preventing muscle aches from overuse, tension, or fibromyalgia.

Neck pain and stiffness

Common neck pain is from muscle strain or tension. Usually, everyday activities are responsible. Such activities include bending over a desk for hours, having poor posture while watching TV or reading, placing your computer monitor too high or too low, sleeping in an uncomfortable position, or twisting and turning the neck in a jarring manner while exercising.

Traumatic accidents or falls can cause severe neck injuries like vertebral fractures, whiplash, blood vessel destruction, and even paralysis.

Other causes include a herniated disc, fibromyalgia (pain syndrome throughout the body), and arthritis. Meningitis, although much less common, can cause significant neck stiffness.

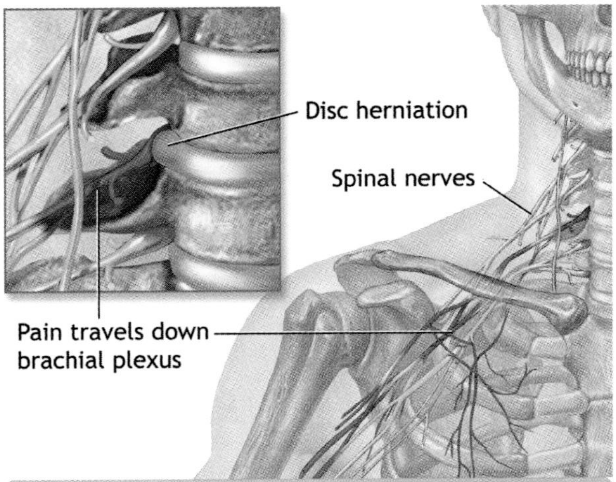

A herniated disc pressing on a spinal nerve can cause neck pain. The pain may also radiate down the arm through a network of nerves called the brachial plexus.

Home care

For minor, common causes of neck pain:

- Take acetaminophen or ibuprofen.
- Apply heat or ice to the painful area. One good method is to use ice for the first 48 to 72 hours, then use heat after that. Heat may be applied with hot showers, hot compresses, or a heating pad. Be careful not to fall asleep with a heating pad on.
- Perform slow range-of-motion exercises – up and down, side to side, and from ear to ear – to gently stretch the neck muscles.
- Have a partner gently massage the sore or painful areas.
- Try sleeping on a firm mattress without a pillow or with a special neck pillow.

When to contact a medical professional

- One week of self care hasn't helped.
- You have a fever and headache, and your neck is so stiff that you cannot touch your chin to your chest. (This may be meningitis – call 911 or get to a hospital.)
- You have numbness, tingling, or weakness in your arm or hand.
- Your neck pain was caused by a fall, blow, or injury. (If you cannot move your arm or

hand, someone must call 911.)

- You have swollen glands or a lump in your neck.
- Your pain does not respond to standard doses of over-the-counter pain medication.

Prevention

- Use relaxation techniques and regular exercise to prevent unwanted stress and tension to the neck muscles.
- Learn stretching exercises for your neck and upper body. Stretch every day, especially before and after exercise. A physical therapist can help.
- If you tend to get neck pain from exercise, apply ice to your neck after physical activity.
- Use good posture, especially if you sit at a desk all day. Keep your back supported. Adjust your computer monitor to eye level. This prevents you from continually looking up or down.
- If you work at a computer, stretch your neck every hour or so.
- Use a headset when on the telephone, especially if answering or using the phone is a main part of your job.
- When reading or typing from documents at your desk, place them in a holder at eye level.
- Evaluate your sleeping conditions. Make sure your pillow is properly and comfortably supporting your head and neck. You may need a special neck pillow. Make sure your mattress is firm enough.
- Use seat belts and bike helmets to prevent injuries.

Numbness and tingling

Numbness and tingling are abnormal sensations that can occur anywhere in your body, but are often felt in your hands, feet, arms, or legs.

There are many possible causes:

- Remaining in the same seated or standing position for a long time.
- Injuring a nerve supplying the body part where you feel the sensation. If you have a neck injury, for example, you may feel the sensation anywhere along your arm or hand. Similarly, a low back injury can cause sciatica – a sensation of numbness or tingling down the back of your leg.

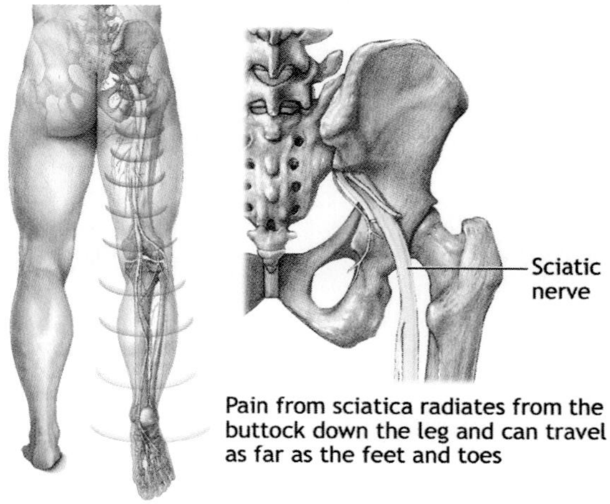

Pain from sciatica radiates from the buttock down the leg and can travel as far as the feet and toes

- Lack of blood supply to the area. For example, plaque buildup from atherosclerosis in the legs can cause pain, numbness, and tingling while walking. (This is called claudication.)

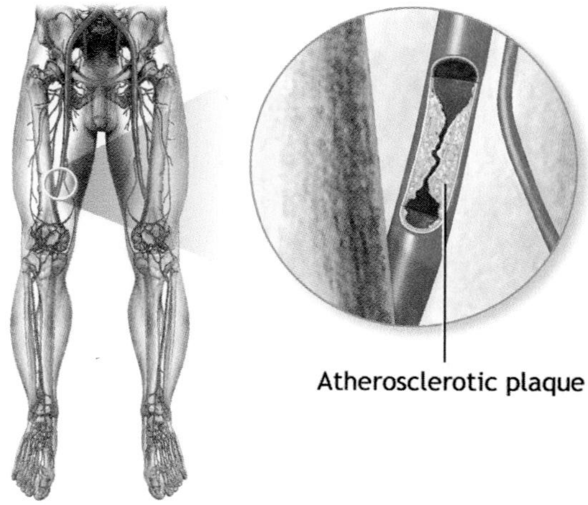

- Pressure on the spinal nerves, like that from a herniated disk.

- Carpal tunnel syndrome. This can cause numbness or tingling in your wrist, fingers, hand, or forearm.

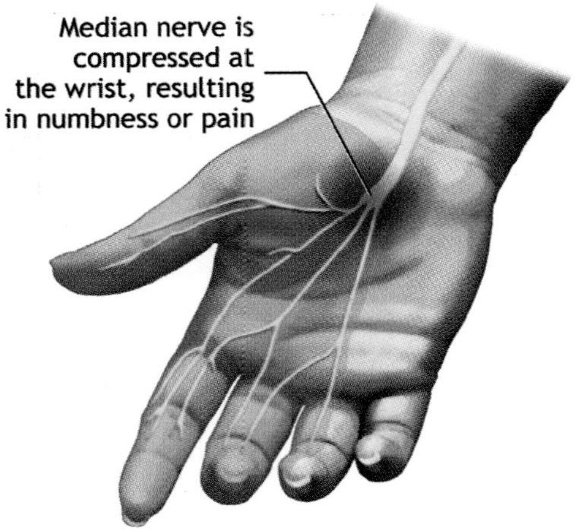
Median nerve is compressed at the wrist, resulting in numbness or pain

- Certain medical conditions, including diabetes, underactive thyroid, multiple sclerosis, seizures, or migraine headaches.
- Abnormal levels of calcium, potassium, or sodium in your body.
- Vitamin B12 deficiency.
- Transient ischemic attack (TIA) or stroke
- Certain medications.
- Toxic action on nerves, such as that from lead, alcohol, or tobacco.
- Radiation therapy.

Home care

The underlying cause of numbness or tingling should be identified and then treated by your doctor. For example, if you have carpal tunnel syndrome or low back pain, certain exercises may be recommended.

If you have diabetes, your doctor will discuss ways to control your blood sugars. Medications that cause numbness or tingling may need to be switched or adjusted. DO NOT make any changes to your medications without instructions from your doctor. Low levels of vitamin B12 will be treated with vitamin supplements.

For multiple sclerosis, these steps can help some of the symptoms:

- Exercise to maintain muscle tone. Your doctor or physical therapist can guide you and design an appropriate program.
- Rest and practice relaxation techniques for improved energy level.
- Avoid temperature extremes.

Because of the decrease in feeling, a numb hand or foot from any cause may be more prone to accidental injury. Take care to protect the area from cuts, bumps, bruises, burns, or other injury.

When to contact a medical professional

Go to a hospital or call 911 if:

- Weakness or paralysis occurs with numbness or tingling.
- Numbness or tingling occur just after a head, neck, or back injury.
- You cannot control the movement of an arm or a leg or you have lost bladder or bowel control.
- You are confused or have lost consciousness, even briefly.
- You have slurred speech, change in vision, difficulty walking, or weakness.

Call your doctor if:

- Numbness or tingling has no obvious cause (like a hand or foot "falling asleep").
- You have pain in your neck, forearm, or fingers.
- You are urinating more often.
- Numbness or tingling is in your legs and worsens when you walk.
- You have a rash.
- You have dizziness, vertigo, muscle spasm, or other unusual symptoms.

Pneumonia

Pneumonia is an inflammation of the lungs caused by an infection. Many different organisms can cause it, including bacteria, viruses, and fungi.

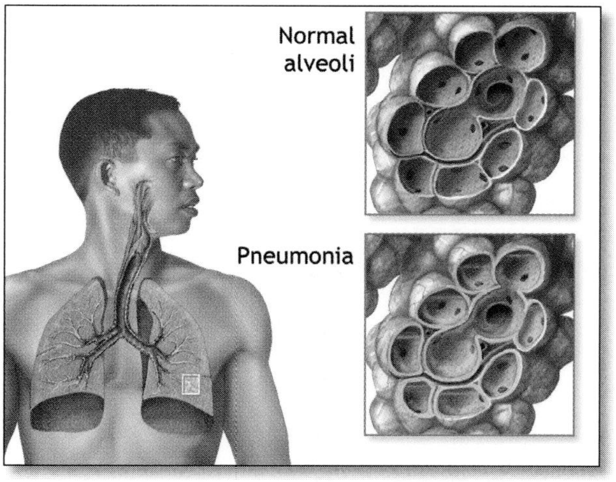

Pneumonia can range from mild to severe, even fatal. The severity depends on the type of organism causing pneumonia as well as your age and underlying health.

Symptoms

The main symptoms of pneumonia are:

- Cough with greenish or yellow mucus; bloody sputum happens on occasion
- Fever with shaking chills
- Sharp or stabbing chest pain worsened by deep breathing or coughing
- Rapid, shallow breathing
- Shortness of breath

Additional symptoms include:

- Headache
- Excessive sweating and clammy skin
- Loss of appetite
- Excessive fatigue
- Confusion in older people

Home care

If the cause is bacterial, the goal is to cure the infection with antibiotics. If the cause is viral, antibiotics will NOT be effective. In some cases it is difficult to distinguish between viral and bacterial pneumonia, so antibiotics may be prescribed.

Many people can be treated at home with antibiotics. If you have an underlying chronic disease, severe symptoms, or low oxygen levels, you will likely require hospitalization for intravenous antibiotics and oxygen therapy. Infants and the elderly are more commonly admitted for treatment of pneumonia.

You can take these steps at home:

- Drink plenty of fluids to help loosen secretions and bring up phlegm.
- Get lots of rest. Have someone else do household chores.
- Control your fever with aspirin or acetaminophen. DO NOT give aspirin to children.

When to contact a medical professional

Call your doctor if:

- You have worsening respiratory symptoms.
- You have shortness of breath, shaking chills, or persistent fevers.
- Your breathing is rapid or painful.
- You cough up bloody or rust-colored mucus.
- You have chest pain that worsens when you cough or inhale.
- You have night sweats or unexplained weight loss.
- You have a weak immune system, as with HIV or chemotherapy.

Infants with pneumonia may not have a cough. Call your doctor if your infant makes grunting noises or the area below the rib cage is retracting while breathing.

Prevention

- Wash your hands frequently, especially after blowing your nose, going to the bathroom, diapering, and before eating or preparing foods.
- Don't smoke. Tobacco damages your lung's ability to ward off infection.
- Wear a mask when cleaning dusty or moldy areas

Vaccines can help prevent pneumonia in children, the elderly, and people with diabetes, asthma, emphysema, HIV, cancer, or other chronic conditions:

- **Pneumococcal vaccine** (Pneumovax, Prevnar) prevents *Streptococcus pneumoniae.*
- **Flu vaccine** prevents pneumonia and other infections caused by influenza viruses. It must be given yearly to protect against new viral strains.
- **Hib vaccine** prevents pneumonia in children from *Haemophilus influenzae* type b.

Poison ivy, oak, and sumac

Poison ivy, oak, and sumac are plants that commonly cause an allergic skin reaction. The result is typically an itching, red rash with bumps or blisters.

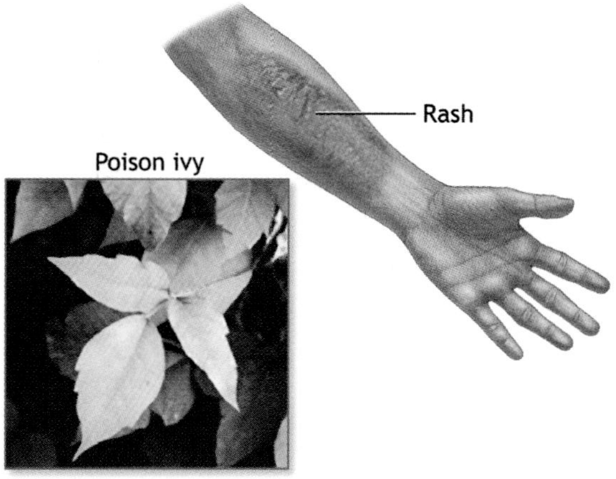

Poison ivy is one of the most frequent causes of skin rash among children and adults who spend time outdoors. The plant can be found throughout the United States, except in the Southwest, Alaska, and Hawaii. It has three shiny green leaves and a red stem. Poison ivy typically grows in the form of a vine, often along riverbanks.

Poison oak is primarily found on the West Coast. It grows in the form of a shrub and has three leaves similar to poison ivy.

Poison sumac grows abundantly along the Mississippi River. It grows as a woody shrub. Each stem contains 7-13 leaves arranged in pairs.

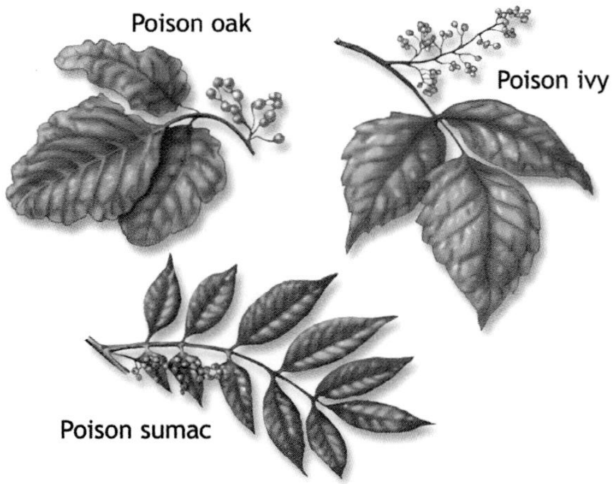

The rash is caused by skin contact with the oily sap (or resin) of these plants. Smoke from burning these plants can cause the same reaction. The oily resin usually enters the skin rapidly, and is seldom transferred from person to person. The rash is NOT caused by the fluid from the blisters. Thus, once the person has washed the oil off the skin, the rash is usually not contagious.

Keep in mind that the resin may last for long periods on contaminated clothing, pets, tools, shoes, and other surfaces. These contaminated items can cause future rashes long after the initial exposure.

First Aid

- Wash the skin thoroughly with soap and warm water. Because the resin enters skin quickly, try to wash it off within 30 minutes. A product called Tecnu, available in camping stores and some pharmacies, is very effective at removing the oils.

- Scrub under the fingernails with a brush to prevent the resin from spreading to other parts of the body.
- Wash clothing and shoes with soap and hot water. Resin can linger on them.
- Promptly bathe animals to remove the oils from their fur.
- Body heat and sweating can aggravate the itching. Stay cool and apply cool compresses to your skin.
- Calamine lotion and hydrocortisone cream can be applied to the skin to reduce itching and blistering. Bathing in lukewarm water with an oatmeal bath product, available in drugstores, may soothe itchy skin. Aluminum acetate (Domeboro solution) soaks can also help to dry the rash and reduce itching.
- If creams, lotions, or bathing do not stop the itching, antihistamines may be helpful.
- In severe cases, especially rash around the face or genitals, your doctor may prescribe oral or injected steroids.

Do Not

- DO NOT touch skin or clothing that still have the resins.
- DO NOT burn poison ivy, oak, or sumac to get rid of it. The resins can be spread via smoke, and can cause severe reactions in people who are far downwind.

When to contact a medical professional

Call 911 or go to an emergency room if:

- Someone is suffering a severe allergic reaction, such as swelling or difficulty breathing, or has had a severe reaction in the past.
- Someone has been exposed to the smoke of a burning plant.

Call your provider if:

- Itching is severe and cannot be controlled.
- The rash affects your face, lips, eyes, or genitals.
- The rash shows signs of infection, such as pus, yellow fluid leaking from blisters, odor, or increased tenderness.

Prevention

- Wear long sleeves, long pants, and socks when walking in areas where these plants may grow.
- Skin products such as Ivy Block lotion can be applied beforehand to reduce the risk of a rash.

Prostate enlargement

The prostate gland produces the fluid that carries sperm during ejaculation. As the prostate enlarges, which happens to almost all men as they get older, it can press on the urethra (the tube that empties urine from the bladder). This causes problems with urination.

Prostate enlargement is often called benign prostatic hypertrophy or hyperplasia (BPH). It is not cancer and it does not put you at increased risk for prostate cancer.

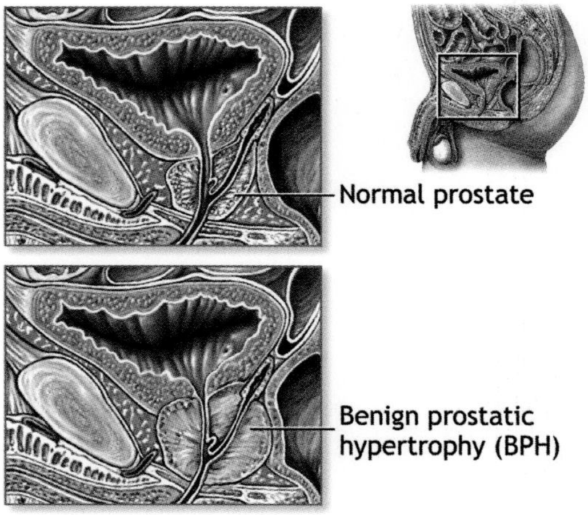

Symptoms

Less than half of all men with BPH have symptoms of the disease, which include:

- Slowed or delayed start of the urinary stream
- Weak urine stream
- Dribbling after urinating
- Straining to urinate
- Strong and sudden urge to urinate
- Incomplete emptying of your bladder
- Needing to urinate 2 or more times per night
- Urinary retention (complete inability to urinate)
- Incontinence
- Pain with urination or bloody urine (these may indicate infection)

> **Key point**
>
> If you are like most men with an enlarged prostate, you are hoping to avoid drugs or surgery. Both are possible. Read on to find out how.

Home care

The choice of a treatment is based on the severity of your symptoms, the extent to which they affect your daily life, and the presence of any other medical conditions. Treatment options include "watchful waiting," lifestyle changes, medication, or surgery.

If you are over 60, you are more likely to have symptoms. But many men with an enlarged prostate have only minor symptoms. Self-care steps are often enough to make you feel better.

If you have BPH, you should have a yearly exam to monitor the progression of your symptoms and determine if any changes in treatment are necessary.

For mild symptoms:

- Urinate when you first get the urge. Also, go to the bathroom when you have the chance, even if you don't feel a need to urinate.
- Avoid alcohol and caffeine, especially after dinner.
- Don't drink a lot of fluid all at once. Spread out fluids throughout the day. Avoid drinking fluids within 2 hours of bedtime.
- Try NOT to take over-the-counter cold and sinus medications that contain decongestants or antihistamines. These medications can increase BPH symptoms.
- Keep warm and exercise regularly. Cold weather and lack of physical activity may worsen symptoms.
- Learn and perform Kegel exercises (pelvic strengthening exercises).
- Reduce stress. Nervousness and tension can lead to more frequent urination.

Saw palmetto may ease prostate symptoms. Look for fat-soluble saw palmetto extract with 85-95% fatty acids and sterols.

Sit in an aisle seat at the theatre or on an airplane. This won't reduce your symptoms, but it may relieve your anxiety about having to urinate often or suddenly.

If these measures are not enough to ease your symptoms, talk to your doctor, who may consider medications or surgery.

When to contact a medical professional

Call your doctor right away if you have:

- Less urine than usual.
- Fever or chills.
- Back, side, or abdominal pain.
- Blood or pus in your urine.

Also call your doctor if:

- Your bladder does not feel completely empty after you urinate.

- You take medications that may cause urinary problems, like diuretics, antihistamines, antidepressants, or sedatives. DO NOT stop or adjust your medications on your own without talking to your doctor.
- You have taken self-care measures for 2 months without relief.

Rashes

A simple rash is called dermatitis, meaning inflammation of the skin.

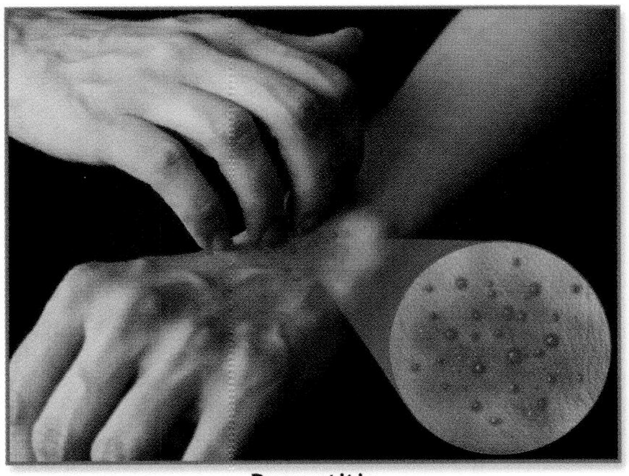

Dermatitis

Contact dermatitis is caused by things your skin touches, such as:

- Dyes and other chemicals in clothing
- Chemicals in elastic, latex, and rubber products
- Cosmetics, soaps, and detergents
- Poison ivy, oak, or sumac

Seborrheic dermatitis is a rash that appears in patches of redness and scaling around the eyebrows, eyelids, mouth, nose, the trunk, and behind the ears. If it happens on your scalp, it is called dandruff in adults and cradle cap in infants.

Age, stress, fatigue, weather extremes, oily skin, infrequent shampooing, and alcohol-based lotions aggravate this harmless but bothersome condition.

Other common causes of a rash include:

- **Eczema (atopic dermatitis)** – tends to happen in people with allergies or asthma. The rash is generally red, itchy, and scaly.
- **Psoriasis** – tends to occur as red, scaly, itchy patches over joints and along the scalp. Fingernails may be affected.
- **Impetigo** – common in children, this infection is from bacteria that live in the top layers of the skin. Appears as red sores that turn into blisters, ooze, then crust over.
- **Shingles** – a painful blistered skin condition caused by the same virus as chickenpox. The virus can lie dormant in your body for many years and re-emerge as shingles.

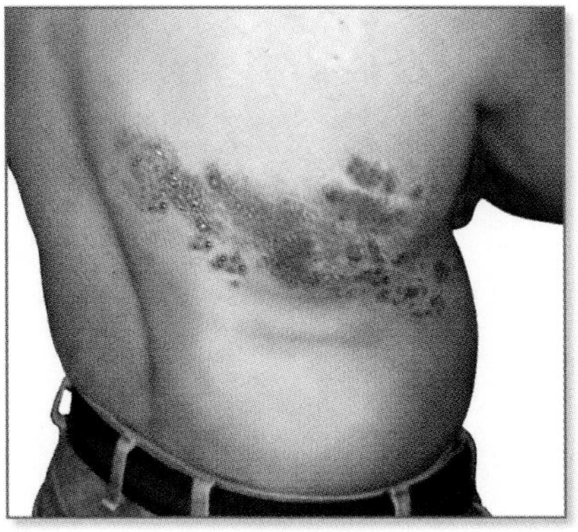

Shingles

- Childhood illnesses like chickenpox, measles, roseola, rubella, hand-foot-mouth disease, fifth disease, and scarlet fever.
- Medications and insect bites or stings.

Home care

Most simple rashes will improve with gentle skin care and avoiding irritating substances. Follow these general guidelines:

- Avoid scrubbing your skin.
- Use as little soap as possible. Use gentle cleansers instead.
- Avoid applying cosmetic lotions or ointments directly on the rash.
- Use warm (not hot) water for cleaning. Pat dry, don't rub.

- Eliminate any newly added cosmetics or lotions.
- Leave the affected area exposed to the air as much as possible.
- Try calamine medicated lotion for poison ivy, oak, or sumac as well as other types of contact dermatitis.

Hydrocortisone cream (1%) is available without a prescription and may soothe many rashes. If you have eczema, apply moisturizers over your skin. Try oatmeal bath products, available at drugstores, to relieve symptoms of eczema, psoriasis, or shingles.

For psoriasis, you may need a prescription. You could also talk to your doctor about ultraviolet (UV) light therapy. It is safest to have such treatment under medical supervision. However, not all clinics or hospitals offer light therapy. Home units are available, but the cost is not always covered by insurance. If you do purchase a home unit, look for a device that delivers narrow band UVB light.

For seborrheic dermatitis, try applying small amounts of anti-dandruff shampoo to patches of this scaly rash on your skin, especially near hairy areas like your eyebrows. Leave on for 10 minutes and then carefully rinse off. If the shampoo feels irritating or your skin becomes redder, STOP use.

For impetigo, an antibacterial cream or oral antibiotic is generally prescribed.

See article on poison ivy, oak, and sumac to learn how to treat and prevent this type of contact dermatitis.

When to contact a medical professional

Call 911 if:

- You are short of breath, your throat is tight, or your face is swollen.
- Your child has a purple rash that looks like a bruise.

Call your provider if:

- You have joint pain, fever, or a sore throat.
- You have streaks of redness, swelling, or very tender areas. These may indicate an infection.
- You are taking a new medication. DO NOT change or stop any of your medications without talking to your doctor.
- You may have a tick bite.
- Home treatment is ineffective, or your symptoms get worse.

Prevention

- Identify and then stay away from products that irritate your skin. If allergies are suspected, your doctor may want to consider skin testing.
- Receive appropriate vaccines for childhood illnesses, like the varicella vaccine for chickenpox and MMR immunization (a combination vaccine that protects against measles, mumps, and rubella).
- Get strep throat treated right away to prevent scarlet fever.
- Wash your hands frequently to prevent spreading viruses like roseola, hand-foot-mouth disease, and fifth disease.
- Learn relaxation methods like yoga, meditation, or tai chi. Stress aggravates many rashes, including eczema, psoriasis, and seborrheic dermatitis.

Rashes in infants and toddlers

Even though baby skin brings to mind freshness and smoothness, most babies will get at least one, and probably several, rashes before they toddle off to preschool. Here are some of the most common.

Erythema toxicum is a common, splotchy rash of newborns. It seems to be a result of the skin adjusting to life outside the uterus. It is found in about half of all babies. Some have splotchy red patches. Some have firm yellow or white bumps surrounded by a flare of red. The rash tends to come and go, shifting its location across the body. The palms and soles are often left out. It is most common on day 2 of life, but can first show up at birth or within the first 2 weeks. The individual splotches may remain in place for only a few hours, or for a number of days. The entire rash may come and go over a couple of weeks.

Milia are little plugs of keratin in the skin glands of the face. The resulting bumps are found on up to half of newborns' faces. The tiny bumps of milia are no larger than a millimeter or two. They are most common on the tip of the nose or chin, and are frequently seen on the cheeks and forehead. These bumps are yellow or white (unlike the red bumps of baby acne). Most milia disappear within the first few weeks of life. Sometimes they last for the first 3 months.

Baby acne can be present at birth, but typically appears at 3 to 4 weeks of age. Fleshy or red pimples occur predominately on the cheeks, but are also quite common on the forehead and chin. Whiteheads are sometimes present. The acne will be most prominent when the baby is hot or fussy, or when the skin is irritated. If the skin comes into contact with cloth laundered in harsh detergents, or becomes wet from spit-up saliva or milk, the condition may appear worse for several days. This condition tends to come and go until the baby is between 4 and 6 months old. Usually, no treatment is necessary.

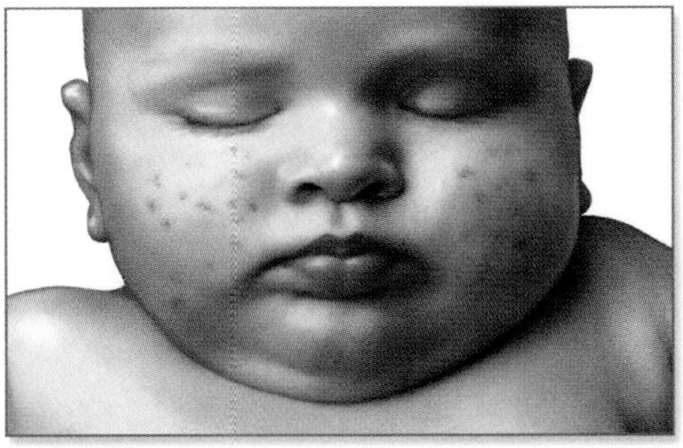

Baby acne

Miliaria is a type of heat rash. It is most common in the first few weeks of life. The pores of a newborn's immature sweat glands plug easily, leading to tiny pink bumps or water blisters. Miliaria is especially common in hot, humid weather but almost any baby can get it. It is more common in babies who are bundled too warmly. Older children can also get miliaria, in which case it is often called "prickly heat." Miliaria should disappear within 2 or 3 days. **Note:** Fever is NOT caused by a rash. If your child has a fever, see the article *Fever*.

Pustular melanosis is a common, benign skin condition seen in newborns, where small blisters peel open, revealing a small "freckle" inside. The blisters are usually already present at birth. When the blister roof is gone, a small white collar of skin may surround this dark spot for a while. Some babies have only the spots (the blister happened before birth). These flat, dark spots are most common under the chin, at the back of the neck, on the forehead, the lower back, or the shins. The blisters peel open within the first 48 hours of life. The "freckles" fade within 3 weeks to 3 months.

Diaper rash has been the most common skin disorder of infancy ever since children began to wear diapers. Almost all children in diapers will get some diaper rashes, no matter how careful the parents are. Breastfed babies get fewer diaper rashes than formula-fed babies. Anytime a baby sits too long in a wet diaper or a stool-soaked diaper, a rash can result.

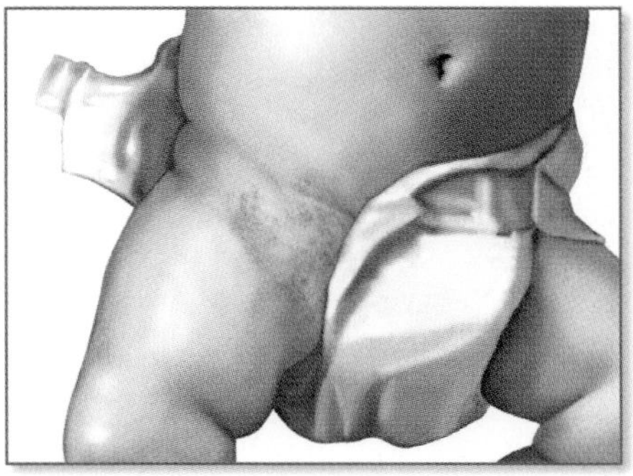

Diaper rash

Eczema can occur at any age, but when it happens in young children it is more likely to be triggered by an allergy to a food. If eczema appears before solids are started, the reaction is likely to be a protein in cow's milk or soy formula. In nursing babies, it could be to a similar protein in the mother's diet. If it starts around the time of the first solid foods, consider whether one of these may be the trigger.

Hand-foot-mouth disease is a common childhood illness featuring mouth sores, fever, and a rash. It is usually caused by a virus called coxsackievirus. Most infections occur in the summer or early fall, with the peak between August and October in the northern hemisphere. Often, the first thing parents notice is their children's decreased appetite for solids. Children may also have a fever and a sore throat. A day or two later, many children develop sores in the mouth. A skin rash may also develop over a day or two, with flat or raised red spots. Unlike with many rashes, the spots are often found on the palms and soles. Also, it is common to have the rash on the buttocks. Often, the red spots will form tender blisters (although not on the buttocks). Unlike with chickenpox, the rash does not itch. Usually the rash disappears and the child feels better within about 1 week.

Roseola is a mild viral illness with a fever followed by a rash. Almost all cases of roseola occur in children before their third birthdays. The peak age is between 6 and 15 months. Classic roseola features a high fever (average 103°F) that lasts for 3 to 5 days (worse at night). Most children behave normally, even with the high fevers. In most, the fever ends abruptly, although it can disappear slowly over a day or so. A rash appears within hours of the fever subsiding. The rash is rose-colored, as the name *roseola* suggests. The rash may be present on the upper arms, legs, and face, but is most prominent on the neck and trunk, where it usually begins. It consists of numerous, small, slightly raised patches that blanch when pressed. The rash does not itch and does not cause blisters.

The rash typically lasts for 24 to 48 hours. In some children, the rash may be fleeting—gone in minutes or hours.

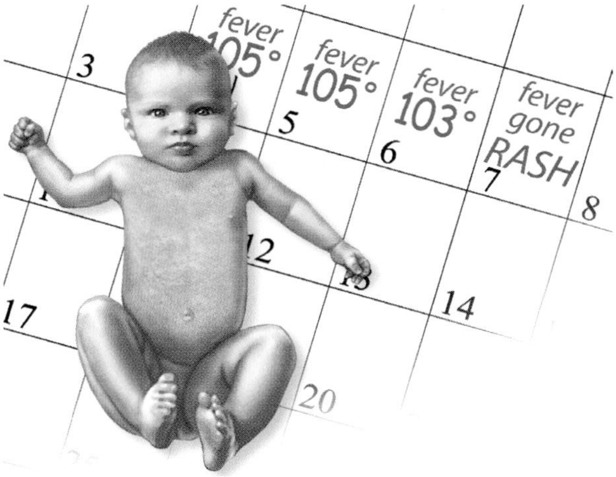

RINGWORM

Ringworm is a skin infection caused by a fungus. Ringworm can affect skin on your body (tinea corporis), scalp (tinea capitis), groin area (tinea cruris, also called jock itch), or feet (tinea pedis, also called athlete's foot).

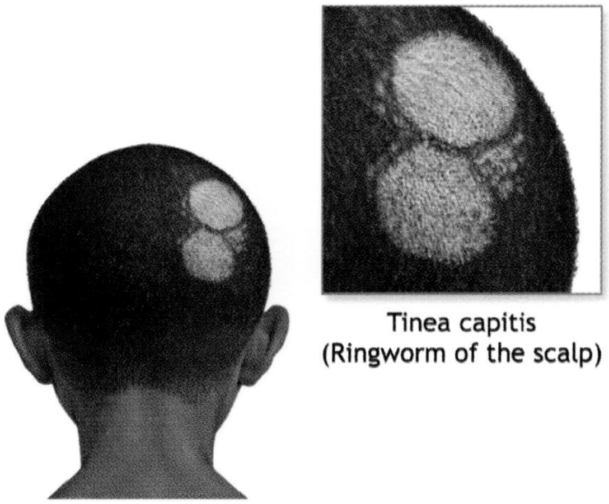

Tinea capitis
(Ringworm of the scalp)

Often, there are several patches of ringworm on your skin at once.

Ringworm is a common skin disorder, especially among children, but it may affect people of all ages. Although its name suggests otherwise, it is caused by a fungus, not a worm.

Many bacteria and fungi live on your body. Some of these are useful to you and your body. Others can multiply rapidly and form infections. Ringworm occurs when a particular type of fungus grows and multiplies anywhere on your skin, scalp, or nails.

Ringworm is contagious. It can be passed from one person to the next by direct skin-to-skin contact or by contact with contaminated items such as combs, unwashed clothing, and shower or pool surfaces. You can also catch ringworm from pets that carry the fungus. Cats are common carriers.

The fungi that cause ringworm thrive in warm, moist areas. Ringworm is more likely when you have frequent wetness (such as from sweating) and minor injuries to your skin, scalp, or nails.

Symptoms

The symptoms of ringworm include:

- Itchy, red, raised, scaly patches that may blister and ooze. The patches often have sharply-defined edges. They are often redder around the outside with normal skin tone in the center. This may create the appearance of a ring. Your skin may also appear unusually dark or light.
- When your scalp or beard is infected, you will have bald patches.
- If nails are infected, they become discolored, thick, and even crumble.

Home care

Ringworm usually responds well to self-care within 4 weeks without having to see a doctor.

- Keep your skin clean and dry.
- Apply over-the-counter antifungal or drying powders, lotions, or creams. Those that contain miconazole, clotrimazole, or similar ingredients are often effective.
- Wash sheets and nightclothes every day while infected.

Infected pets also should be treated.

When to contact a medical professional

Call your doctor right away if you have any signs of a bacterial infection, which can result from scratching. These signs include swelling, warmth to the touch, sudden worsening in redness of the patches, red streaking, pus, discharge, and fever.

Call your doctor if:

- Ringworm infects your scalp or beard.
- Your skin does not improve after 4 weeks of self-care.

Prevention

To prevent ringworm:

- Keep your skin and feet clean and dry.
- Shampoo regularly, especially after haircuts.
- Do not share clothing, towels, hairbrushes, combs, headgear, or other personal care items. Such items should be thoroughly cleaned and dried after use.
- Wear sandals or shoes at gyms, lockers, and pools.
- Avoid touching pets with bald spots.

> **How long will it take to treat?**
>
> Ringworm can usually be treated at home with over-the-counter remedies, although it may be 4 weeks before the infection is gone.

Rosacea

Rosacea is a chronic skin condition involving inflammation of the cheeks, nose, chin, forehead, or eyelids. It may appear as redness, prominent spider-like blood vessels, swelling, or skin eruptions similar to acne.

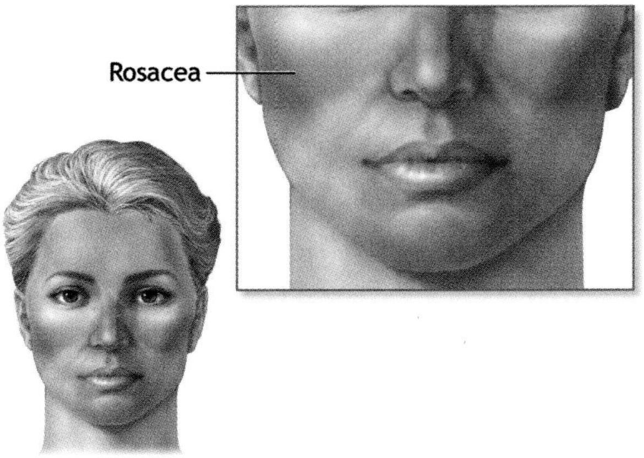

Although the cause of rosacea is unknown, you are more likely to develop this harmless skin condition if:

- You are fair skinned.
- You blush easily.
- You are a woman. However, men are usually more severely affected.
- You are between the ages of 30 and 50.

Home care

There is no known cure for rosacea. The goal is to identify and avoid possible triggers, and thus reduce flare-ups. In fact, the National Rosacea Society strongly recommends that you keep a symptom diary to identify the specific triggers you may have. As you keep track of your symptoms, you should start to see a pattern within several weeks of what makes your rosacea worse. Use this information to avoid future flare-ups.

Here are some steps that may help:

- Avoid sun exposure. Use sunscreen every day.
- Avoid prolonged exertion in hot weather.
- Try to reduce stress. Try deep breathing, yoga, or other relaxation techniques.
- Limit spicy foods, alcohol, and hot beverages.

Triggers vary from person to person. Other triggers may include wind, hot baths, cold weather, specific skin products, exercise, or other factors. Booklets and a symptom diary containing more detailed management tips can be found at www.rosacea.org.

Runny or stuffy nose

Your nose runs when there is excess mucus. The mucus and other secretions may drain from the front of the nose, or down the back (post-nasal drip).

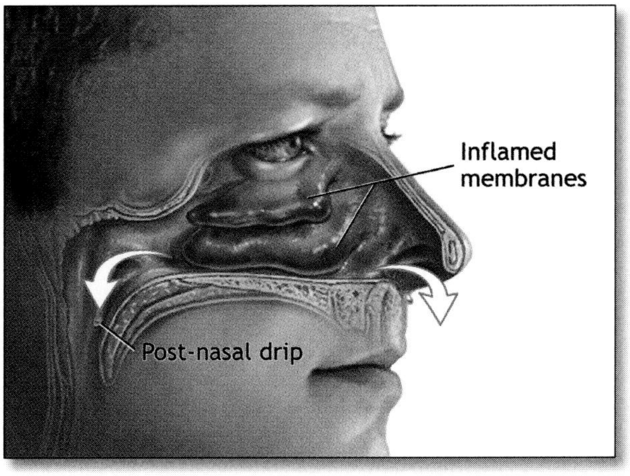

A runny nose may be caused by colds, allergies, sinus infections, or the flu. It can also be caused by head injuries, and by small objects placed in the nose (especially in young children).

Many people think that a nose gets **congested** (stuffy) from too much thick mucus. Not so! A congested nose happens when the membranes lining the nose become swollen from inflamed blood vessels. Congestion can be caused by most of the same reasons as a runny nose – including colds, allergies, sinus infections, and the flu. Overuse of some nasal sprays or drops can also lead to congestion.

Allergy, cold, or sinus infection?

Allergies involve a clear nasal discharge with sneezing. There may be itchy, watery eyes and a dry cough. With colds, sneezes tend to be more productive, and coughs sound wetter than with allergies. A sinus infection often begins like a cold but then lasts for greater than 10 to 14 days with no period of improvement.

When are you contagious?

If the nasal secretions are caused by a viral or bacterial infection, they may be teeming with live germs. This is especially true for the first 2 to 3 days of symptoms. Covering the nose with the inside of your elbow when sneezing or coughing helps reduce the spread of germs. Also, frequent hand cleaning is wise.

Home care

To relieve a runny or stuffy nose, the following over-the-counter medicines may help:

- **Decongestants** – these may help relieve congestion by shrinking the blood vessels in the lining of the nose. They only help with stuffiness, not a runny nose or other symptoms. Decongestant nasal sprays and drops should not be used for more than 3 days. After that, continued use can make the congestion worse.
- **Antihistamines** – these may reduce the amount of mucus. Be careful, because some antihistamines can make you drowsy.

These medicines help you breathe, but do not treat the underlying condition. Also, many over-the-counter allergy and cold medicines contain multiple ingredients, so look carefully to see what is in the one you choose. If you have heart disease, thyroid disease, high blood pressure, or other serious condition, talk to your provider before using them.

Medicines are not the only way to relieve a stuffy or runny nose. Often, gentler solutions are better. Try these steps to thin the mucus, which can help you breathe easier and get your nasal secretions back to normal:

- Use gentle saline nasal sprays.
- Increase the humidity in the air with a vaporizer or humidifier.
- Drink extra fluids. Hot tea, broth, or chicken soup may be especially helpful.

For a baby too young to blow his or her nose, an infant nasal aspirator (bulb) can help remove the mucus. If the mucus is thick and sticky, loosen it by putting 2 or 3 saline nose drops into each nostril.

Congestion is often worse when you are lying down. Keep upright, or at least keep the head elevated. This is especially helpful for young children.

Pharmacies and supermarkets sell adhesive strips that can be placed on the nose when you are congested. These help widen the nasal passages, making breathing easier.

Overuse of antibiotics

Many people think that a green or yellow nasal discharge means a bacterial infection, which requires antibiotics. This is NOT true. Colds will often begin with a clear nasal discharge, but after several days it usually turns creamy, yellow, or green for a time. Colds are caused by viruses, and antibiotics will not help. A green or nasal discharge is not a sign that you need antibiotics.

The bottom line

In most cases, an office visit to a doctor won't help a stuffy nose or other cold symptoms. The doctor will probably just suggest the self-care steps outlined here.

Shoulder pain

The shoulder is the most mobile joint in the human body. The joint includes four tendons. The purpose of a tendon is to hold muscle to bone.

Together, these four "rotator cuff" tendons stabilize the upper arm bone to the shoulder socket and allow a wide range of motion in the shoulder.

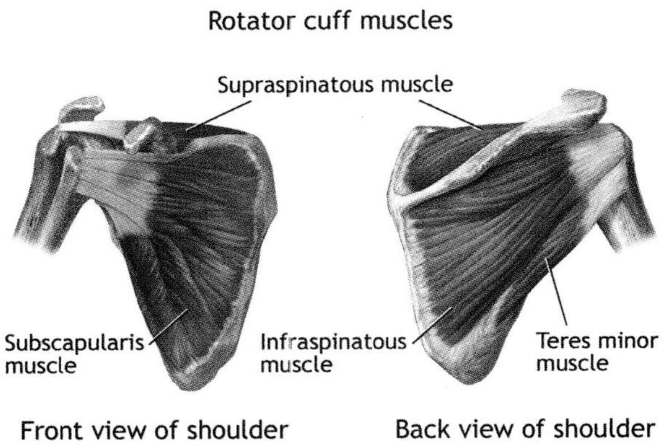

Any swelling, inflammation, tearing, or bony changes around these tendons causes pain when a person tries to move the arm above the head, behind the back, or straight out in front.

The tendons pass underneath a rigid bony arch in the shoulder called the acromion.

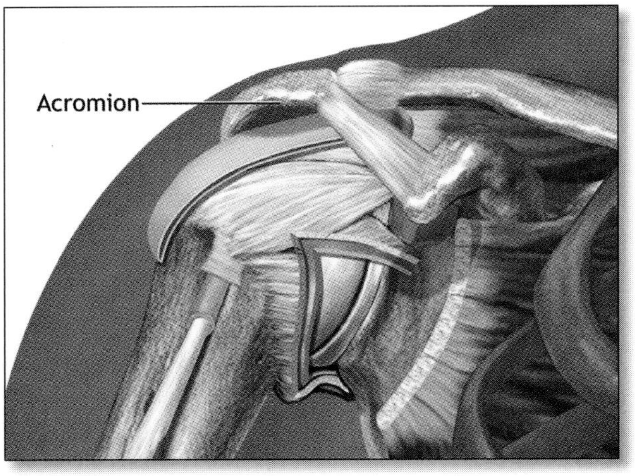

The most common cause of shoulder pain is when the tendons become trapped under this arch. The compressed tendons become inflamed or damaged, a condition called rotator cuff tendinitis. This can occur from general wear and tear as you get older, an activity that requires constant shoulder use like baseball pitching, or an injury.

Shoulder pain can also be due to:

- **Arthritis** in the joints about the shoulder (gradual narrowing of the joints and loss of protective cartilage).
- **Fractures** of the shoulder bones.
- **Frozen shoulder syndrome** occurs when you don't move your shoulder because of pain or injury. The muscles or connective structures stiffen up inside the shoulder and make motion painful and difficult.
- **Bursitis** (inflammation of a fluid-filled sac, or bursa, that lies between tendon and skin or between tendon and bone). Normally a bursa protects the joint and helps make movement more fluid.

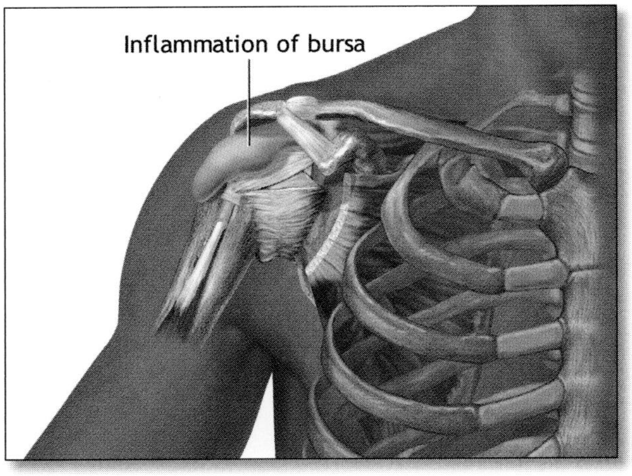

- **Inflammation of nearby tendons**, such as those connected to the bicep muscles of your arms, from overuse or injury.

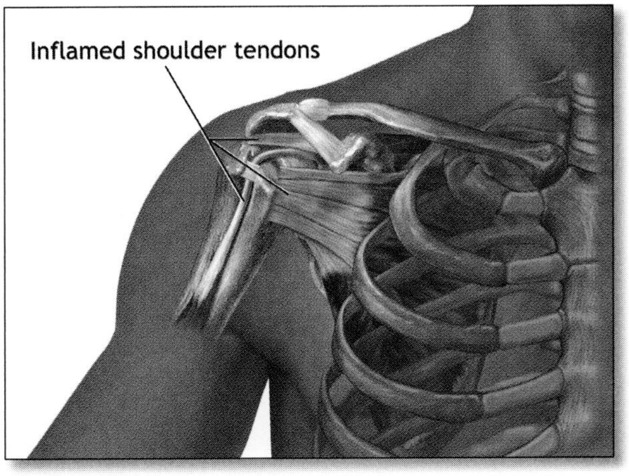

- **Dislocation of your shoulder**, which is when the ball-shaped head of your arm comes out of the socket.

Home care

When you first feel shoulder pain, apply ice for up to 15 minutes, then leave it off for 15 minutes. Repeat this cycle for several hours.

Wrap the ice in a cloth, DO NOT apply ice directly to the skin. Then, continue to ice 3 to 4 times a day for 2 to 3 days.

Rest the shoulder from strenuous activity for the next few days. When the pain and swelling have subsided, gradually begin to strengthen the shoulder muscles. Perform light weight lifting, using a full range of motion. Consider seeing a physical therapist for help doing this safely.

Ibuprofen may help reduce inflammation and pain.

When to contact a medical professional

Call 911 if you feel sudden pressure or crushing pain in your shoulder, especially if it extends from your chest, jaw, or neck, or occurs with shortness of breath, dizziness or sweating. Very sudden shoulder pain can, occasionally, be a sign of a heart attack.

If you just had a severe blow or injury and your painful shoulder is swollen, badly bruised, or bleeding, get safely to an emergency room where they will check for a fracture or dislocation.

Contact your doctor if :

- You have fever, swelling, or redness.
- You are unable to use the joint.
- Your pain lasts more than 1-2 weeks despite self-care measures.

Prevention

- If you have had shoulder pain in the past, use ice and ibuprofen after exercising.
- Learn proper exercises to stretch and strengthen your rotator cuff tendons and shoulder muscles. A doctor or physical therapist can help.
- If you are recovering from tendinitis, continue to perform range-of-motion exercises to avoid "frozen shoulder."

In sports-related activities, learn proper technique to prevent painful and expensive shoulder problems.

Sinus pain

Sinusitis refers to inflammation of the sinuses. This is generally caused by a viral, bacterial, or fungal infection.

The sinuses are air-filled spaces around the forehead, cheeks, and eyes that are lined with mucous membranes. Healthy sinuses are sterile (meaning that they contain no bacteria or other organisms) and open, allowing mucus to drain and air to circulate.

When inflamed, the sinuses become blocked with mucus and can become infected. Each year, over 30 million adults and children get sinusitis.

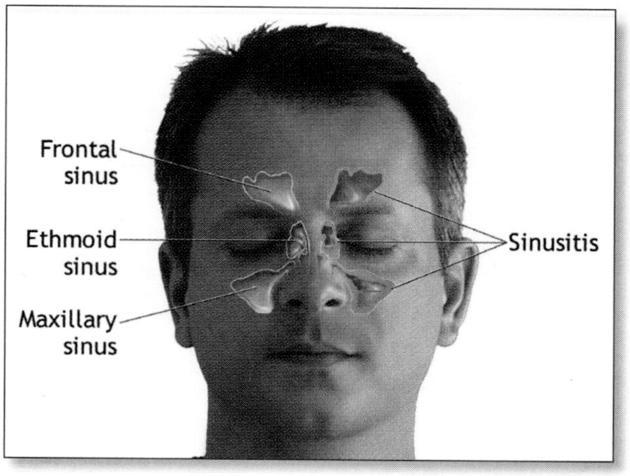

Sinusitis can be acute (lasting anywhere from 2 to 8 weeks) or chronic, with symptoms lingering much longer.

Sinusitis usually follows respiratory infections, such as colds, or an allergic reaction. Some people never get sinusitis, and others develop sinusitis frequently.

Other risks for developing sinusitis include:

- Having asthma
- Overuse of nasal decongestants (rather than continuing to relieve congestion, the

problem gets worse when these are used too often or for too long)

- Having a deviated nasal septum, nasal bone spur, or polyp

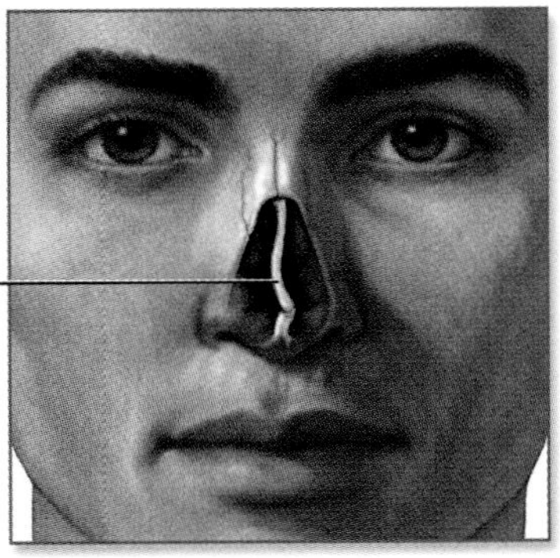

- Presence of a foreign body in your nose
- Frequent swimming or diving
- Dental work
- Pregnancy
- Changes in altitude (flying or climbing)
- Air pollution and smoke
- Gastroesophageal reflux disease (GERD)

Symptoms

The classic symptoms of acute sinusitis usually follow a cold that does not improve, or one that worsens after 5 to 7 days of symptoms. They include:

- Nasal congestion and discharge
- Sore throat and postnasal drip (fluid dripping down the back of your throat, especially at night or when lying down)
- Headache – pressure-like pain, pain behind the eyes, toothache, or facial tenderness
- Cough, often worse at night
- Fever (may be present)
- Bad breath or loss of smell
- Fatigue and generally not feeling well

Symptoms of chronic sinusitis are the same as acute sinusitis, but tend to be milder and last longer than 8 weeks.

Home care

Try the following measures to help reduce congestion in your sinuses:

- Use a humidifier.
- Spray with nasal saline several times per day.
- Inhale steam 2 to 4 times per day (for example, sitting in the bathroom with the shower running).
- Drink plenty of fluids to thin the mucus.
- Apply a warm, moist wash cloth to your face several times per day.

Be careful with over-the-counter spray nasal decongestants. They can help initially, but using them beyond 3-5 days can actually worsen nasal congestion.

Also, for sinus pain or pressure:

- Avoid temperature extremes, sudden changes in temperature, and bending forward with your head down.
- Try acetaminophen or ibuprofen.
- Avoid flying when you are congested.

If self-care measures are not working, your doctor will consider prescription medications, antibiotics, further testing, or referral to an Ear, Nose, and Throat (ENT) specialist.

When to contact a medical professional

Call your doctor if:

- Your symptoms last longer than 10 to 14 days or you have a cold that gets worse after 7 days.
- You have a severe headache, unrelieved by over-the-counter pain medicine.
- You have a fever.
- You still have symptoms after taking all of your antibiotics properly.

A green or yellow discharge does not necessarily indicate a sinus infection or the need for antibiotics.

Prevention

The best way to prevent sinusitis is to avoid or quickly treat flus and colds:

- Receive an influenza vaccine each year.
- Wash your hands frequently, particularly after shaking hands with others.
- Eat plenty of fruits and vegetables, which are rich in antioxidants and other chemicals that could boost your immune system and help your body resist infection.
- Reduce stress.

Additional tips for preventing sinusitis:

- Avoid smoke and pollutants.
- Use a humidifier to increase moisture in your nose and sinus areas.
- Drink plenty of fluids to increase moisture within your body.
- Take decongestants during an upper respiratory infection.
- Treat allergies promptly and appropriately.

> **Key point**
>
> Don't rush to antibiotics for sinus pain. Read this article to learn gentler solutions that help without antibiotics.

Skin - dry

Dry skin is common. It happens more often in the winter when cold air outside and heated air inside cause low humidity. Forced-air furnaces make skin even drier.

The skin loses moisture and may crack and peel, or become irritated and inflamed.

Bathing too frequently, especially with harsh soaps, may contribute to dry skin. Eczema may cause dry skin.

Home care

It may help to change your bathing habits:

- Keep baths or showers short.
- Use warm (not hot) water.
- Use as little soap as possible. Limit its use to face, armpits, and genitals if you can. Try mild cleansers like Aveeno or Cetaphil or mild soaps like Neutrogena or Dove.
- Dry your skin thoroughly but gently – pat, DON'T rub.
- Take baths or showers less often.

Also, increase skin and body moisture:

- Use bath oils and moisturizers at least daily. Thick, greasy moisturizers work best. Avoid products with alcohol. Apply just after a bath or shower, when your skin is still damp.
- Use a humidifier if the air is dry.
- Drink plenty of water throughout the day.

Apply cool compresses to itchy areas, and try over-the-counter cortisone creams or lotions if your skin is inflamed. If this is not enough, talk to your doctor about possible prescription lotions.

Sleeping problems

Everyone needs to get a good night's rest on a regular basis. Although sleep requirements vary somewhat from person to person, an average adult needs around 8 hours of sleep each night. Unfortunately, about 1 out of 3 people in the United States has insomnia. Insomnia can take several forms:

- Difficulty falling asleep when you first go to bed at night.
- Waking up too early in the morning.

- Waking up frequently throughout the night.

As a result, you may feel unrefreshed after sleep. You may feel drowsy, fatigued, and irritable during the day. Insomnia can make it difficult to concentrate and can contribute to headaches. You may be unable to sleep despite being tired, and become anxious as bedtime approaches.

Prevention and treatment

Simple lifestyle changes can help you improve your sleep habits. In fact, the majority of people improve WITHOUT medication. Most sleep medications, both over-the-counter and by prescription, make you feel drowsy the next day. You can become dependent on them, requiring higher and higher amounts to fall and stay asleep. This disrupts your sleep pattern even further. The insomnia becomes a vicious cycle. Medication, therefore, should be considered a last resort.

The first step in treating insomnia is to develop and maintain healthy sleep habits. This means that you should:

- Go to bed and wake up at a consistent time each day. Try to keep this same schedule even on the weekends, especially when you are first treating insomnia.
- Do not read, work, watch television, or use a computer in bed.
- Avoid naps, especially late in the afternoon or evening.
- Keep your bedroom cool, well-ventilated, quiet, and dark. If you hear distracting noises, try a white-noise machine in the background.
- Avoid looking at the clock. This promotes anxiety and obsession about falling asleep.
- If sleep does NOT occur within 15 to 20 minutes in bed (or upon awakening in the middle of the night), move to another room with dim lighting. Don't lie there and fret about the fact that you are not asleep.

Here are some other steps you could take:

- Exercise regularly. It is best to do so before dinnertime. Exercise can make you feel more awake if done too close to bedtime.
- Avoid caffeine, especially after 3 PM.
- Don't smoke.
- Get regular exposure to late afternoon sun. (Use sun block). This stimulates the release of a hormone called melatonin, which helps regulate your circadian rhythm. Circadian rhythm can be thought of as your internal clock that governs the timing of hormone production, sleep, body temperature, and other important functions.
- Practice a stress-reduction technique each day, like yoga, meditation, or deep relaxation (progressive contraction and relaxation of muscle groups throughout your body). Using one of these methods just before bedtime can help you fall asleep more readily.
- Try a hot bath before bedtime.
- Avoid fluids just before going to bed.
- Eat a light, carbohydrate snack (like cereal or crackers) just before going to bed. Avoid large, heavy meals within two hours of bedtime.

Short-term use of melatonin supplements may be useful for temporary forms of insomnia like jet lag or shift work. The safety and effectiveness of using melatonin for a long-period of time, however, is NOT known.

When to contact a medical professional

Very few people actually talk to their doctor about sleeping problems. But it is important to tell your doctor:

- If you think you have a medical or psychological condition contributing to insomnia.
- Before using any kind of over-the-counter medication, herb, or supplement for insomnia.

- If self-care measures have NOT helped after about one month.
- If your partner or roommate tells you that you snore or have periods at night that you stop breathing.

At your doctor's appointment, come prepared with the following information:

- The average amount of total sleep you get each night.
- The length of time it takes you to fall asleep.
- The quality of your sleep.
- Your usual number of awakenings throughout the night
- Any impact insomnia has had on your daytime functioning.
- Attempted self-treatments and how well they have worked.
- Your mood and stress level.

KEY POINT

Behavioral and lifestyle changes are the first line of treatment for insomnia and other sleeping difficulties. Medication is often considered a "last resort," use only if non-drug treatments aren't working.

SNORING

Snoring is common in adults and usually not an indication of an underlying disorder.

Sometimes, however, snoring can be a sign of a serious sleep disorder called sleep apnea. This means you have periods when you are not breathing for more than 10 seconds while you sleep. These periods of "apnea" are indicated by a long period of silence just after you have been snoring. They are followed by a sudden snort or gasp when breathing resumes. Then, snoring starts all over again. If you have sleep apnea, this cycle generally happens several times a night.

The major risk from this condition is stroke due to episodes when your brain is not getting enough oxygen. If sleep apnea is suspected, your doctor (or a sleep specialist) can test you for it by doing a sleep study either at home or in a hospital setting.

In most people, the reason for snoring is not known. The following are potential causes other than sleep apnea:

- Sleeping pills, antihistamines, or alcohol at bedtime
- Nasal congestion from colds or allergies, especially if it lasts a long time
- Enlarged adenoids and tonsils that block the airway

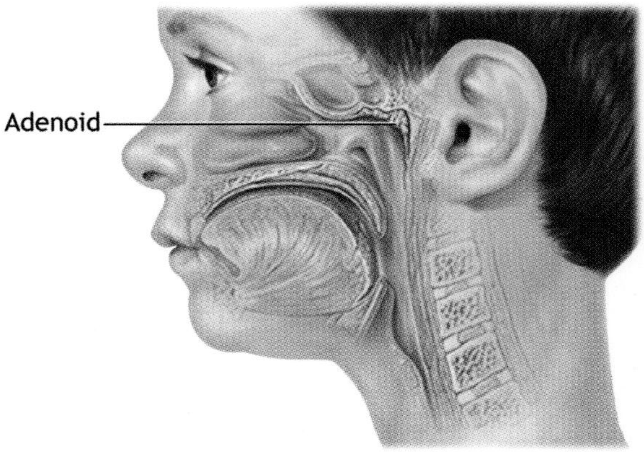

- Being overweight, which leads to excessive neck tissue that puts pressure on the airway
- Last month of pregnancy

HOME CARE

The following can reduce snoring:

- Lose weight if you are overweight.
- Cut down or eliminate alcohol and other sedatives at bedtime.
- Avoid sleeping flat on your back. Sleep on your side if possible. Some doctors even suggest sewing a golf or tennis ball into the back of your night clothes. Then, if you roll over onto your back, you are reminded to stay on your side because of

the discomfort. Eventually, sleeping on your side is a habit and you don't need to be reminded.

When to contact a medical professional

Call your doctor right away if you awaken at night confused. Also call your doctor if you have:

- Excessive daytime drowsiness, morning headaches, recent weight gain, awakening in the morning not feeling rested, or change in your level of attention, concentration, or memory.
- Episodes of no breathing (apnea). Your partner may need to tell you if this is happening.

Children with chronic snoring should also be evaluated for apnea. Sleep apnea in children has been linked to growth problems, ADHD, poor school performance, learning difficulties, bedwetting, and high blood pressure. Most children who snore do NOT have apnea, but a sleep study is the only reliable way to tell for sure.

Sore throat

A sore throat is discomfort, pain, or scratchiness in the throat. A sore throat often makes it painful to swallow.

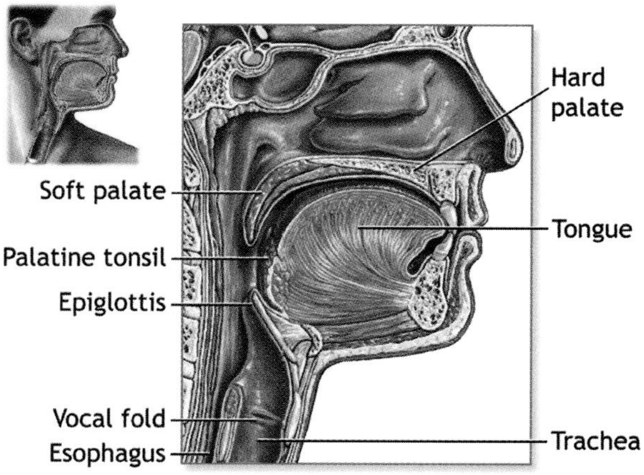

Anatomy of the throat and mouth.

Sore throats are common. Most of the time the soreness is worse in the morning and improves as the day progresses.

Like colds, the vast majority of sore throats are caused by viral infections. This means most sore throats will NOT respond to antibiotics. Many people have a mild sore throat at the beginning of every cold. When the nose or sinuses become infected, drainage can run down the back of the throat and irritate it, especially at night. Or, the throat itself can be infected.

Strep throat is the most common bacterial cause of sore throat. Because strep throat can occasionally lead to rheumatic fever, antibiotics are given. Strep throat often includes a fever (greater than 101°F), white draining patches on the throat, and swollen or tender lymph glands in the neck. Children may have a headache and stomach pain.

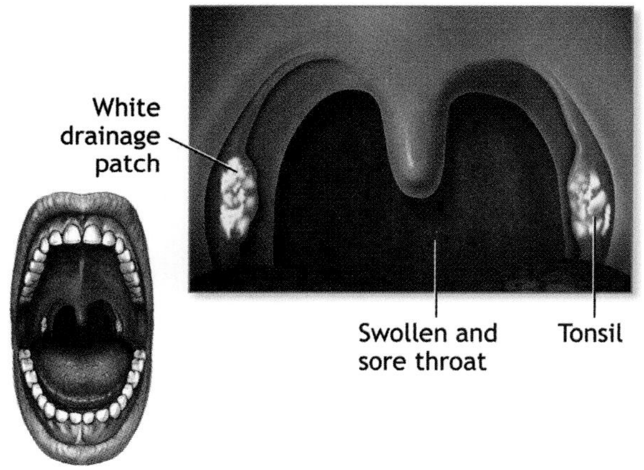

A sore throat is less likely to be strep throat if it is a minor part of a typical cold (with runny nose, stuffy ears, cough, and similar symptoms). Strep can't be accurately diagnosed by looking at the throat alone. It requires a laboratory test.

Sometimes breathing through the mouth will cause a sore throat in the absence of any infection. During the months of dry winter air, some people will wake up with a sore throat most mornings. This usually disappears after having something to drink.

Home care

Most sore throats are soon over. In the meantime, the following remedies may help:

- Drink warm liquids. Honey or lemon tea is a time-tested remedy.
- Gargle several times a day with warm salt water. (1/2 tsp of salt in 1 cup water.)
- Cold liquids or popsicles help some sore throats.
- Sucking on hard candies or throat lozenges can be very soothing, because it increases saliva production. This is often as effective as more expensive remedies, but should not be used in young children because of the choking risk.
- Use a cool-mist vaporizer or humidifier to moisten and sooth a dry and painful throat.
- Try over-the-counter pain medications, such as acetaminophen. DO NOT give aspirin to children.

When to contact a medical professional

Call your provider if there is:

- Severe difficulty swallowing or breathing
- Excessive drooling in a young child
- A fever, especially 101°F or greater
- Tender or swollen lymph glands in the neck
- Pus in the back of the throat
- A red rash that feels rough, and increased redness in the skin folds

Prevention

Clean your hands frequently, especially before eating. This is a powerful way to help prevent many sore throat infections. You might avoid some sore throats by reducing contact with people with sore throats, but often these people are contagious even before they have symptoms, so this approach is less effective.

Not too long ago, tonsils were commonly removed in an attempt to prevent sore throats. This is no longer recommended in most circumstances.

> **It's important to know...**
>
> Most sore throats are from a virus and will NOT get better with antibiotics. Antibiotics should only be used if you test positive for strep throat.

Spitting up (infants)

Spitting up is the gentle sloshing of stomach contents up and out of the mouth in babies, sometimes accompanied by a burp. It is an entirely different process than vomiting, which is the forceful expulsion of contents from the stomach by a fierce contraction of the diaphragm.

Most babies spit up milk out of their mouths or noses. This is because the sphincter at the top of the stomach is often loose.

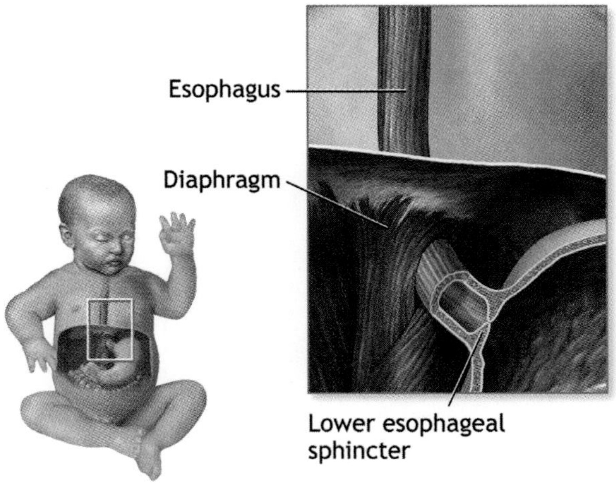

In otherwise healthy, happy babies who are growing well, the spit-up is mostly milk, rather than stomach acid, and nothing needs to be done. (Except a lot of laundry.)

Babies gaining at least 6 ounces a week and with wet diapers at least every 6 hours are usually growing well. On average, spitting up peaks at 4 months and is over by about 7 months of age, though it can take longer.

Spitting up is not likely to be a formula intolerance or allergy to something in a nursing mother's diet. The sphincter at the top of the stomach may be too loose (so it can't hold things in), the valve at the bottom of the stomach may be too tight (so the stomach gets too full), or big air bubbles may take up too much room. Sometimes babies just drink too much, too fast.

Some babies do reflux enough acid that the lining of the esophagus becomes tender, red, and swollen. They might arch their backs in pain. The acid can be inhaled into the lungs, irritating the sensitive linings. These children might not gain weight well, or might cry a lot from discomfort. Some might develop a chronic cough, wheezing, or recurrent pneumonia. A few even stop breathing (apnea) to try to protect their lungs. All of these children need relief from their reflux.

To reduce spitting up, burp your baby several times during and after feeding. Sit the baby upright, with your hand supporting the head. Let the baby lean over slightly, bending at the waist.

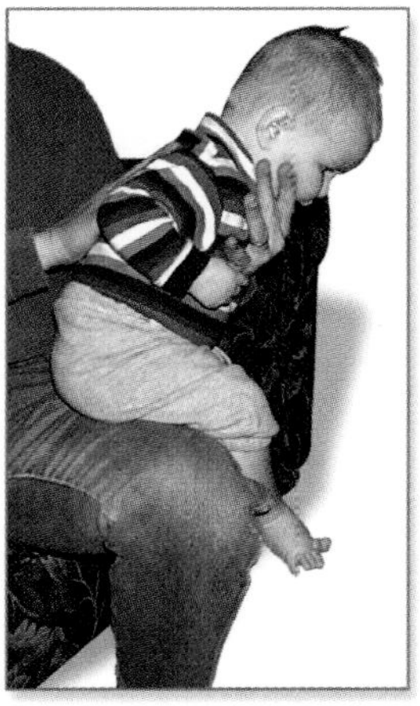

Recommended burping position

The upright posture moves air to the top of the stomach, and the forward lean puts a little pressure on the stomach to eject the air, helping the baby to burp. Avoid pressure on the abdomen, which occurs when holding your baby over your shoulder – this just causes more expulsion of stomach contents.

Here are other ways to reduce spitting up:

- For breastfed babies, try limiting nursing to just one breast per feeding.
- For bottle-fed babies, avoid feeding large amounts. Instead, feed smaller amounts more frequently. Be sure the nipple doesn't have too large a hole.
- Try holding the baby upright for 15 to 30 minutes after feedings.
- Avoid excessive movement and jiggling during and immediately after feeding.
- When it's time to lay your baby down, try keeping the head of his bed slightly elevated.
- Sometimes, switching formulas or removing a food from the mother's diet (usually cow's milk) will help.

If "projectile" spit-up shoots across the room, it's important to consider a condition called pyloric stenosis. Here, the too-tight valve at the bottom of the stomach needs to be treated.

Stomachaches

Belly pain is a common symptom throughout life, especially in children. Infants and toddlers won't report their pain, but may signal the abdominal discomfort with increased crying, gas, pulling up of the legs, vomiting, or stool changes. Common causes of tummy aches in infants include colic, cow's milk protein allergies, constipation, and viral infections.

Older children may tell you they have a tummy ache. Constipation and viral infection remain common causes. In older children, these causes are joined by urinary tract infections, strep throat, lactose intolerance, food poisoning, and emotional upset. Celiac disease should be considered when a child has recurring abdominal pain without a known cause.

In adults, other causes to consider include ulcers, gallstones, reflux disease and hepatitis. Intense abdominal pain, in children or adults, might signal a problem that requires surgery, such as appendicitis.

Most stomachaches are not serious and will fade away on their own. If the pain intensifies over three to five hours, then it's important to contact your doctor. Also contact the doctor if there are accompanying symptoms that would prompt a call, such as a fever or sore throat.

If stomachaches become an ongoing problem it is wise to work with your doctor to find the underlying cause.

Stool - black or bloody

Blood in the stool can originate from anywhere along your digestive tract, from mouth to anus.

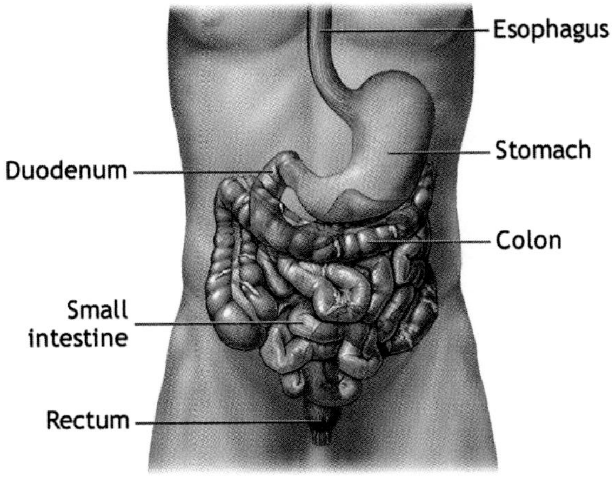

It may be present in such small amounts that you cannot actually see it, but is only detect-

Appendectomy (removal of appendix)

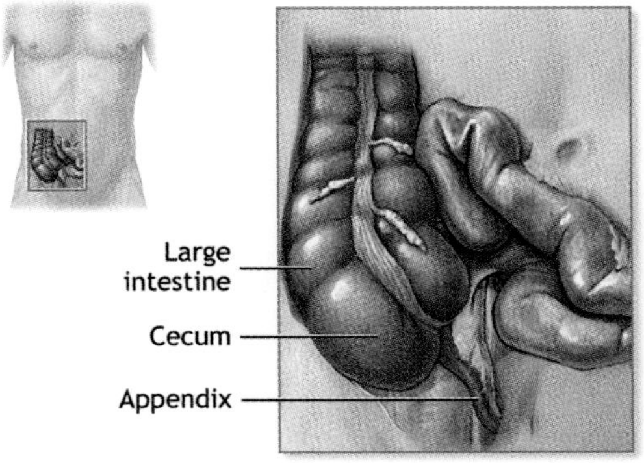

The appendix is a small, finger-shaped pouch of intestinal tissue arising from the cecum near its junction with the small intestine.

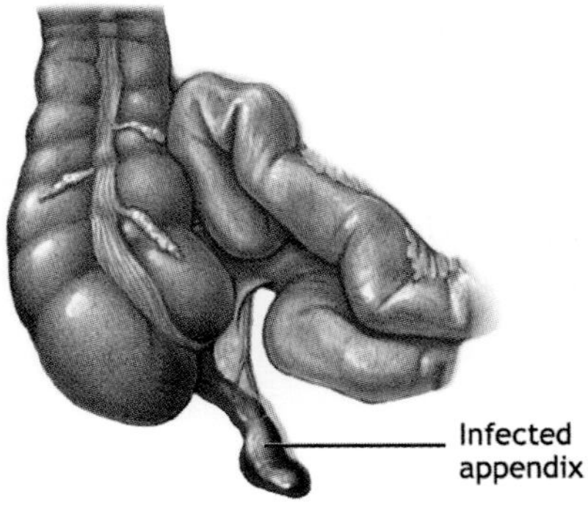

An infected appendix may cause intense abdominal pain. An appendectomy is completed before the appendix ruptures and spreads the infection into the abdominal cavity.

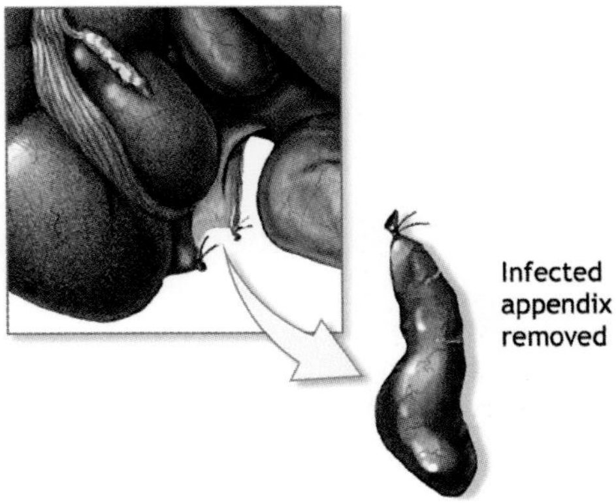

The infected appendix is surgically removed, typically by a laparoscopic procedure in which surgical instruments and lighted camera are passed through tiny incisions in the abdomen.

able by a fecal occult blood test.

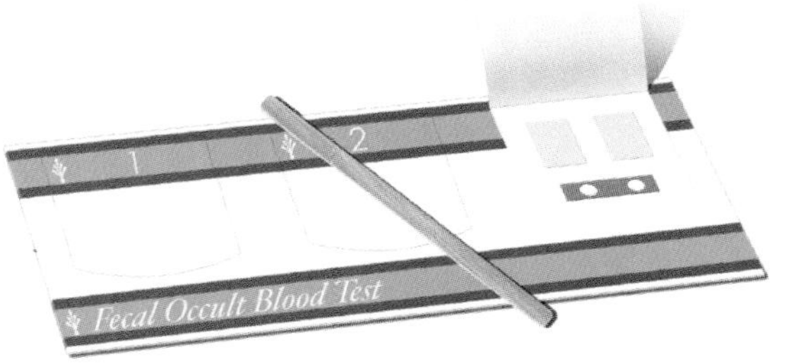

Stool samples from 3 consecutive bowel movements are collected, smeared on a sample card, then mailed to a laboratory for analysis.

When there IS enough blood to change the appearance of your stools, the doctor will typically want to know the exact color to try to estimate the site of bleeding.

To make a definite diagnosis, however, endoscopy or special x-ray studies are needed.

A black stool usually means that the blood is coming from the upper part of the gastrointestinal (GI) tract. This includes the esophagus, stomach, or first part of the small intestine.

Blood will typically appear like tar after it has been exposed to the body's digestive juices. Stomach ulcers caused by ibuprofen, naproxen, or aspirin are common causes of upper GI bleeding.

Maroon-colored stools or bright red blood usually suggest that the blood is coming from the lower part of the GI tract (large bowel or rectum).

Hemorrhoids and diverticulitis (inflammation of an abnormal pouch in the colon called a diverticulum) are the most common causes of lower GI bleeding. However, sometimes massive or rapid bleeding in the stomach causes bright red stools.

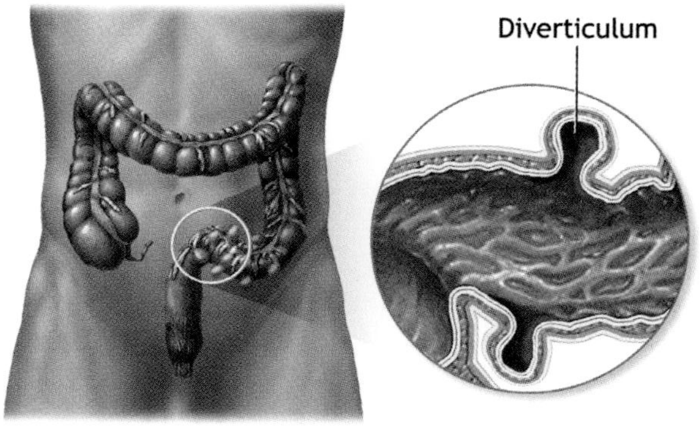

When to contact a medical professional

Call your doctor if you notice blood or changes in the color of your stool. Even if you think that hemorrhoids are causing blood in your stool, your doctor should examine you in order to make sure that there is no other, more serious cause present at the same time.

In children, a small amount of blood in the stool is usually not serious. The most common causes are constipation and milk allergies. But it is still worth reporting to your doctor, even if no workup is necessary.

Prevention

- Eat vegetables and foods rich in natural fiber and low in saturated fat. These may reduce constipation, hemorrhoids, diverticulosis, and colon cancer.
- Avoid prolonged, excessive use of anti-inflammatory drugs like ibuprofen, naproxen, and aspirin. These can irritate the stomach and cause ulcers.
- Avoid drinking excessive alcohol. This can irritate the lining of the esophagus and stomach.
- Don't smoke. It is linked to peptic ulcers and cancers of the GI tract.
- Try to avoid too much stress – a possible factor in peptic ulcer disease.
- If your doctor diagnoses you with a Helicobacter infection (often related to ulcers),

he may recommend antibiotics to prevent a bleeding ulcer in the future.

The earlier you detect colon cancer, the more likely that treatment will be successful. The American Cancer Society recommends one or more of the following screening tests after age 50 for early detection of colon cancer and pre-cancer:

- Fecal occult blood testing every year.
- Flexible sigmoidoscopy or barium enema every five years.
- Colonoscopy every 10 years.

Screening tests should be started earlier if you have a family history of colon cancer or polyps. Tests should also be performed more often if you have had polyps, colon cancer, or inflammatory bowel disease.

Strep throat

Strep throat is caused by Streptococcus bacteria. It is the most common bacterial infection of the throat.

Strep throat is most common in children between the ages of 5 and 15, although it can happen in younger children and adults. Children younger than 3 can get strep infections, but these usually don't affect the throat.

Strep throat is most common in the late fall, winter, and early spring. The infection is spread by person-to-person contact with nasal secretions or saliva, often among family or household members.

People with strep throat get sick 2–5 days after they are exposed. The illness usually begins suddenly, with a fever that peaks on the second day. Many also have sore throat, headache, stomachache, nausea, or chills.

In some people, strep throat is very mild, with only a few of these symptoms. In others, strep throat is severe. There are many strains of strep. Some strains produce toxins that can lead to a scarlet fever rash. This rash is thought to be an allergic reaction to the toxins. Untreated, strep throat can sometimes lead to rheumatic fever. Kidney complications are among the other possibilities.

Home care

Even though the sore throat usually gets better on its own, people who have strep throat SHOULD take antibiotics to prevent more serious complications of this infection, including rheumatic fever. Penicillin has been traditionally recommended. However, resistance to penicillin is increasing, and cephalosporins may be more effective in some situations.

Be aware that most sore throats are caused by viruses, not strep. The Centers for Disease Control and Prevention (CDC) recommends AGAINST treating sore throats with antibiotics unless the strep test is positive. Strep cannot be diagnosed by symptoms or a physical exam alone.

Ibuprofen can help people feel much better while the antibiotic is taking effect. Gargling with warm salt water (one half teaspoon of salt in a glass of warm water) several times a day may also help.

When to contact a medical professional

See *Sore Throat* for guidelines on when to call your health care provider. Call if you develop the symptoms of strep throat and you think you were exposed to someone with strep throat. Also, call if you are being treated for strep throat and are not feeling better within 24 to 48 hours.

Key point

Strep is diagnosed with a strep test, not by looking in the throat. If you have strep, antibiotics are required. Good old-fashioned penicillin is generally the best – not one of the newer, more expensive, broad-spectrum antibiotics.

Prevention

Most people with strep are contagious until they have been on antibiotics 24-48 hours. Thus, they should stay home from school, daycare, or work until they have been on antibiotics for at least a day.

Get a new toothbrush after you are no longer contagious, but before finishing the antibiotics. Otherwise the bacteria can live in the toothbrush and re-infect when the antibiotics are done. Also, keep your family's toothbrushes and utensils separate, unless they have been washed.

If repeated cases of strep still occur in a family, you might check to see if someone is a strep carrier. Carriers have strep in their throats, but the bacteria do not make them sick. Sometimes, treating them can prevent others from getting strep throat.

Stress and anxiety

Stress can come from any situation or thought that makes you feel frustrated, angry, or anxious. What is stressful to one person is not necessarily stressful to another.

Stress is a normal part of life. In small quantities, stress is good – it can motivate you and help you be more productive. However, too much stress, or a strong response to stress, is harmful. It can set you up for general poor health as well as specific physical or psychological illnesses like infection, heart disease, or depression. Persistent and unrelenting stress often leads to anxiety and unhealthy behaviors like overeating and abuse of alcohol or drugs.

Emotional states like grief or depression and health conditions like an overactive thyroid, low blood sugar, or heart attack can also cause stress.

Anxiety is a feeling of apprehension or fear. The source of this uneasiness is not always known or recognized, which can add to the distress you feel. Anxiety is often accompanied by physical symptoms, including:

- Twitching or trembling
- Muscle tension, headaches
- Sweating
- Dry mouth, difficulty swallowing
- Abdominal pain (may be the only symptom of stress, especially in a child)

Sometimes other symptoms accompany anxiety:

- Dizziness
- Rapid or irregular heart rate
- Rapid breathing
- Diarrhea or frequent need to urinate
- Fatigue
- Irritability, including loss of your temper
- Sleeping difficulties and nightmares
- Decreased concentration
- Sexual problems

Home care

The most effective solution is to find and address the source of your stress or anxiety. Unfortunately, this is not always possible. A first step is to take an inventory of what you think might be making you "stress out":

- What do you worry about most?
- Is something constantly on your mind?
- Does anything in particular make you sad or depressed?

Then, find someone you trust (friend, family member, neighbor, clergy) who will listen to you. Often, just talking to a friend or loved one is all that is needed to relieve anxiety. Most communities also have support groups and hotlines that can help. Social workers, psychologists, and other mental health professionals may be needed for therapy and medication.

Also, find healthy ways to cope with stress. For example:

- Eat a well-balanced, healthy diet. Don't overeat.
- Get enough sleep.
- Exercise regularly.
- Limit caffeine and alcohol.
- Don't use nicotine, cocaine, or other recreational drugs.
- Learn and practice relaxation techniques like guided imagery, progressive muscle relaxation, yoga, tai chi, or meditation. Try biofeedback, using a certified professional to get you started.
- Take breaks from work. Make sure to balance fun activities with your responsibilities. Spend time with people you enjoy.

When to contact a medical professional

Call 911 if:

- You have crushing chest pain, especially with shortness of breath, dizziness, or sweating. A heart attack can cause feelings of anxiety.
- You have thoughts of suicide.
- You have dizziness, rapid breathing, or racing heartbeat for the first time or it is worse than usual.

Call your health care provider if:

- You are unable to work or function properly at home because of anxiety.
- You do not know the source or cause of your anxiety.
- You have a sudden feeling of panic.
- You have an uncontrollable fear – for example, of getting infected and sick if you are out, or a fear of heights.
- You repeat an action over and over again, like constantly washing your hands.
- You have an intolerance to heat, weight loss despite a good appetite, lump or swelling in the front of your neck, or protruding eyes. Your thyroid may be overactive.
- Your anxiety is elicited by the memory of a traumatic event.
- You have tried self care for several weeks without success or you feel that your anxiety will not resolve without professional help.

Ask your pharmacist or health care provider if any prescription or over-the-counter drugs you are taking can cause anxiety as a side effect. Do not stop taking any prescribed medicines without your provider's instructions.

Deciding on a treatment option

Self-care steps help whether your doctor recommends medication or not. In fact, for many people who have an anxiety disorder, therapy alone can improve anxiety even without medication. Talk to your doctor about a referral to a therapist, especially if you are unable to work or function properly at home.

Swimmer's ear

Swimmer's ear is an infection of the skin lining the ear canal. Bacteria normally live on the surface of this skin with no ill effect. If there is a break in the skin's normal barrier, however, the bacteria can get inside and cause an infection called external otitis or swimmer's ear (this is different from an "ear infection" or otitis media).

If the ear is wet for long, the skin in the canal can become prune-like in the same way one's fingers and toes become soft and wrinkled. Bacteria can easily move into the soft skin. Tiny scratches in the ear canal (usually from sticking a finger or some other object into the ear) also leave the skin vulnerable to infection. The skin can also be breached as a result of the ear's becoming extraordinarily dry, causing the skin to crack. Ironically, swimmer's ear can be the result of spending time in desert conditions.

Swimmer's ear is more common in people who spend time in swimming pools than in people who swim in lakes. The chlorine in swimming pools kills the beneficial bacteria in the ear fairly effectively, but is not as effective against the harmful bacteria hiding there. This does not mean the water in the swimming pool is infected – the wetness is the problem. For unclear reasons, swimmer's ear is not common in infants, but it is particularly prevalent in pre-school and school-age children.

There are a couple of ways to prevent swimmer's ear. One is to make sure the ears get dry after being in the water by turning the head and gently pulling the ear in different directions to help drain the water out of the ear. It is also helpful to dry the opening of the ear very carefully as far as you can reach with a towel. If swimmer's ear becomes a recurrent problem, you can put a few drops of rubbing alcohol in the ear each time it becomes wet, to help kill bacteria and dry the skin. Another good alternative is instilling a few drops of white vinegar. This gently slows the growth of bacteria in the skin.

The symptoms of swimmer's ear are an itchy or painful ear. This is often accompanied by a small amount of clear discharge.

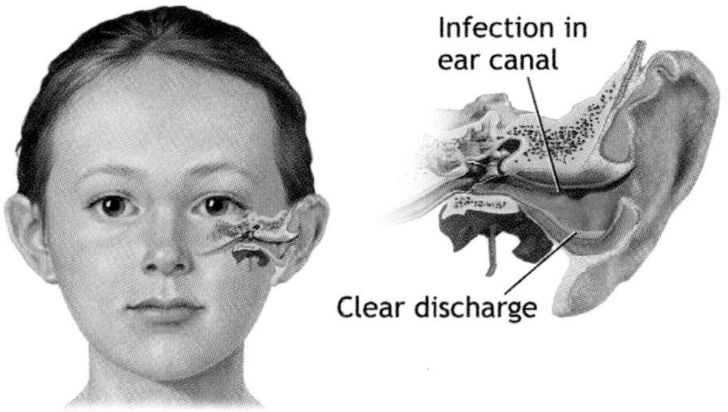

Signs and symptoms of swimmer's ear.

The ear is particularly sensitive to the ear lobe's being moved up and down. If someone does develop swimmer's ear, it can often be treated with a few drops of white vinegar placed in both ears. Put the vinegar in one ear and leave it for about five minutes before turning that ear down in order to drain the vinegar solution. Repeat this twice a day for three days. If the symptoms worsen or persist for over three days, prescription antibiotic drops may be necessary.

Swimming is generally not associated with the other type of ear infection (otitis media). This is true even if a child has ear tubes.

Swollen glands

Lymph nodes are glands that play an important part in your body's defense against infection. They produce lymph, which travels throughout your body in the lymph system, and filters impurities in your body.

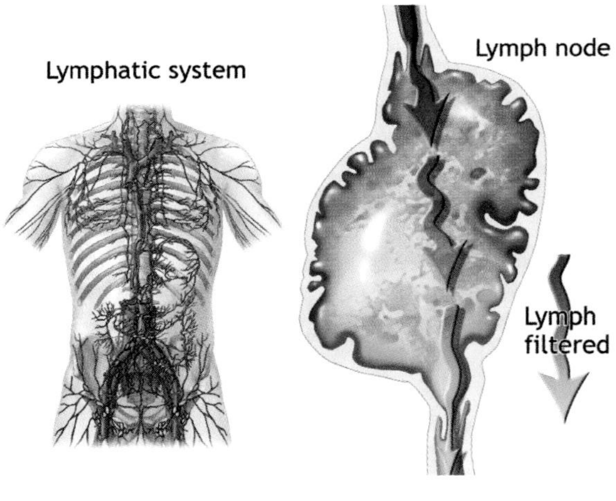

Common areas where the lymph nodes can be felt include:

- Groin
- Armpit
- Neck (there is a chain of lymph nodes on either side of the front of the neck, both sides of the neck, and down each side of the back of the neck)
- Under the jaw and chin

- Behind the ears
- On the back of the head

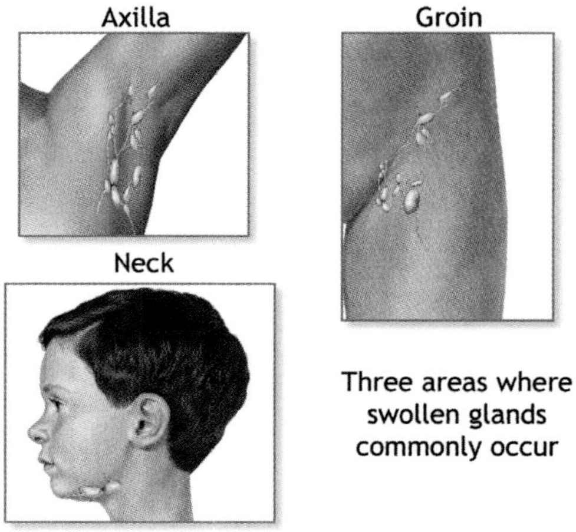

Three areas where swollen glands commonly occur

Lymph nodes can become swollen from infection, inflammatory conditions, an abscess, or cancer. Other causes of enlarged lymph nodes are rare. By far, the most common cause of swollen lymph nodes is infection.

When swelling appears suddenly and is painful, it is usually caused by injury or an infection. Enlargement that comes on gradually and painlessly may result from cancer or a tumor.

Infections that commonly cause swollen lymph nodes include mononucleosis, German measles, tuberculosis, mumps, ear infection, tonsillitis, abscessed or impacted tooth, gingivitis (swelling of the gums), mouth sores, and sexually transmitted diseases.

Immune or autoimmune disorders that can cause swollen lymph nodes include rheumatoid arthritis and HIV. Cancers that can cause swollen glands include leukemia, Hodgkin's disease, or non-Hodgkin's lymphoma.

Which lymph nodes are swollen depends on the type of problem and the body parts involved. Identifying the location can help determine the possible cause.

Home care

Soreness in lymph glands usually disappears in a couple of days without treatment, but the nodes may not return to normal size for several weeks after the infection has cleared. Generally, if glands are painful, it is because they swell rapidly in the early stages of fighting an infection.

When to contact a medical professional

Call your doctor if:

- Your glands don't get smaller after several weeks or continue to get larger.
- Your swollen glands are red and tender.
- Your glands feel hard, irregular, or fixed in place.
- You have a fever, night sweats, or unexplained weight loss.
- Any node is larger than 1cm in diameter in a child.

Testicle pain

The testicles, which sit inside the scrotum, are very sensitive.

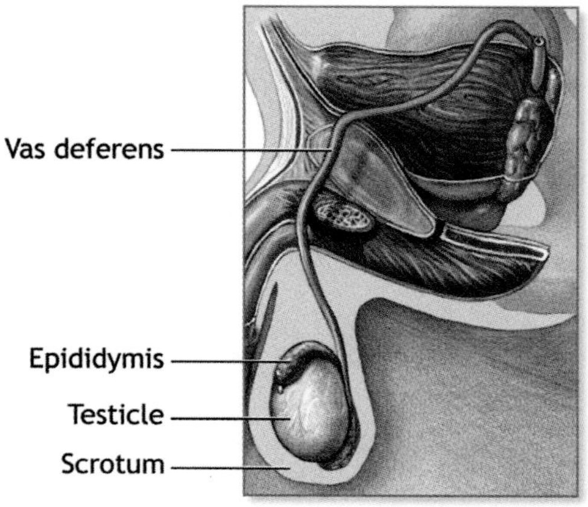

Even a minor injury can cause pain or discomfort. When severe testicle pain begins suddenly, however, it is an emergency.

If a young man has abdominal pain, the scrotum should always be carefully examined. Abdominal pain may occur before testicle pain in some conditions, such as testicular torsion. This is a twisting of the testicles that can cut off their blood supply, causing tissue to die within hours. If tissue does die, then fertility may be affected, and the testicle may have to be removed.

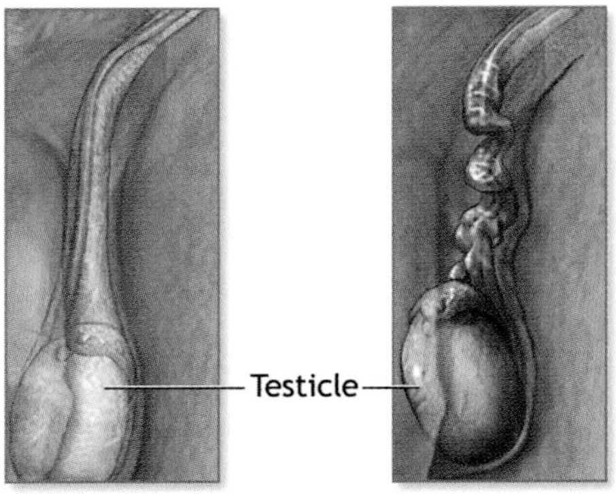

Testicular cancer is usually painless. But any testicle lump should be evaluated by your doctor, whether or not there is pain.

Common causes of testicle pain include:

- Injury
- Infection or inflammation
- Testicular torsion – most common in young men between 10 and 20 years old

Possible infections include:

- **Epididymitis** – inflammation of the ducts through which sperm leaves the testicle. This is often caused by bacteria like chlamydia, a sexually transmitted disease.
- **Orchitis** – inflammation of one or both testicles, which may be caused by bacteria or a virus like mumps. Orchitis can occur at the same time as epididymitis or prostatitis (inflammation of the prostate gland).

Fluid in the testicles often causes painless swelling, but may cause mild discomfort. There are several main types of fluid collection:

- **Varicocele** – enlarged veins in the scrotum that carry blood away from the testicles.

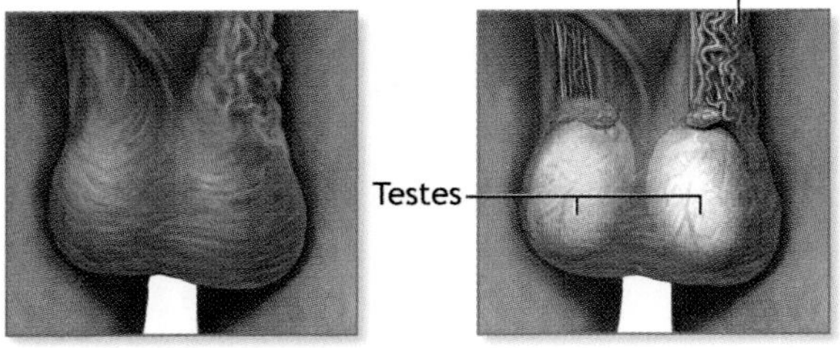

A varicocele can be felt and sometimes seen as a tortuous mass on the surface of the scrotum

A varicocele has veins that contain inadequate valves

- **Spermatocele** – fluid in the epididymis that forms a cyst and often contains dead sperm cells.

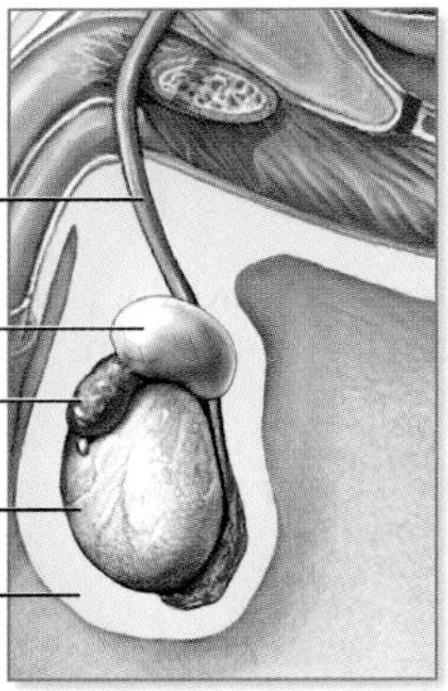

- **Hydrocele** – fluid in the area inside the scrotum, surrounding the testicle; common in newborns.

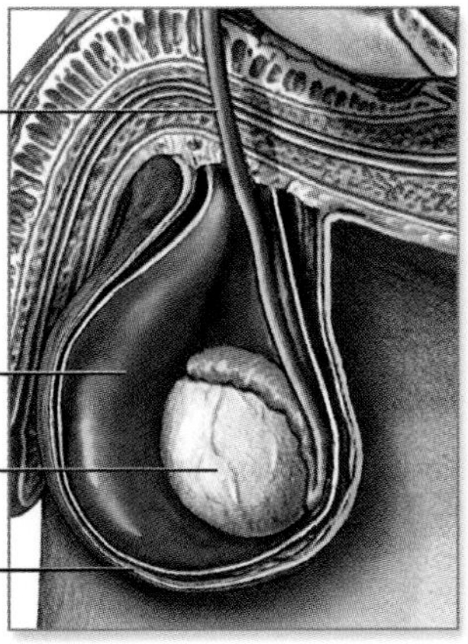

Pain may also be caused by a hernia or an unrelieved erection.

Home care

Some causes of testicle pain can lead to infertility if not treated promptly. Testicular torsion is an emergency, and needs to be treated within a few hours. Infections also should be examined and treated right away as well. If the infection is caused by a bacteria, your doctor will prescribe an antibiotic.

For non-urgent causes of testicle pain, including minor injuries and fluid collection, the following home care steps may reduce discomfort and swelling. These steps will also help if you have an infection.

- Provide support to the scrotum by wearing an athletic supporter.
- Apply ice to the scrotum.
- Take warm baths if there are signs of inflammation.
- While lying down, place a rolled towel under your scrotum.
- Try over-the-counter pain relievers, like acetaminophen or ibuprofen. DO NOT give aspirin to children.

When to contact a medical professional

Call your doctor immediately or go to an emergency room if:

- Your pain is severe or sudden.
- You have had an injury or trauma to the scrotum, and you still have pain or swelling after one hour.
- Your pain is accompanied by nausea or vomiting.

Also call your doctor right away if:

- You feel a lump in the scrotum.
- You have a fever.
- Your scrotum is warm, tender to the touch, or red.
- You have been in contact with someone who has the mumps.

Prevention

- Prevent injury by wearing an athletic supporter during physical activities.
- Prevent sexually transmitted diseases by wearing condoms. See *Safe Sex*.
- Perform testicular self-exams monthly if you are at risk for testicular cancer. See *Testicular Self-Exam*.
- Make sure that children have received the MMR vaccine (a combination vaccine for mumps, measles, and rubella).

Thrush

Thrush is caused by a fungus called *Candida albicans*. This organism lives in your mouth and is usually kept in check by healthy organisms that also live there. However, when your resistance to infection is low, the fungus can grow, leading to lesions in your mouth and on your tongue.

Oral thrush

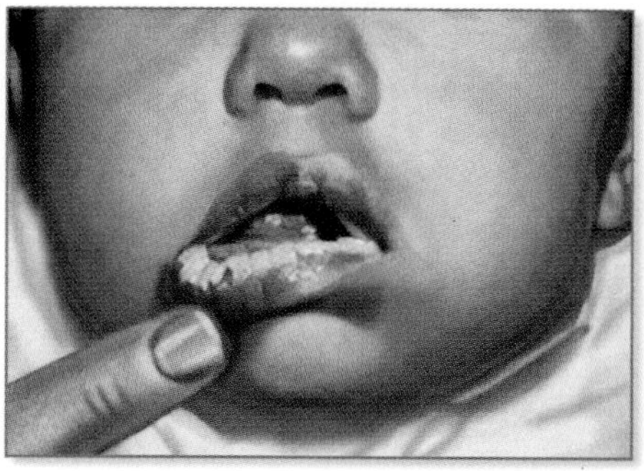

The following can lessen your resistance to infection and increase your chances of getting thrush:

- Taking antibiotics or steroid medications
- Having HIV or AIDS
- Receiving chemotherapy for cancer or drugs to suppress your immune system following an organ transplant
- Being very old or very young

- Being in poor health
- Having diabetes

Thrush is commonly seen in infants. It is not considered abnormal in infants unless it lasts longer than a couple weeks.

Symptoms

Thrush appears as whitish, velvety plaques in the mouth and on the tongue. Underneath the whitish material, there is red tissue that may bleed. The lesions can slowly increase in number and size.

Home care

For thrush in infants, treatment is often NOT necessary. It generally resolves on its own within two weeks.

There are two goals when treating oral thrush in adults. The first is to improve your immune system's ability to function. For example, in diabetics, good control of the diabetes may be enough to clear the infection without other treatment.

The second is to directly treat the infection. For this purpose, your doctor may prescribe an antifungal mouthwash or lozenges to suck on. These are usually used for 5-10 days. If they don't work, other medication may be prescribed.

When to contact a medical professional

Call your doctor if:

- Your infant has had lesions in the mouth consistent with thrush for at least 2 weeks.
- Your infant is eating poorly due to the lesions.
- You are a teen or adult with lesions that are consistent with thrush.
- You have pain or difficulty swallowing.
- You are HIV positive, are receiving chemotherapy, or take medications to suppress your immune system.

Prevention

If you have frequent outbreaks of thrush, your doctor may recommend taking antifungal medication on a regular basis to avoid recurrent infections.

If an infant with thrush is breast-feeding, talk to your doctor about ways to prevent future infections, such as an antifungal medication. Sterilize or discard any pacifiers. For bottle-fed babies with thrush, discard the nipples and buy new ones as the baby's mouth begins to clear.

Tired, lack of energy

Fatigue is a feeling of weariness, tiredness, or lack of energy.

Fatigue is different from drowsiness. In general, drowsiness is feeling the need to sleep, while fatigue is a lack of energy and motivation. Drowsiness and apathy (a feeling of indifference or not caring about what happens) can be symptoms of fatigue.

Fatigue can be a normal and important response to physical exertion, emotional stress, boredom, or lack of sleep. However, it can also be a nonspecific sign of a more serious psychological or physical disorder. When fatigue is not relieved by enough sleep, good nutrition, or a low-stress environment, it should be evaluated by your doctor. Because fatigue is a common complaint, sometimes a potentially serious cause may be overlooked.

Home care

Here are some tips for reducing fatigue:

- Get adequate, regular, and consistent amounts of sleep each night.
- Eat a healthy, well-balanced diet and drink plenty of water throughout the day.
- Exercise regularly.
- Learn better ways to relax. Try yoga or meditation.

- Maintain a reasonable work and personal schedule.
- Change your stressful circumstances, if possible. For example, switch jobs, take a vacation, and deal directly with problems in a relationship.
- Take a multivitamin. Talk to your doctor about what is best for you.
- Avoid alcohol, nicotine, and drug use.

If you have chronic pain or depression, treating either often helps address the fatigue. However, some antidepressant medications may cause or worsen fatigue. Your medication may have to be adjusted to avoid this problem. DO NOT stop or change any medications without instruction from your doctor.

Stimulants (including caffeine) are NOT effective treatments for fatigue, and can actually make the problem worse when the drugs are stopped. Sedatives also tend to worsen fatigue in the long run.

When to contact a medical professional

Call your doctor right away if:

- You are confused or dizzy.
- You have blurred vision.
- You have little to no urine, or recent swelling and weight gain.

Call your doctor if:

- You have ongoing, unexplained weakness or fatigue, especially if accompanied by fever or unintentional weight loss.
- You have constipation, dry skin, weight gain, or intolerance to cold.
- You wake up and fall back to sleep multiple times through the night.
- You have headaches.
- You are taking any medications, prescription or non-prescription, or using drugs that may cause fatigue or drowsiness.
- You feel sad or depressed.
- You have insomnia.

TMJ disorders

The temporomandibular joints (TMJs) connect your lower jaw to your skull.

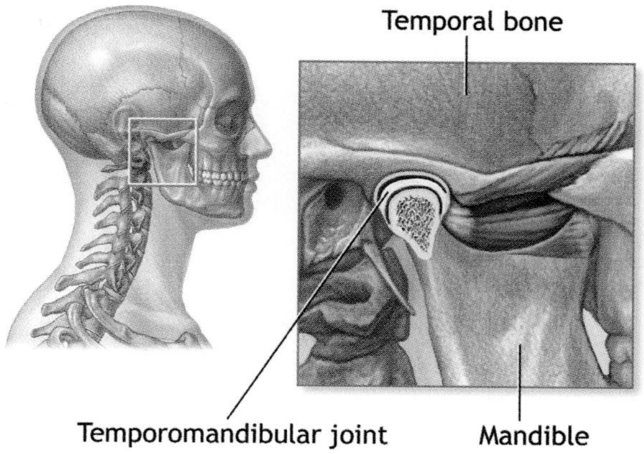

There are two matching joints – one on each side of your head, located just in front of your ears. The abbreviation "TMJ" literally refers to the joint but is often used to refer to any disorders or symptoms of this region. Such problems include popping sounds in the jaw, inability to fully open the mouth, jaw pain, headaches, earaches, toothaches, and various other types of facial pain.

Many TMJ-related symptoms are caused by the effects of physical and emotional stress on the structures around the joint. These structures include the muscles of the jaw, face, and neck; the teeth; the cartilage disc at the joint; and nearby ligaments, blood vessels, and nerves.

For example, daily stress can lead you to clench and grind your teeth, both during the day and at night while you sleep. Clenching means you tightly clamp your top and bottom teeth together, especially the back teeth. The stressful force of clenching causes pressure on the muscles, tissues, and other structures around your jaw.

Many people who clench also grind their teeth. Grinding is when you slide your teeth over each other, generally in a sideways, back-and-forth movement. This action may wear down your teeth and be noisy enough at night to bother sleeping partners.

Poor posture can also be an important factor. For example, holding your head forward while looking at a computer all day strains the muscles of the face and neck.

Other factors that might aggravate TMJ symptoms are inability to relax, poor diet, and lack of sleep.

All of these stresses can result in trigger points – contracted muscles and pinched nerves in your jaw, head, and neck. Trigger points can refer pain to other areas, causing a headache, earache, or toothache.

Home care

Simple, gentle therapies are usually recommended first. If those don't work, mouth guards and more aggressive treatments may be considered. Surgery is generally considered a last resort. Fortunately, there are many steps you can take at home long before that point.

Try massaging the various muscles that may be involved. Probe all of the muscles of the face, shoulders, and back of the neck (avoid the area around the throat). Press on the muscles to identify extremely painful points. Remember that muscles may refer pain to another location, and the muscle itself may not be painful until it is actually pressed hard. Massage the painful area with hard, slow, short strokes. Do this several times a day until the muscle is no longer painful when pressed.

To massage the masseter muscles on each side of your jaw, place your thumb inside your mouth and squeeze the thick muscle in your cheek (toward the back of your mouth) with your fingers. To get at the harder-to-reach jaw muscles inside your mouth, use your index finger to probe for tender areas behind the teeth, and use the finger to massage these spots. (The masseter muscle is illustrated on page 215.)

Here are some other steps to consider:

- Maintain good posture while working at a computer, watching TV, and reading. Take frequent breaks to relieve stressed muscles.
- Make a habit of relaxing your facial and jaw muscles throughout the day.
- Avoid eating hard foods, like nuts, candies, and steak.
- Drink plenty of water every day and get plenty of sleep.
- Learn relaxation techniques to reduce overall stress and muscle tension in your back, neck, and body.

Two excellent books are *Taking Control of TMJ* by Robert Uppgaard and *The Trigger Point Therapy Workbook* by Clair Davies.

When to contact a medical professional

See a TMJ specialist immediately if you are having trouble eating or opening your mouth. Keep in mind that a wide variety of possible conditions can cause TMJ symptoms, from arthritis to whiplash injuries. Therefore, see a TMJ specialist for a full evaluation if self-care measures do not help within several weeks.

TMJ problems do not fall clearly into one medical discipline, and TMJ specialists have a wide variety of treatment approaches. If you are interested in a massage-based approach, look for a massage or physical therapist trained in trigger point therapy, neuromuscular therapy (NMT), clinical massage or pain relief, particularly as it applies to TMJ pain.

Dentists who specialize in evaluating and treating TMJ disorders will typically perform x-ray exams and prescribe a mouth guard. Surgery is now considered a last resort by the vast majority of TMJ experts.

Tremors

A tremor is an involuntary movement or shaking of any body part (even your head or voice may be involved). It is often most noticeable in your hands. There are three main types of tremors:

- Resting or static tremors – occur when your hand or affected body part is at rest.
- Intention tremors – occur when you are moving your hand or affected body part and disappear at rest.
- Postural tremors – occur when you are holding your hand or affected body part in a particular position for a period of time.

Tremors may be caused by:

- Too much coffee or other caffeinated drink
- Excessive alcohol consumption, alcoholism, or alcohol withdrawal
- Stress, anxiety, or fatigue – these can cause a postural tremor
- Normal aging
- A variety of drugs and prescription medicines
- Low blood sugar
- Parkinson's disease – this is the classic cause of a resting tremor and is often accompanied by slowness of movement, muscle rigidity, and an abnormal gait
- Multiple sclerosis – can cause an intention tremor
- Over active thyroid – can cause a postural tremor

Home care

For tremors caused by stress, try relaxation techniques like meditation, deep relaxation, or breathing exercises. For tremors of any cause, avoid caffeine and get enough sleep.

For tremors caused by a medication, consult with your doctor about stopping the drug, reducing the dosage, or switching medications. DO NOT change or stop medications on your own.

For tremors caused by alcohol abuse, seek treatment and support to help you avoid alcohol.

Severe tremors may interfere with your ability to perform daily activities. Assistance with these activities may be necessary. Precautions should be taken to avoid injury during activities such as walking or eating.

When to contact a medical professional

Call your doctor if:

- Your tremor is worse at rest and gets better with movement, like when you reach for something.
- Your tremors are prolonged, severe, or interfere with your life.
- Your tremors occur with other symptoms, like headache, weakness, abnormal tongue motion, or other types of involuntary movements.

Ulcers

Ulcers are erosions in the lining of the stomach or duodenum (the first part of the small intestines). An ulcer in the stomach is called a **gastric ulcer**. An ulcer in the duodenum is called a **duodenal ulcer**. Together, ulcers of the stomach and duodenum are referred to as **peptic ulcers**.

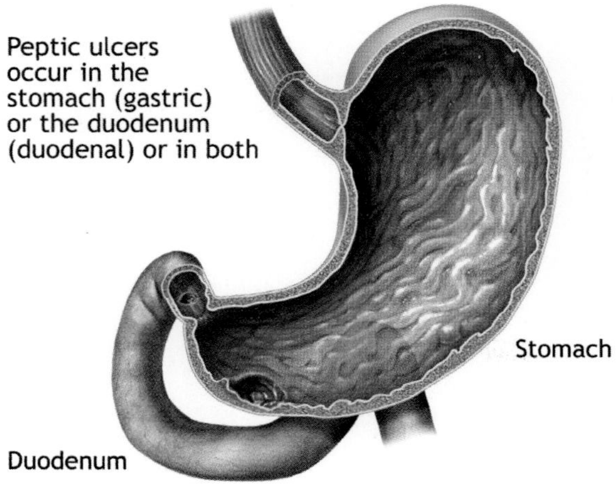
Peptic ulcers occur in the stomach (gastric) or the duodenum (duodenal) or in both
Stomach
Duodenum

Most ulcers are erosions of the first layer of the inner lining. If the hole goes all the way through, this is called a perforation of the intestinal lining. This can cause shock and is a medical emergency.

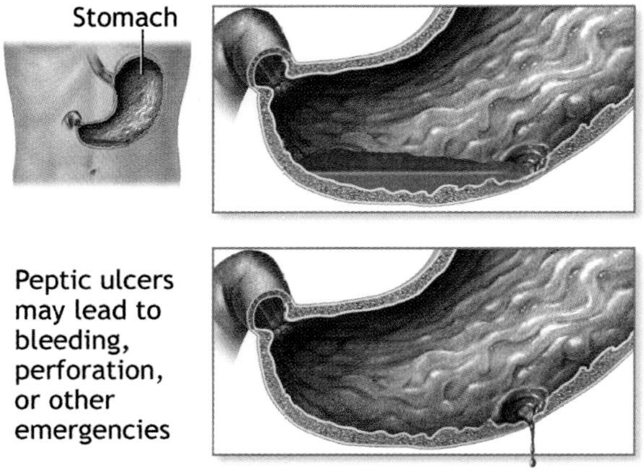

Stomach
Peptic ulcers may lead to bleeding, perforation, or other emergencies

Normally, the lining of the stomach and small intestines have protection against the irritating acids produced in your stomach. For a variety of reasons, the protective mechanisms may become faulty, leading to a breakdown of the lining. This results in inflammation (gastritis) or an ulcer.

The most common cause of such damage is a bacterium called *Helicobacter pylori*. Most people with peptic ulcers have this organism living in their gastrointestinal (GI) tract. On the other hand, many people have this organism living in their GI tract but they don't get an ulcer.

> **KEY POINT**
>
> Most ulcers are caused by a bacterium called *H. pylori*. Do what it takes to treat the organism correctly now. (In other words, follow your doctor's instructions carefully and take all of the recommended medication.) It's more effective than partially treating it now, and having to treat it again later on.

Other factors can make it more likely for you to get an ulcer, including:

- Using aspirin, ibuprofen, or naproxen
- Drinking alcohol excessively
- Smoking cigarettes and using tobacco

A once popular belief was that stress causes ulcers. This is not true. Stress may make you experience more pain from an ulcer and it may make it more difficult to heal from an ulcer. But, stress does not cause an ulcer.

SYMPTOMS

Abdominal pain is the main symptom. It may awaken you at night, occur 2-3 hours after you eat, or get worse if you skip a meal. The pain may be relieved by antacids or milk.

Other possible symptoms include:

- Nausea, vomiting
- Weight loss
- Fatigue
- Heartburn, indigestion, belching
- Chest pain
- Vomiting blood
- Bloody or dark tarry stools

It is important to note that you may have no symptoms at all from an ulcer.

HOME CARE

You should see a doctor if you have symptoms of an ulcer. Treatment often involves a combination of medications to kill the *Helicobacter pylori* bacteria, reduce acid levels, and protect the GI tract. This combination strategy allows your ulcer to heal and reduces the chance it will come back. Take all of your medications exactly as prescribed.

WHEN TO CONTACT A MEDICAL PROFESSIONAL

Call 911 if you:

- Suddenly develop sharp abdominal pain.
- Have symptoms of shock like fainting, excessive sweating, or confusion.

- Are vomiting blood or have blood in your stool (especially if maroon or dark, tarry black)
- Have a rigid, hard abdomen that is tender to touch.

Call your doctor if:

- You have ulcer symptoms.
- You feel dizzy or lightheaded.
- Your symptoms worsen with antacids.

Prevention

- Don't smoke or chew tobacco.
- Limit alcohol.
- Avoid aspirin, ibuprofen, and naproxen. Try acetaminophen instead.
- Eat several small meals a day at regular intervals.
- Limit coffee (both caffeinated and decaffeinated), black tea, and cola.

Urinary Tract Infections

A urinary tract infection, or UTI, is an infection that can happen anywhere along the urinary tract – the kidneys, the ureters (the tubes that take urine from each kidney to the bladder), the bladder, or the urethra (the tube that empties urine from the bladder to the outside).

Normal anatomy of the urinary tract

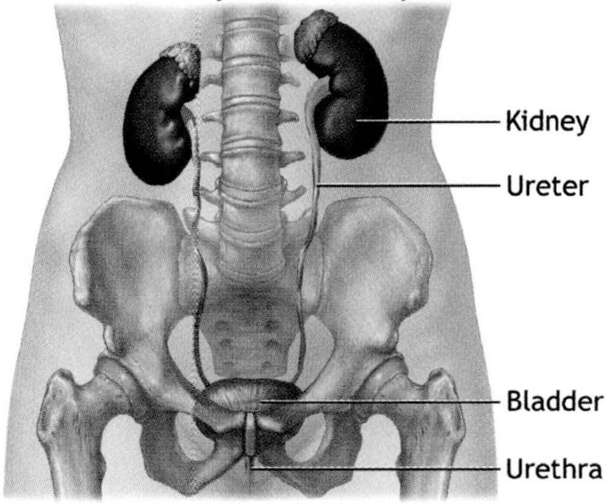

Cystitis, a common condition, is usually caused by a bacteria from the anus entering the urethra and then the bladder. This leads to inflammation and infection in the lower urinary tract.

Certain people are more likely to get UTIs. Women tend to get them more often because their urethra is shorter and closer to the anus. Elderly people (especially those in nursing homes) and people with diabetes also get more UTIs.

In addition, the following risk factors increase the chances of getting a UTI:

- Pregnancy and menopause
- Kidney Stones
- Sexual intercourse, especially if you have multiple partners or use a diaphragm for birth control
- Prostate inflammation or enlargement
- Narrowed urethra
- Immobility (for example, during recovery from a hip fracture)
- Not drinking enough fluids
- Bowel incontinence
- Catheterization

Some children develop UTIs. In boys, they are most common before the first birthday. UTIs are more common among uncircumcised boys. In young girls, UTIs are most common around age 3, overlapping with the toilet training period.

Cystitis in children can be promoted by abnormalities in the urinary tract. Therefore, children with cystitis, especially those under age 5, deserve special follow-up to prevent later kidney damage.

Symptoms

The symptoms of a UTI include:

- Pressure in the lower pelvis
- Pain or burning with urination

- Frequent or urgent need to urinate
- Need to urinate at night
- Cloudy urine
- Blood in the urine
- Foul or strong urine odor

Young children with UTIs may only have a fever, or even no symptoms at all.

> **Tip**
>
> If UTIs happen frequently, first determine with your doctor if there is an underlying reason. Then, follow the steps in the Prevention section of this article to avoid getting them so often.

Home care

A mild case of cystitis may resolve on its own without treatment. Because of the risk of the infection spreading to the kidneys, however, antibiotics are usually recommended. It is important that you finish the entire course of prescribed antibiotics.

In children, cystitis should be treated promptly with antibiotics to protect their developing kidneys. In the elderly, prompt treatment is recommended due to the greater chances of fatal complications.

When to contact a medical professional

Call your doctor if you, or your child, have symptoms of a UTI. Call right away if there is fever or chills, back or side pain, or vomiting. These symptoms suggest a possible kidney infection.

Also call if:

- You have diabetes or are pregnant.
- There is discharge from the penis or vagina.
- The penis or vagina is painful, or sexual intercourse is painful.
- You suspect a child may have been sexually abused.
- There is blood or pus in the urine.
- The symptoms come back a short time after treatment with antibiotics.

Prevention

- Keep your genital area clean.
- Wipe from front to back.
- Drink plenty of fluids.
- Urinate after sexual intercourse.
- Avoid fluids that irritate the bladder, like alcohol and caffeine.
- Drink cranberry juice, but NOT if you have a personal or family history of kidney stones.
- DO NOT douche or use similar feminine hygiene products.
- Wear cloth undergarments.

If you are prone to UTIs, your doctor may recommend taking antibiotics more regularly to prevent infection.

Urination - difficulty with flow

Difficulty starting or maintaining a urinary stream is called urinary hesitancy.

This problem affects people of all ages and occurs in both sexes, but it is most common in older men with enlarged prostate glands.

Almost all older men have some degree of difficulty in starting urination, dribbling, or decreased force of the urinary stream.

Urinary hesitancy can be caused by:

- Benign prostatic hyperplasia (enlarged prostate)
- Urinary tract infection, especially if chronic and recurrent

- Prostatitis (inflammation or infection of the prostate gland)
- Drugs (some cold remedies, some nasal decongestants, tricyclic antidepressants, and anticholinergics which may be used for incontinence)
- Shy or bashful bladder syndrome in younger people (unable to urinate when another person is in the room)
- Neurologic disorders

Home care

- Monitor, record, and report your urination patterns to your doctor.
- Apply heat to your lower abdomen (below your belly button and above the pubic bone). This is where the bladder lies. The heat relaxes muscles and aids urination.
- Massage or place light pressure over your bladder to stimulate emptying.
- Drink plenty of fluid, especially fruit juices like cranberry.
- For infections, antibiotics from your doctor will be needed. Symptoms that suggest a possible infection include burning or pain with urination, frequent urination, cloudy urine, and a sense of urgency (strong, sudden urge to urinate.)

When to contact a medical professional

If you have not been evaluated for this problem previously, you should call your doctor for urinary hesitancy, dribbling, or weak urine stream.

Call your doctor right away if you have fever, vomiting, side or back pain, shaking chills, or passing little urine for 1-2 days.

Call if you have blood in your urine, cloudy urine, frequent or urgent need to urinate, or a discharge from the penis or vagina.

Urination - frequent or urgent

Frequent urination means needing to urinate more often than usual. Urgent urination is a sudden, compelling urge to urinate, along with discomfort in your bladder.

A frequent need to urinate at night is called nocturia. Most people can sleep for 6 to 8 hours without having to urinate. Middle aged and older men often wake to urinate once in the early morning hours.

Together, frequent and urgent urination are classic signs of a urinary tract infection. Since inflammation reduces the bladder's capacity to hold urine, even small amounts of urine cause discomfort.

Diabetes, pregnancy, and prostate problems are other common causes of these symptoms.

Other causes include:

- Interstitial cystitis (an ongoing inflammation of the bladder that is much more common in women than men; often difficult to diagnose and treat)
- Diuretics and many other medications

Common causes of nighttime urination:

- Drinking too much before bedtime, especially caffeine or alcohol
- Enlarged prostate

Home care

Follow the therapy recommended by your doctor to treat the underlying cause of your urinary frequency or urgency. It may help to keep a diary of times and amounts of urine voided to bring with you to the doctor.

In some cases, you may experience some urinary incontinence for a period of time. You may need to take steps to protect your clothing and bedding.

When to contact a medical professional

Call your doctor right away if:

- You have fever, back or side pain, vomiting, or shaking chills.
- You have increased thirst or appetite, fatigue, or sudden weight loss.

Also call your doctor if:

- You have urinary frequency or urgency, but you are not pregnant and you are not drinking excessive amounts of fluid.
- You have incontinence or have altered your lifestyle because of your symptoms.
- You have bloody or cloudy urine.
- There is a discharge from the penis or vagina.

Urinary incontinence

Incontinence is the inability to control the passage of urine. This can range from an occasional leakage of urine, to a complete inability to hold any urine.

The two main types of urinary incontinence are:

- **Stress incontinence** – occurs during certain activities like coughing, sneezing, laughing, or exercise.
- **Urge incontinence** – involves a strong, sudden need to urinate followed by instant bladder contraction and involuntary loss of urine. You don't have enough time between when you recognize the need to urinate and when you actually do urinate.

Bowel incontinence, a separate topic, is the inability to control the passage of stool.

Incontinence is most common among the elderly. Women are more likely than men to have urinary incontinence.

Infants and children are not considered incontinent, but merely untrained, up to the time of toilet training. Occasional accidents are not unusual in children up to age 6 years. Young (and sometimes teenage) girls may have slight leakage of urine when laughing.

Nighttime urination in children is normal until the age of 5 or 6.

Incontinence may be sudden and temporary, or ongoing and long-term. Causes of sudden or temporary incontinence include:

- Urinary tract infection or inflammation
- Prostate infection or inflammation
- Stool impaction from severe constipation, causing pressure on the bladder
- Side effects of medications (such as diuretics, tranquilizers, some cough and cold remedies, certain antihistamines for allergies, and antidepressants)
- Increased urine amounts, like with poorly controlled diabetes
- Pregnancy
- Weight gain
- Short-term bedrest – for example, when recovering from surgery
- Mental confusion

Causes that may be more long-term:

- Spinal injuries
- Urinary tract anatomical abnormalities
- Neurological conditions like multiple sclerosis or stroke
- Weakness of the sphincter, the circular muscles of the bladder responsible for opening and closing it; this can happen following prostate surgery in men, or vaginal surgery in women
- Pelvic prolapse in women – falling or sliding of the bladder, urethra, or rectum into the vaginal space, often related to having had multiple pregnancies and deliveries
- Large prostate in men

- Depression or Alzheimer's disease
- Nerve or muscle damage after pelvic radiation
- Bladder cancer
- Bladder spasms

Home care

See your doctor for an initial evaluation and to come up with a treatment plan. Treatment options vary, depending on the cause and type of incontinence you have. Fortunately, there are many things you can do to help manage incontinence.

The following methods are used to strengthen the muscles of your pelvic floor:

- **Bladder retraining** – this involves urinating on a schedule, whether you feel a need to go or not. In between those times, you try to wait to the next scheduled time. At first, you may need to schedule 1 hour intervals. Gradually, you can increase by 1/2 hour intervals until you are only urinating every 3-4 hours without leakage.
- **Kegel exercises** – contract the pelvic floor muscles for 10 seconds, then relax them for 10 seconds. Repeat 10 times. Do these exercises 3 times per day. You can do Kegel exercises any time, any place.

To find the pelvic muscles when you first start Kegel exercises, stop your urine flow midstream. The muscles needed to do this are your pelvic floor muscles. DO NOT contract your abdominal, thigh, or buttocks muscles. And DO NOT overdo the exercises. This may tire the muscles out and actually worsen incontinence.

Two methods called biofeedback and electrical stimulation can help you learn how to perform Kegel exercises. Biofeedback uses electrodes placed on the pelvic floor muscles, giving you feedback about when they are contracted and when they are not. Electrical stimulation uses low-voltage electric current to stimulate the pelvic floor muscles. It can be done at home or at a clinic for 20 minutes every 1 to 4 days.

Biofeedback and electrical stimulation will no longer be necessary once you have identified the pelvic floor muscles and mastered the exercises on your own.

Vaginal cones enhance the performance of Kegel exercises for women. Other devices for incontinence are also available.

For leakage, wear absorbent pads or undergarments. There are many well-designed products that go completely unnoticed by anyone but you.

Other measures include:

- Regulate your bowels to avoid constipation. Try increasing fiber in your diet.
- Quit smoking to reduce coughing and bladder irritation. Smoking also increases your risk of bladder cancer.
- Avoid alcohol and caffeinated beverages, particularly coffee, which can overstimulate your bladder.
- Lose weight if you need to.
- Avoid foods and drinks that may irritate your bladder like spicy foods, carbonated beverages, and citrus fruits and juices. Keep blood sugars under good control if you have diabetes.

Your doctor may recommend medication or surgery, especially if home care measures are not helping or if your symptoms are getting worse.

Performing Kegel exercises while you are pregnant and soon after delivery may help prevent incontinence related to childbirth.

When to contact a medical professional

Discuss incontinence with your doctor. Gynecologists and urologists are the specialists most familiar with this condition. They can evaluate the causes and recommend treatment approaches.

Call 911 or go to an emergency room if any of the following accompany a sudden loss of urine control:

- Difficulty talking, walking, or speaking
- Sudden weakness, numbness, or tingling in an arm or leg
- Loss of vision
- Loss of consciousness or confusion
- Loss of bowel control

Call your doctor if:

- You have been constipated for more than one week.
- You have difficulty starting your urine flow, dribbling, nighttime urination, pain or burning with urination, increased frequency or urgency, or cloudy or bloody urine.
- You are taking medications that may be causing incontinence. DO NOT adjust or stop any medications without talking to your doctor.
- You are over 60 years old and your incontinence is new, especially if you are also having trouble with your memory or caring for yourself.
- You have the urge to go often, but are only passing small amounts of urine.
- Your bladder feels full even after you have just urinated.
- Incontinence persists for more than 2 weeks even with exercises to strengthen your pelvic muscles.

URINE - BLOODY

Blood in your urine can turn toilet water pale pink or bright red. Or, you may just see spots of blood in the water after urinating.

In women, blood may appear to be in the urine when it is actually coming from the vagina. In men, what may be mistaken for urinary bleeding is sometimes a bloody ejaculation, usually due to a prostate problem.

Discoloration from certain drugs, beets, or other foods can mimic blood in the urine.

You may not see blood in your urine. In some cases, it is found microscopically when your doctor checks your urine during a routine exam. Your doctor will follow up on this problem to see if it persists and identify the cause.

When blood is visible to the naked eye, prompt and thorough evaluation is always needed. In children, hospitalization is often necessary to complete the work up.

There are many potential causes of blood in the urine. Often, bloody urine is from a problem in your kidneys or other parts of the urinary tract. If your kidneys, urinary tract, prostate, and genitals turn out to be fine, your doctor may check to see if you have a bleeding disorder.

WHEN TO CONTACT A MEDICAL PROFESSIONAL

Blood in the urine should never be ignored. Tell your doctor about this symptom and get an appropriate evaluation, especially if you have unexplained weight loss, burning with urination, frequent urination, or urgent urination.

Call your doctor right away if:

- You have fever, nausea, vomiting, shaking chills, or pain in your abdomen, side, or back.
- You are unable to urinate.
- You are passing blood clots.

VAGINAL DISCHARGE

Substances emitted from the vagina can vary in consistency (thick, pasty, thin), color (clear, cloudy), and smell (normal, odorless, bad odor).

Having some amount of vaginal discharge is normal, especially if you are of childbearing age. Glands in the cervix produce a clear mucus. These secretions may turn white or yellow when exposed to the air. These are all normal variations.

The amount of mucus produced by the cervical glands varies throughout the menstrual cycle. This is normal and depends on the amount of estrogen circulating in your body.

Vaginal discharge that suddenly differs in color, odor, or consistency, or significantly increases or decreases in amount, may indicate an underlying problem like an infection. If abnormal vaginal discharge is due to a sexually transmitted disease (STD), your sexual partner(s) will likely require treatment as well.

The following situations can increase the amount of normal vaginal discharge:

- Sexual excitement
- Emotional stress
- Ovulation (when you produce and release an egg from your ovary in the middle of your menstrual cycle)

These conditions can lead to abnormal vaginal discharge:

- Vaginal yeast infection – the discharge is generally cheesy white with redness and itching. Vaginal yeast infections may be related to antibiotics, birth control or other estrogen pills, pregnancy, diabetes, or a weakened immune system.
- Bacterial vaginosis – an infection that causes a grey discharge and fishy odor that worsen after sexual intercourse.
- Trichomonas – a sexually-transmitted parasite that causes yellowish-grey or green discharge and intense itching.
- Other infections and sexually transmitted diseases like chlamydia or gonorrhea.
- Forgotten tampon or foreign body.

Home care

To help prevent and treat vaginal discharge:

- Keep your genital area clean and dry.
- Avoid douching. While many women feel cleaner if they douche after menstruation or intercourse, it may actually worsen vaginal discharge because it removes healthy bacteria lining the vagina that are there to protect you from infection.
- Use an over-the-counter cream or vaginal suppository, IF you know that you have a yeast infection.
- Try to reduce stress.
- Eat yogurt with live cultures or take *Lactobacillus acidophilus* tablets when on antibiotics to avoid a yeast infection.
- Use condoms to avoid catching or spreading sexually transmitted diseases.
- Keep your blood sugars under good control if you have diabetes.

If the discharge is caused by a sexually transmitted disease, your sexual partner (or partners) must be treated as well, even if they have no symptoms. Failure of partners to accept treatment can cause continual reinfection which may lead to a serious problem like infertility.

When to contact a medical professional

Call your doctor right away if:

- Your discharge is associated with fever or pain in your pelvis or abdomen.
- You have been exposed to a sexual partner with gonorrhea, chlamydia, or other sexually transmitted disease.
- You have increased thirst or appetite, unexplained weight loss, increased urinary frequency, or fatigue – these may be signs of diabetes.

Also call if:

- A child who has not reached puberty has vaginal discharge.

- You think that your discharge may be related to a medication.
- You are concerned that you may have a sexually transmitted disease or you are unsure of possible exposure.
- Your symptoms worsen or last longer than 1 week despite home care measures.
- You have blisters or other lesions on your vagina or vulva.
- You have burning with urination or other urinary symptoms – you may have a urinary tract infection.

Vaginal itching

Common causes of vaginal itching include:

- **Chemical irritants** – such as detergents, fabric softeners, feminine sprays, ointments, creams, douches, and contraceptive foams or jellies.
- **Vaginal yeast infection** – often includes a discharge that is white and curd-like. Vaginal yeast infections can be caused by antibiotics, birth control pills, pregnancy, diabetes, and weakened immune system.
- **Vaginitis** – inflammation, itching, discharge, and odor caused by other infections (including sexually transmitted diseases). Vaginitis in girls before puberty is common. If a young girl has a sexually transmitted vaginal infection, however, sexual abuse must be considered and addressed.
- **Menopause** – the drop in estrogen causes thinning of the vaginal wall and less lubrication.
- **Stress** – may increase vaginal itching and make you more susceptible to infections.

Home care

To prevent and treat vaginal itching:

- Keep your genital area clean and dry. Use plain, unscented soap.
- Avoid colored or perfumed toilet tissue and bubble bath.
- Wear cotton panties or pantyhose with a cotton crotch. Avoid panties made from synthetic materials. For infants and toddlers, change diapers often.
- Change out of wet clothing, especially wet bathing suits or exercise clothing, as soon as possible.
- Avoid feminine hygiene sprays and douches.
- Eat yogurt with live cultures or take *lactobacillus acidophilus* tablets when using antibiotics. Check with your doctor.
- Cleanse by wiping or washing from front to back (vagina to anus) after urinating or having a bowel movement.
- Lose weight if you are over weight.
- Keep your blood sugars under good control if you have diabetes.

It is also helpful to:

- Avoid scratching, which will only aggravate the problem.
- Avoid overexertion, heat, and excessive sweating.
- Delay sexual activity until your symptoms get better or at least use a lubricant during intercourse.
- Use condoms to avoid catching or spreading sexually transmitted diseases.

If you know that you have a yeast infection because your symptoms are exactly the same as those in the past, try over-the-counter creams or vaginal suppositories.

Yeast infections are not considered sexually transmitted. However, sometimes men also develop itching and redness following sexual contact. If this is the case or you get recurrent infections for unclear reasons, both you and your partner may require treatment. Talk to your doctor.

For itching related to menopause, your doctor may consider estrogen cream or tablets to insert vaginally.

When to contact a medical professional

Call your doctor right away if:

- You have pelvic or lower abdominal pain or fever.
- You have increased thirst or appetite, unexplained weight loss, frequent urination, or fatigue – these may be signs of diabetes.

Call your doctor if:

- Your symptoms worsen, last longer than 1 week, or recur despite self-care.
- You have unusual vaginal bleeding, swelling, or discharge.
- Your partner also has symptoms or you think you may have a sexually transmitted disease.
- You have burning with urination or other urinary symptoms – you may have a urinary tract infection.
- You have blisters or ulcers on your vagina or vulva.

Vision problems

Changes in vision, blurriness, blind spots, halos around lights, or dimness of vision should always be evaluated by a medical professional. Such changes may represent an eye disease, aging, eye injury, or a condition like diabetes that affects many organs in your body.

Whatever the cause, vision changes should never be ignored. They can get worse and significantly impact the quality of your life. Professional help is always necessary. As you determine which professional to see, the following descriptions may help:

- **Opticians** dispense glasses and do not diagnose eye problems.
- **Optometrists** perform eye exams and may diagnose eye problems. They prescribe glasses and contact lenses. In some states they prescribe eye drops to treat diseases.
- **Ophthalmologists** are doctors who diagnose and treat diseases that affect the eyes. These doctors may also provide routine vision care services, such as prescribing glasses and contact lenses.

Sometimes an eye problem is part of a general health problem. In these situations, your primary care provider should also be involved.

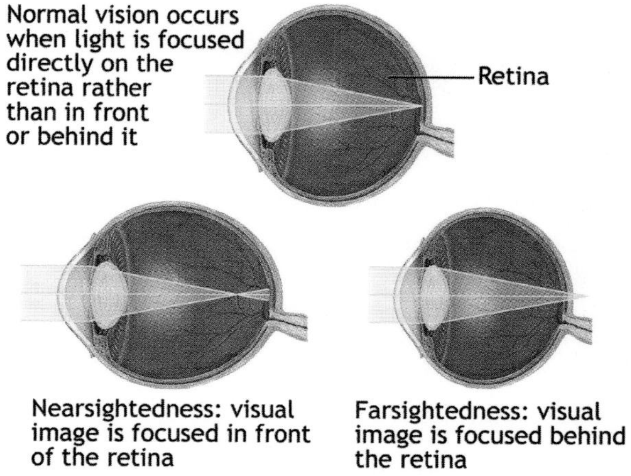
Normal vision occurs when light is focused directly on the retina rather than in front or behind it
Retina
Nearsightedness: visual image is focused in front of the retina
Farsightedness: visual image is focused behind the retina

Nearsightedness (myopia) and farsightedness (presbyopia) are vision conditions in which light is not focused correctly on the retina. Eyeglasses and contacts may be prescribed to correct these problems.

Vision changes and problems can be caused by many different conditions:

- **Presbyopia** – difficulty focusing on objects that are close. Common in the elderly.
- **Cataracts** – cloudiness over the eye's lens, causing poor nighttime vision, halos around lights, and sensitivity to glare. Daytime vision is eventually affected. Common in the elderly.
- **Glaucoma** – increased pressure in the eye, causing poor night vision, blind spots, and loss of vision to either side. A major cause of blindness. Glaucoma can happen gradually or suddenly – if sudden, it's a medical emergency.

- **Diabetic retinopathy** – this complication of diabetes can lead to bleeding into the retina. Another common cause of blindness.
- **Macular degeneration** – loss of central vision, blurred vision (especially while reading), distorted vision (like seeing wavy lines), and colors appearing faded. The most common cause of blindness in people over age 60.
- **Eye infection, inflammation, or injury.**
- **Floaters** – tiny particles drifting across the eye. Although often brief and harmless, they may be a sign of retinal detachment.
- **Retinal detachment** – symptoms include floaters, flashes of light across your visual field, or a sensation of a shade or curtain hanging on one side of your visual field.
- **Optic neuritis** – inflammation of the optic nerve from infection or multiple sclerosis. You may have pain when you move your eye or touch it through the eyelid.
- **Stroke or TIA.**
- **Brain tumor.**
- **Bleeding into the eye.**
- **Temporal arteritis** – inflammation of an artery in the brain that supplies blood to the optic nerve.
- **Migraine headaches** – spots of light, halos, or zigzag patterns are common symptoms prior to the start of the headache. An ophthalmic migraine is when you have only visual symptoms without a headache.

When to contact a medical professional

Call 911 if:

- You experience partial or complete blindness in one or both eyes, even if it is only temporary.
- You experience double vision, even if it is temporary.
- You have a sensation of a shade being pulled over your eyes or a curtain being drawn from the side.

Common causes of vision problems

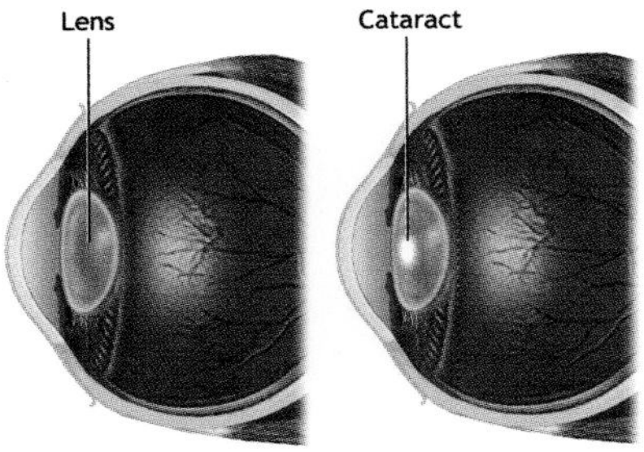

Cataract

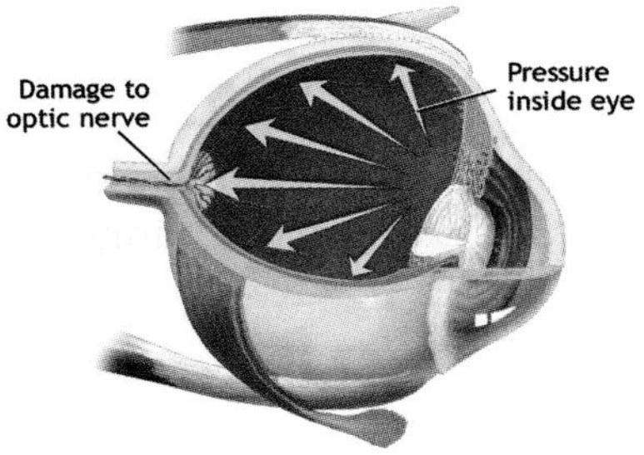

Glaucoma

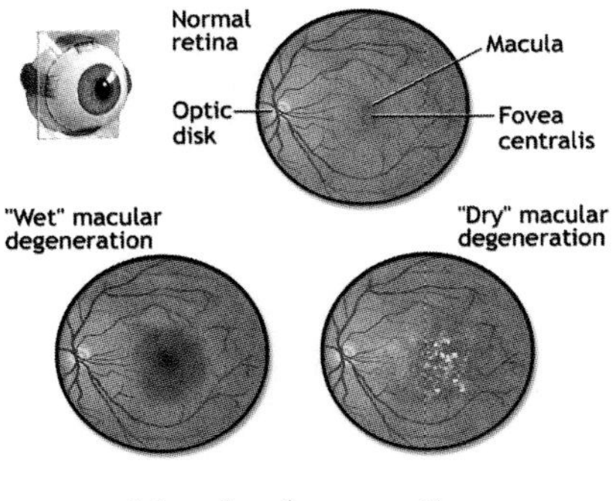

Macular degeneration

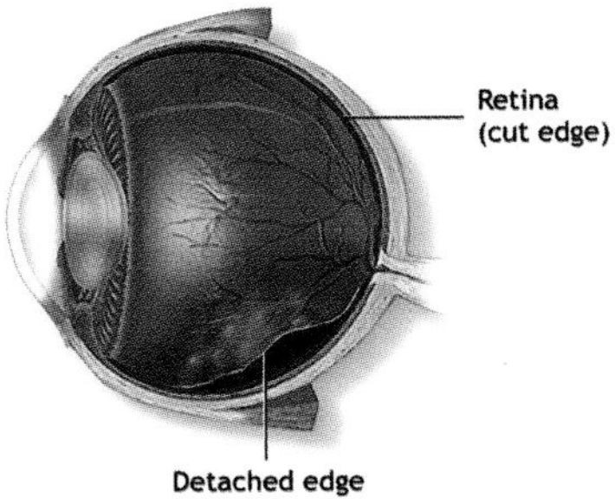

Retinal detachment

- Blind spots, halos around lights, or areas of distorted vision appear suddenly.
- You have eye pain, especially if also red. A red, painful eye is a medical emergency.

Call your provider if you have:

- Trouble seeing objects to either side
- Difficulty seeing at night or when reading
- Gradual loss of the sharpness of your vision
- Difficulty distinguishing colors
- Blurred vision when trying to view objects near or far
- Diabetes or family history of diabetes
- Eye itching or discharge
- Vision changes that seem related to medication (DO NOT stop or change a medication without talking to your doctor)

Prevention

Regular eye checkups from an ophthalmologist or optometrist are important. They should be done once a year if you are over age 65. Your doctor will recommend earlier and more frequent exams if you have diabetes or if you are already showing early signs of eye problems from diabetes, high blood pressure, or other causes.

The pressure in your eyes will be measured at some visits to test for glaucoma. Periodically, your eyes will be dilated to examine the retina for any signs of problems from aging, high blood pressure, or diabetes.

These important steps can prevent eye and vision problems:

- Wear sunglasses to protect your eyes.
- Don't smoke.
- Limit how much alcohol you drink.
- Keep your blood pressure and cholesterol under control.
- Keep your blood sugars under control if you have diabetes.
- Eat foods rich in antioxidants, like green leafy vegetables.

Vomiting and upset stomach

Nausea is the sensation of having an urge to vomit. Vomiting is forcing the contents of the stomach up through the esophagus and out of the mouth.

Your body has a few main ways to respond to an ever-changing, wide variety of invaders and irritants. Sneezing ejects the intruders from the nose, coughing from the lungs and throat, diarrhea from the intestines, and vomiting from the stomach.

Vomiting is a forceful action accomplished by a fierce, downward contraction of the diaphragm. At the same time, the abdominal muscles tighten against a relaxed stomach with an open sphincter. The contents of the stomach are propelled up and out.

Vomiting is a complex, coordinated reflex orchestrated by the vomiting center of the brain. It responds to signals coming from:

- The mouth, stomach, and intestines
- The bloodstream, which may contain medicines or infections
- The balancing systems in the ear (motion sickness)
- The brain itself, including unsettling sights, smells, or thoughts

An amazing variety of stimuli can trigger vomiting, from migraines to kidney stones. Sometimes, just seeing someone else vomit will start you vomiting, in your body's effort to protect you from possible exposure to the same danger.

Vomiting is common. Almost all children will vomit several times during their childhood. In most cases, it is due to a viral gastrointestinal infection.

"Spitting up," the gentle sloshing of stomach contents up and out of the mouth, sometimes with a burp, is an entirely different process. Some spitting up is normal for babies, and usually gets gradually better over time. Worsening spit up might be reflux disease. Discuss this with your child's doctor.

Most of the time, nausea and vomiting do not require urgent medical attention. However, if the symptoms continue for days, they are severe, or you cannot keep down any food or fluids, they may be signs of a more serious condition.

Dehydration is the main concern with most vomiting. How fast you become dehydrated depends on your size, frequency of vomiting, and whether you also have diarrhea.

Home care

It is important to stay hydrated. Try steady, small amounts of clear liquids, such as electrolyte solutions. Other clear liquids, such as water, ginger ale, or fruit juices also work unless the vomiting is severe or a baby is vomiting.

For breastfed babies, breastmilk is usually best. Formula-fed babies usually need clear liquids.

Don't drink too much at one time. Stretching the stomach can make nausea and vomiting worse. Avoid solid foods until there has been no vomiting for six hours, and then work slowly back to a normal diet.

An over-the-counter bismuth stomach remedy like Pepto-Bismol is effective for upset stomach, nausea, indigestion, and diarrhea. Because it contains aspirin-like salicylates, it should NOT be used in children or teenagers who might have (or recently had) chickenpox or the flu.

Most vomiting comes from mild viral illnesses. Nevertheless, if you suspect the vomiting is from something serious, the person may need to be seen immediately.

> **Key point**
>
> It's hard to sit in a waiting room while vomiting. Learn when you can manage this at home, when you really need to be seen, and what steps you can take to prevent needing to go to the doctor or emergency room.

When to contact a medical professional

Call 911 or go to an emergency room if you think vomiting is from poisoning or a child has taken aspirin.

Call if the person has:

- Vomiting longer than 24 hours
- Blood or bile in the vomit
- Severe abdominal pain
- Headache and stiff neck
- Signs of dehydration

Signs of dehydration include:

- Increased thirst
- Infrequent urination or dark yellow urine
- Dry mouth
- Eyes that appear sunken
- Crying without tears
- Loss of normal skin elasticity (if you touch or squeeze the skin, it doesn't bounce back the way it usually does)

You should also call if:

- A young child is lethargic or has marked irritability
- An infant is vomiting repeatedly
- A child is unable to retain any fluids for 8 hours or more
- The vomiting is recurrent
- An adult is unable to retain any fluids for 12 hours or more

- Nausea persists for a prolonged period of time (in a person who is not pregnant)

Prevention

A number of medicines are effective at preventing vomiting. Your doctor is unlikely to prescribe these because, in most situations, the vomiting is an important part of getting well. In some situations, however, preventing the vomiting makes life much better.

Warts

Warts are small, usually painless growths on the skin caused by a virus. They are generally harmless. However, warts can be disfiguring and embarrassing, and occasionally they itch or hurt (particularly on the feet).

The different types of warts include:

- **Common warts:** usually appear on the hands, but can appear anywhere.
- **Flat warts:** generally found on the face and forehead. Common in children, less so in teens, and rare in adults.
- **Genital warts:** usually found on the genitals, in the pubic area, and the area between the thighs, but can appear inside the vagina and anal canal.
- **Plantar warts:** found on the soles of the feet.
- **Subungual and periungual warts:** appear under and around the fingernails or toenails

The typical wart is a raised round or oval growth on the skin with a rough surface. Compared with the surrounding normal skin, warts may appear light, dark, or black (rare). Most adults are familiar with the look of a typical wart and have little trouble recognizing them. Unusual warts with smooth surfaces or flat warts in children may be more difficult for parents to recognize.

Common warts tend to cause no discomfort unless they are in areas of repeated friction or pressure. Plantar warts, for example, can become extremely painful. Large numbers of plantar warts on the foot may cause difficulty running and even walking.

Examples of warts

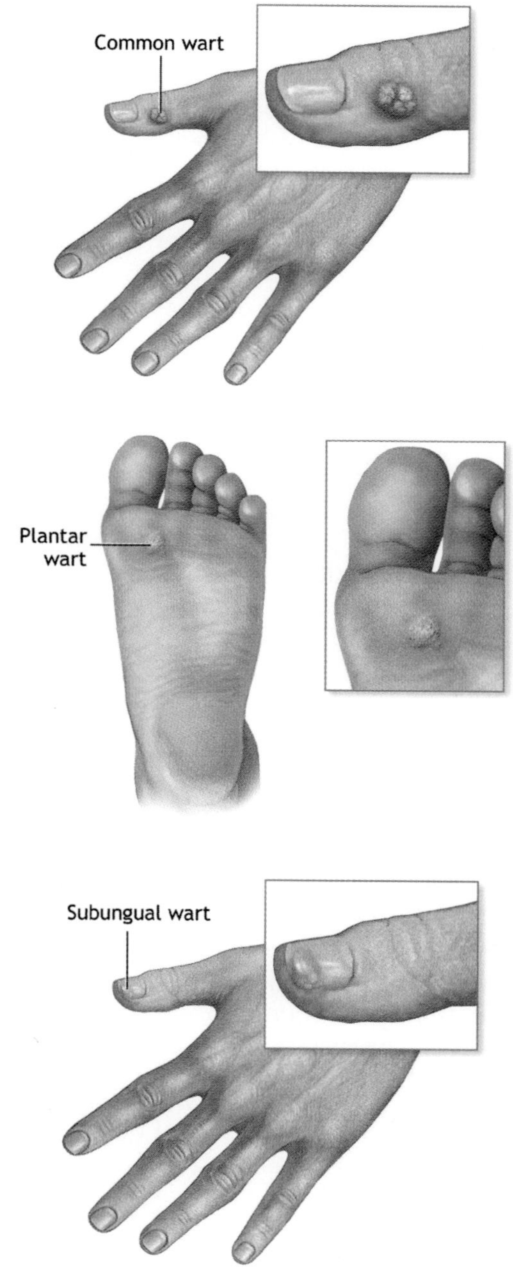

Some warts will disappear without treatment, although it can sometimes take a couple years. Treated or not, warts that go away often reappear. Genital warts are quite contagious, while common, flat, and plantar warts are much less likely to spread from person to person. All warts can spread from one part of your own body to another.

Home care

Over-the-counter medications can remove warts. These are applied to the wart every day for several weeks. DO NOT use these medications on your face or genitals. It helps to file the wart down when damp (for example, after a bath or shower) before applying these medications.

Special cushions are available at drugstores for plantar warts. These pads help relieve any pressure and pain from the warts.

DO NOT attempt to remove a wart yourself by burning, cutting, tearing, picking, or any other method.

Interestingly, placing duct tape over a wart may help it disappear. A small study had people wear duct tape for six straight days, remove it, wet and scrape the wart down using a file, and then reapply the tape the next morning. This was done until the wart disappeared, but no longer than two months. The people wearing the duct tape had as much luck getting rid of their warts as those who had their warts frozen off by a doctor. This method might be worth a try if you have a painless, yet unsightly wart.

When to contact a medical professional

Call for an appointment with your doctor if:

- There are signs of infection (red streaking, pus, discharge, or fever) or bleeding. Warts can bleed a little, but if bleeding is significant or not easily stopped by light pressure, see a doctor.
- Your warts do not respond to self care and you want it removed.
- You have pain associated with the wart.
- You have anal or genital warts.
- You have diabetes or a weakened immune system (for example, HIV) and have developed warts.
- There is any change in the color or appearance of the wart.

Prevention

- Avoid direct skin contact with a wart on someone else.
- After filing your wart, wash the file carefully since you can spread the virus to other parts of your body.
- After touching any of your warts, wash your hands carefully.

Warts - genital

Genital warts are soft wart-like growths on the genitals caused by a viral skin disease. Genital warts are a type of sexually transmitted disease (STD).

The virus responsible for genital warts is called human papilloma virus (HPV). This virus can cause warts on the penis, vulva, urethra, vagina, cervix, and around the anus.

HPV infection around the genitals is common, although most people have no symptoms. Even if you do NOT have symptoms, however, you must be treated to avoid complications and spreading the condition to others.

HPV grows well in the moist genital area. Warts on the outer genitals are easily recognized. They are raised, flesh-colored lesions that may occur singly or in clusters. Left untreated, warts may rapidly enlarge, taking on a "cauliflower-like" appearance.

In women, HPV can invade the vagina and cervix. These warts are flat and not easily visible without special procedures. Because HPV can lead to cancerous and precancerous changes in the cervix, it is important that this condition be diagnosed and treated. Regular pap smears are necessary to detect HPV or other abnormal changes related to this virus. Having both HPV and herpes virus together puts you at particular risk for cervical cancer.

The following factors put you at higher risk for getting genital warts and other complications of HPV:

- Multiple sexual partners
- Not knowing if someone you had sex with had STDs
- Early age when you start to be sexually active
- Tobacco and alcohol use
- Stress and other viral infections (such as HIV or herpes) at the same time

If a child has genital warts, you should suspect sexual abuse as a possible cause.

Home care

Genital warts must be treated by a doctor. DO NOT use over-the counter remedies meant for other kinds of warts. Your doctor may treat genital warts by applying a skin treatment in the office. Or, the doctor may prescribe a medication that you apply at home several times per week.

If you develop genital warts, all of your sexual partners must be examined by a health care provider and treated if genital warts are found.

Women who have had genital warts, and women whose partners ever had genital warts, should have pap smears at least every 6 months. For warts on the cervix, women may be advised to have pap smears every 3 months after initial treatment.

When to contact a medical professional

Call your doctor if a current or past sexual partner is found to have genital warts. Call if you have visible warts on your external genitals, itching, discharge, or abnormal vaginal bleeding. Keep in mind that genital warts may not appear for months to years after having sexual contact with an infected person.

Call your doctor if a young child is thought to possibly have genital warts.

Sexually active teens are very susceptible to HPV and should get screened for HPV infection regularly.

Prevention

Total abstinence is the only fullproof way of avoiding genital warts and other STDs. You can also avoid STDs by having a monogamous sexual relationship with a partner known to be disease-free.

Skin near the warts and around the genitals, anus, and other areas can pass the virus from one person to the next. Therefore, male and female condoms cannot fully protect you.

Nonetheless, condoms should still be used. They reduce your chances of getting or spreading STDs..

These precautions must be taken at all times. HPV can be passed from person to person even when there are no visible warts or other symptoms.

See *Safe Sex*.

Wrist pain

Carpal tunnel syndrome is a common cause of wrist pain. You may feel aching, burning, numbness, or tingling in your palm, wrist, thumb, or fingers. The thumb muscle can become weak, making it difficult to grasp things. Pain may extend up to your elbow.

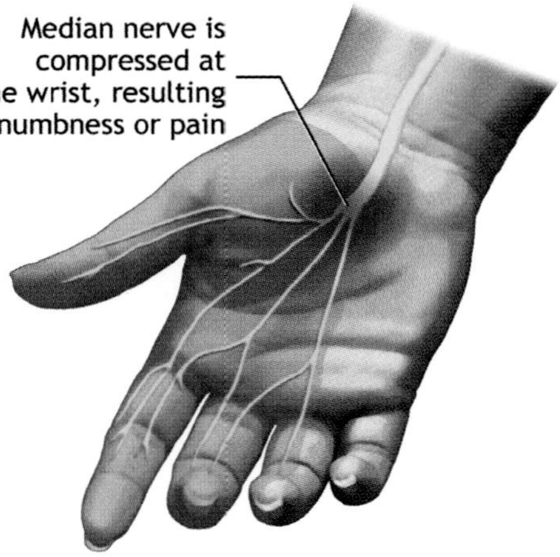
Median nerve is compressed at the wrist, resulting in numbness or pain

Carpal tunnel syndrome occurs when an important nerve (called the median nerve) gets compressed at the wrist because of swelling.

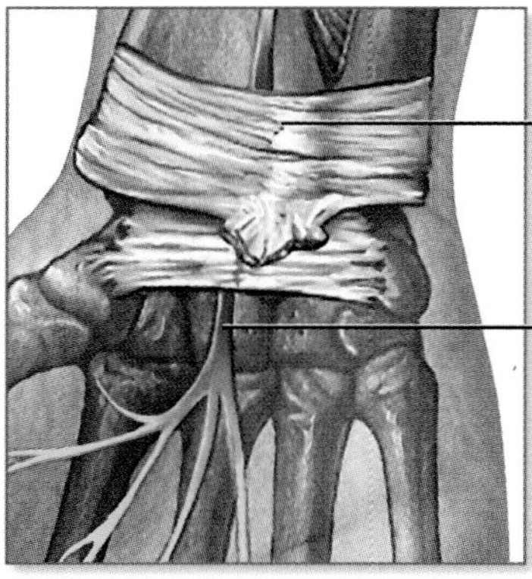
Constriction at carpal ligament
Inflammation of median nerve

Such swelling can occur if you:

- Do a repetitive motion with your wrist like typing on a computer keyboard, using a computer mouse, playing racquetball or handball, sewing, painting, writing, or using a vibrating tool.
- Are pregnant, menopausal, or overweight.
- Have diabetes, premenstrual syndrome, an underactive thyroid, or rheumatoid arthritis.

Wrist pain with bruising and swelling is often a sign of an injury. The signs of a possible broken bone include misshapen joints and inability to move the wrist, hand, or a finger. Other common injuries include sprain, strain, tendinitis, and bursitis.

Arthritis is another common cause of wrist pain, swelling, and stiffness. There are many types of arthritis. Osteoarthritis occurs with age and overuse. Rheumatoid arthritis generally affects both wrists. Psoriatic arthritis accompanies psoriasis.

Infectious arthritis is a medical emergency. The signs of an infection include redness and warmth of the wrist, fever above 100°F, and recent illness.

Other common causes of wrist pain include:

- Gout – this occurs when you produce too much uric acid, a waste product. It forms crystals in joints, rather than being excreted in the urine.
- Pseudogout – this is when calcium deposits in your joints (usually the wrists or knees), causing pain, redness, and swelling.

Home care

For carpal tunnel syndrome, you may need to make adjustments to your work habits and environment:

- Make sure that your keyboard is low enough that your wrists aren't bending upwards while you type.
- Take plenty of breaks from activities that aggravate the pain. When typing, stop often to rest the hands, if only for a moment. Rest your hands on their sides, not the wrists.

- An occupational therapist can show you ways to ease pain and swelling and stop the syndrome from coming back.
- Over-the-counter pain medications like ibuprofen or naproxen can relieve pain and swelling.
- Various mousepads, typing pads, split keyboards, and wrist splints (braces) are designed to relieve wrist pain. Some people find these devices help their symptoms. You may wish to try a few different kinds to see if any help.

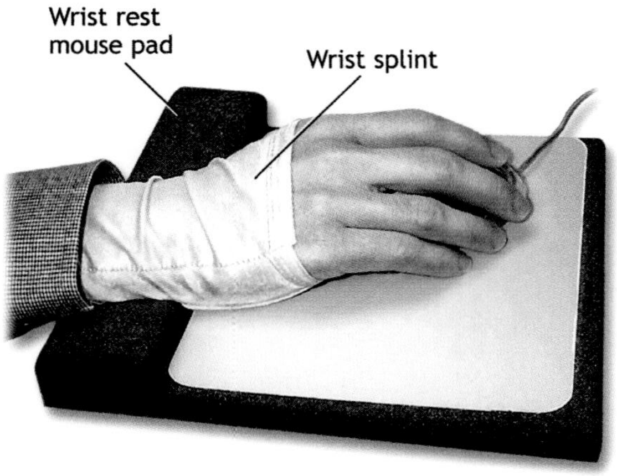

- You may only need to wear a wrist splint at night while you sleep. This helps reduce the swelling. If that alone is not working, wear the splints during the day and apply hot or cold compresses periodically.

For a recent injury:

- Rest your wrist. Keep it elevated.
- Apply ice to the tender and swollen area.
- Take over-the-counter pain medication, like ibuprofen or acetaminophen.
- Wear a splint for several days. Wrist splints can be purchased at many drugstores and medical supply stores.

For non-infectious arthritis:

- Do flexibility and strengthening exercises every day. Work with a physical therapist to learn the best and safest exercises for your wrist.
- Try the exercises after a hot bath or shower so that your wrist is warmed up and less stiff.
- DO NOT perform exercises when your wrist is actively inflamed.
- Make sure that you also rest the joint adequately. Both rest and exercise are important when you have arthritis.

When to contact a medical professional

Get emergency care if:

- You are unable to move your wrist, hand or a finger.
- Your wrist, hand, or fingers are misshapen.
- You are bleeding significantly.

Call your doctor right away if:

- You have a fever over 100°F.
- You have a rash.
- You have swelling and redness of your wrist and you have had a recent illness (like a virus or other infection).

Call your doctor for an appointment if:

- You have swelling, redness or stiffness in one or both wrists.
- You have numbness, tingling, or weakness in the wrist, hand, or fingers with pain.
- You have lost any muscle mass in the wrist, hand, or fingers.
- You have been following self-care treatments for two weeks but still have pain.

Yellow skin (jaundice)

Jaundice is a yellow color in the skin, the mucous membranes, or the eyes. The yellow pigment is from bilirubin, a byproduct of old red blood cells.

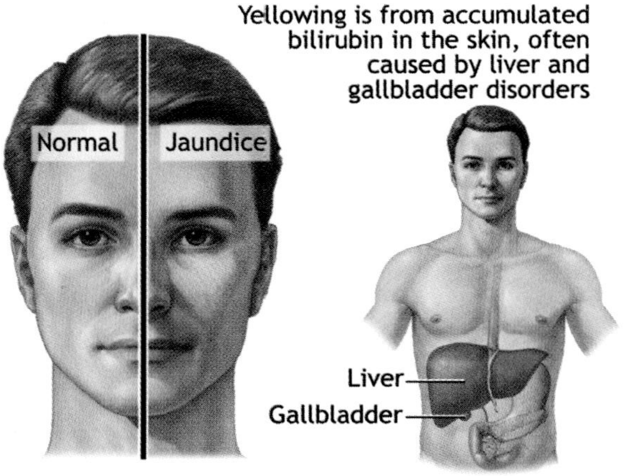

If you've ever had a bruise, you may have noticed that the skin went through a series of color changes as it healed. When you saw yellow in the bruise, you were seeing bilirubin.

Normally, about 1% of our red blood cells retire every day, to be replaced by fresh red blood cells. The old ones are processed in the liver and disposed of. Much of the resulting bilirubin leaves the body in the stool.

If there are too many red blood cells retiring for the liver to handle, yellow pigment builds up in the body. When there is enough to be visible, jaundice results.

Jaundice can be caused by too many red blood cells retiring, by the liver being overloaded or damaged, or by the inability to move processed bilirubin from the liver through the biliary tract to the gut.

Most babies have some jaundice during the first week of life. The ordeal of birth can send many red blood cells to an early retirement (especially if a vacuum is used!), and babies' livers are often unprepared for the load. Before Mom's milk comes in and stooling begins in earnest, bilirubin accumulates more easily. Jaundice is even more common in premature babies.

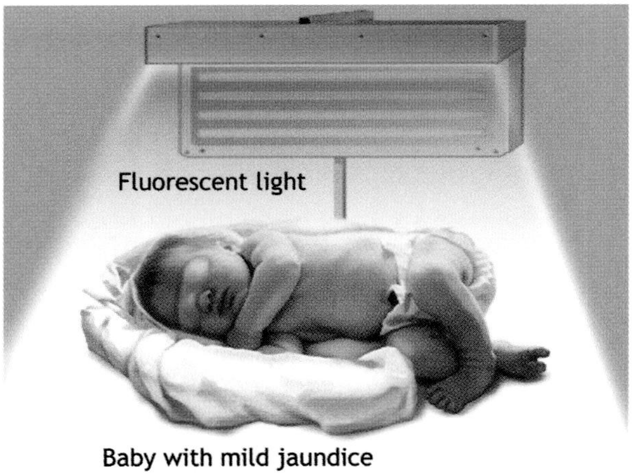

Newborn or premature infants with jaundice may be placed under bili lights to reduce elevated levels of bilirubin.

Physiologic jaundice is the name for normal jaundice commonly seen in healthy babies.

Pathologic jaundice is the name given when jaundice presents a health risk, either because of its degree or its cause. Pathologic jaundice can occur in children or adults. It arises for many reasons, including blood incompatibilities, blood diseases, genetic syndromes, hepatitis, cirrhosis, bile duct blockage, other liver diseases, infections, or medications. The term also applies to physiologic jaundice exaggerated by dehydration, prematurity, difficult delivery, or other reason.

A yellow-to-orange color may be imparted to the skin by consuming too much beta carotene, the orange pigment seen in carrots. In this condition, the whites of the eyes remain white, while people with true jaundice often have a yellowish tinge to the eyes.

Home care

The cause of jaundice must be determined before treatment can be given. Follow prescribed therapy to treat the underlying cause.

When to contact a medical professional

ALL jaundice in an infant, child, or adult should be medically evaluated. ALWAYS call your doctor if jaundice is present.

Prevention

Feed babies frequently and don't let them become dehydrated.

With jaundice, the important thing to prevent is kernicterus – toxic levels of bilirubin accumulating in the brain. Early identification and treatment of jaundice will usually prevent kernicterus, whatever the cause.

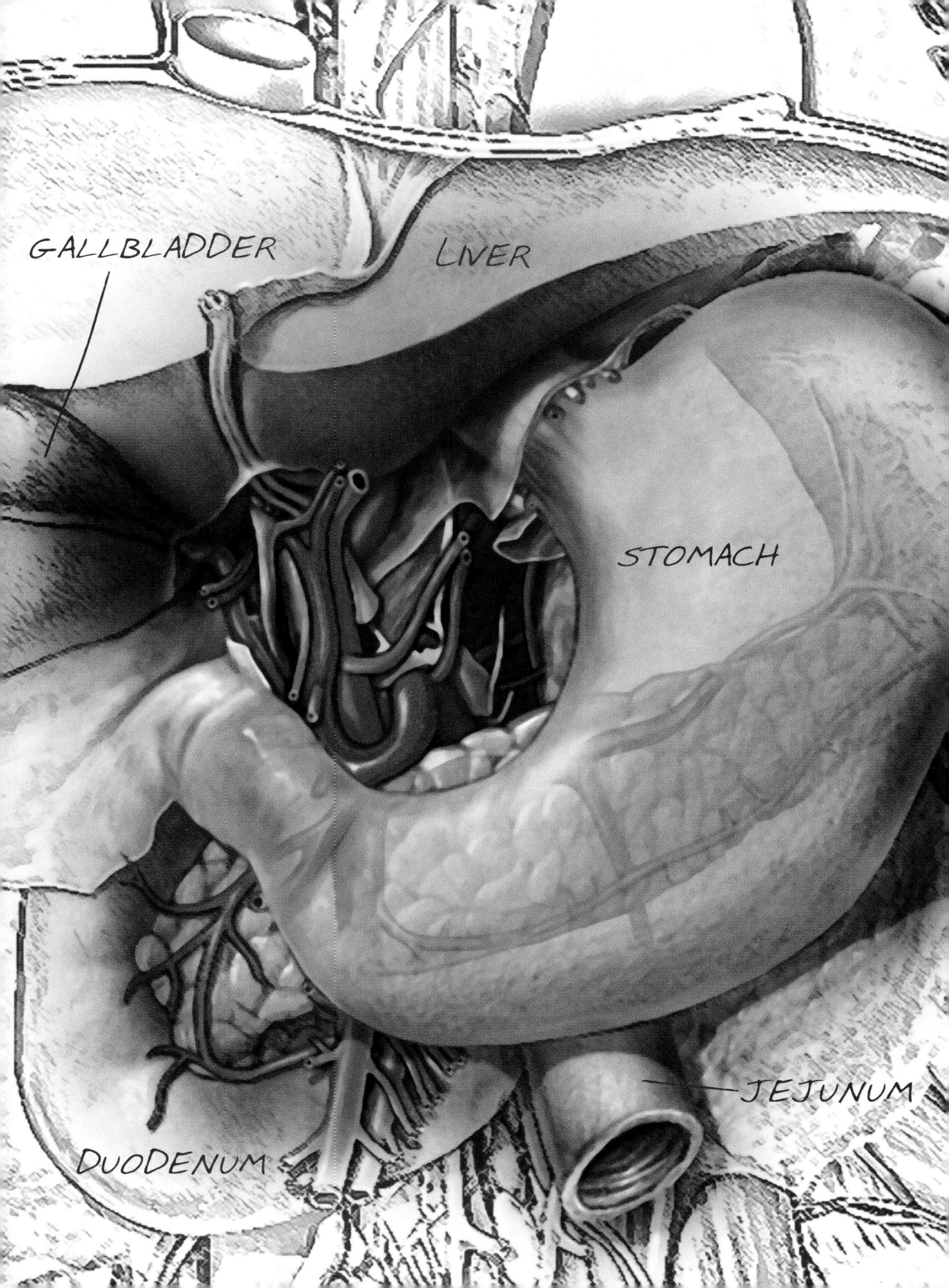

GALLBLADDER
LIVER
STOMACH
JEJUNUM
DUODENUM

BODY ATLAS

SKULL AND SPINE

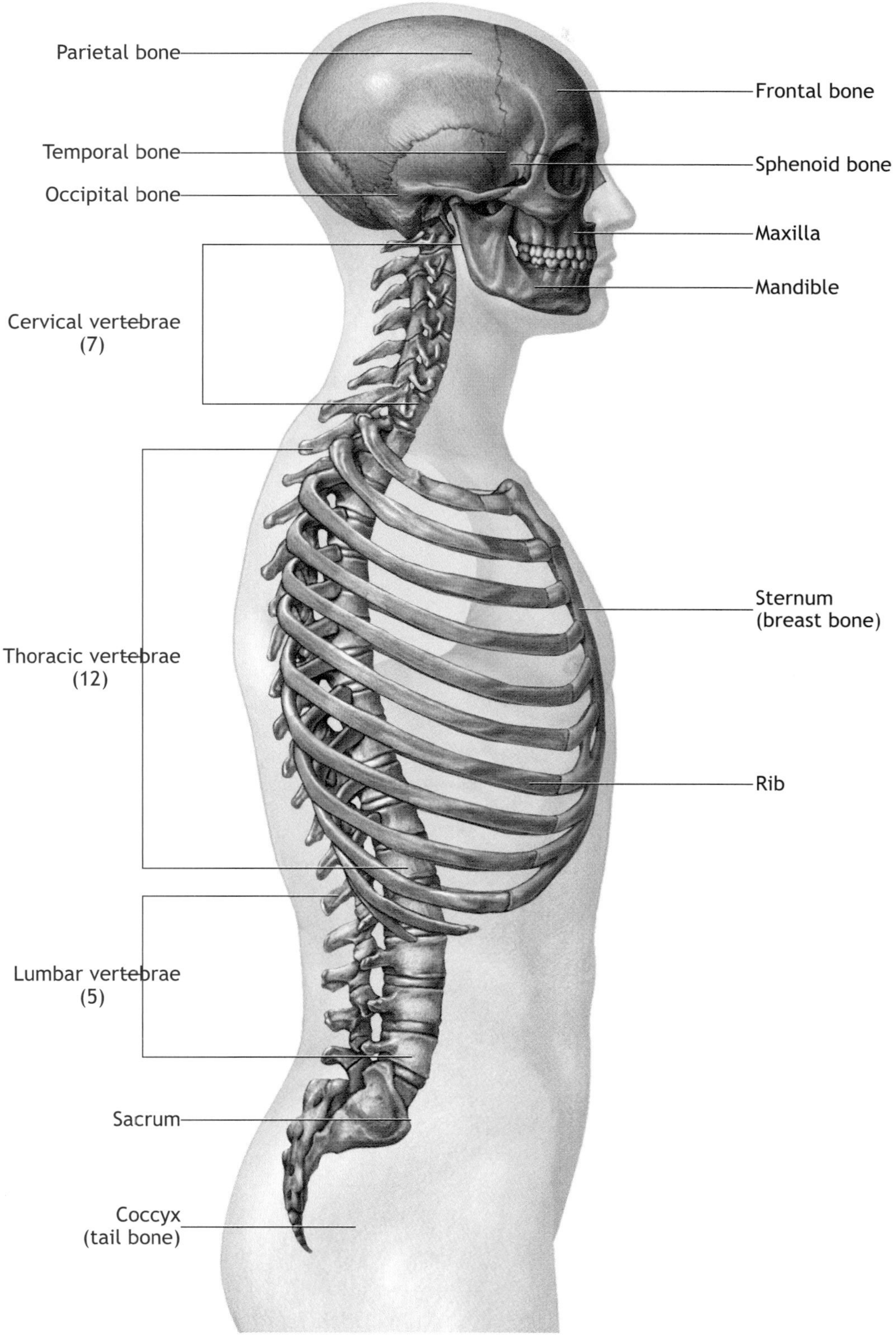

Skeleton: Front View

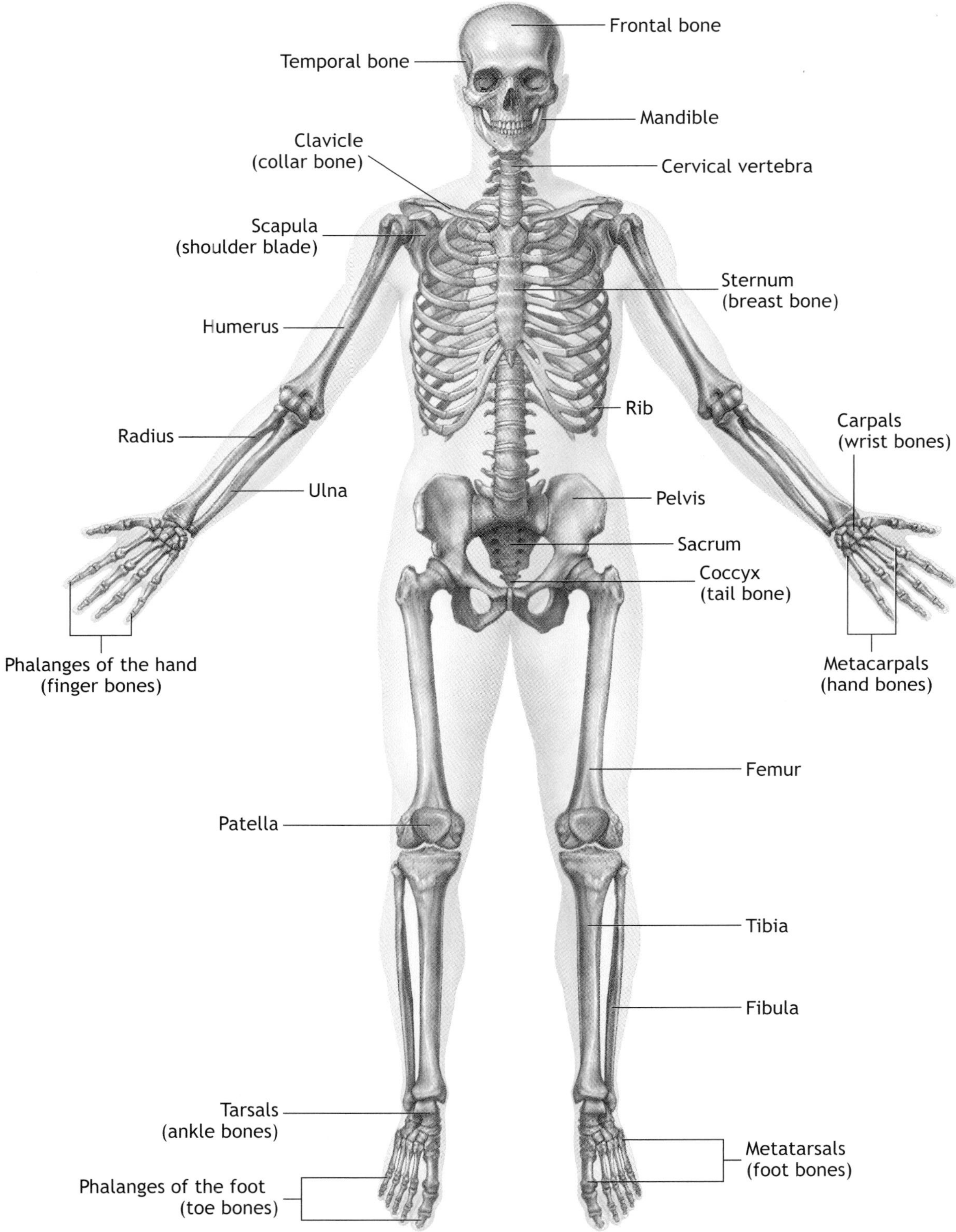
Frontal bone
Temporal bone
Mandible
Clavicle
(collar bone)
Cervical vertebra
Scapula
(shoulder blade)
Sternum
(breast bone)
Humerus
Rib
Radius
Carpals
(wrist bones)
Ulna
Pelvis
Sacrum
Coccyx
(tail bone)
Phalanges of the hand
(finger bones)
Metacarpals
(hand bones)
Femur
Patella
Tibia
Fibula
Tarsals
(ankle bones)
Metatarsals
(foot bones)
Phalanges of the foot
(toe bones)

Skeleton: back view

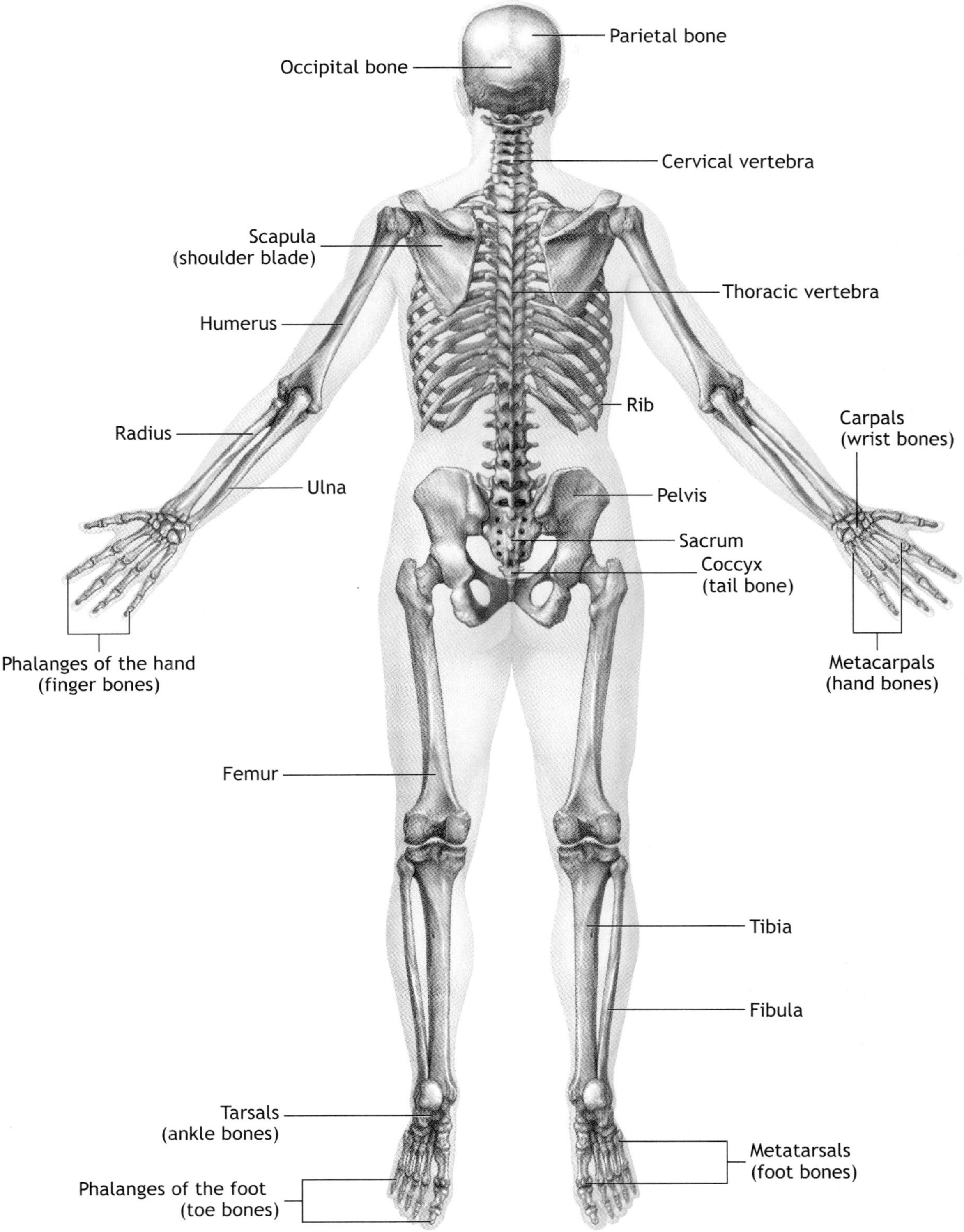

SHOULDER, HIP, AND KNEE JOINTS

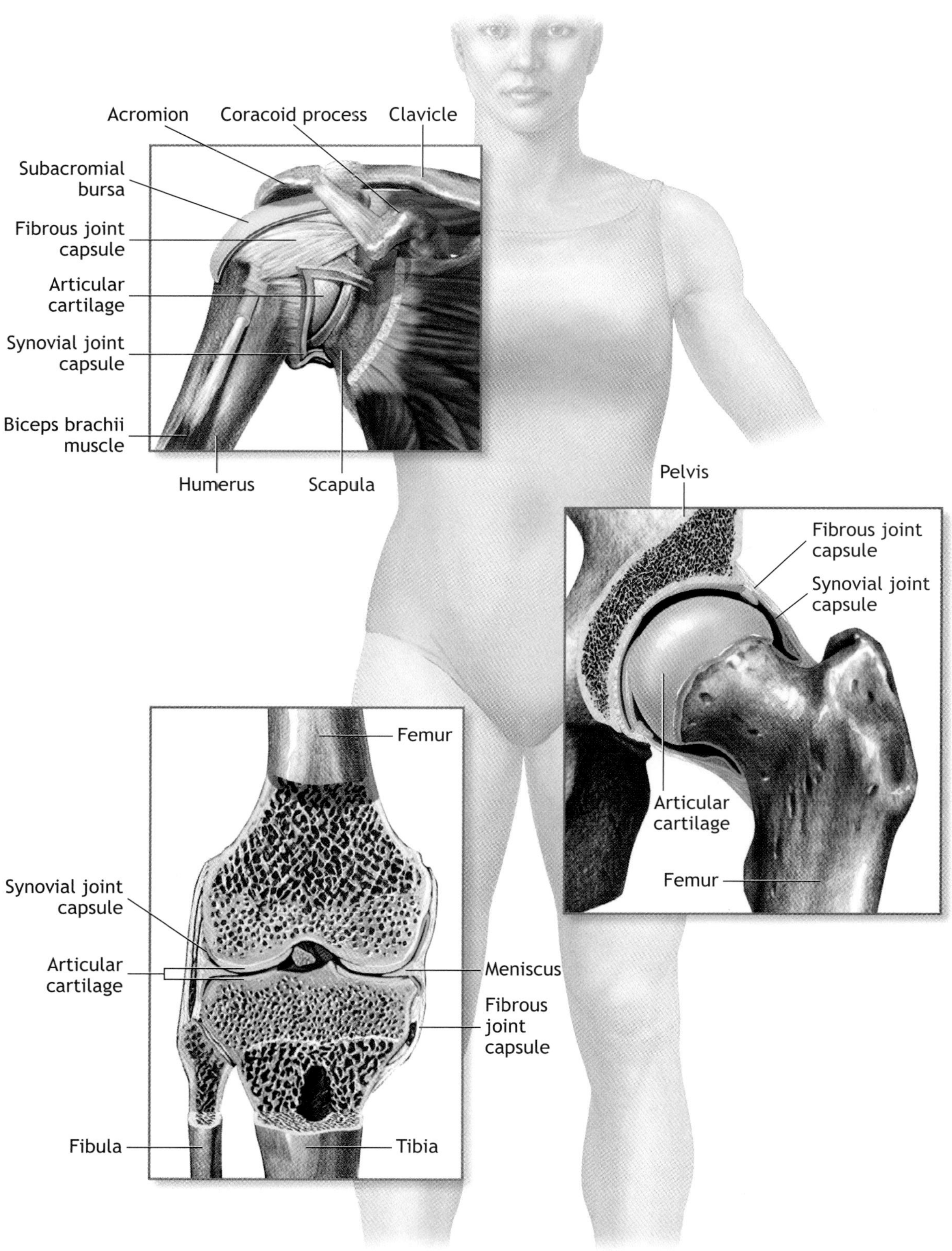
Acromion
Coracoid process
Clavicle
Subacromial bursa
Fibrous joint capsule
Articular cartilage
Synovial joint capsule
Biceps brachii muscle
Humerus
Scapula
Pelvis
Fibrous joint capsule
Synovial joint capsule
Articular cartilage
Femur
Femur
Synovial joint capsule
Articular cartilage
Meniscus
Fibrous joint capsule
Fibula
Tibia

Muscles of the Face

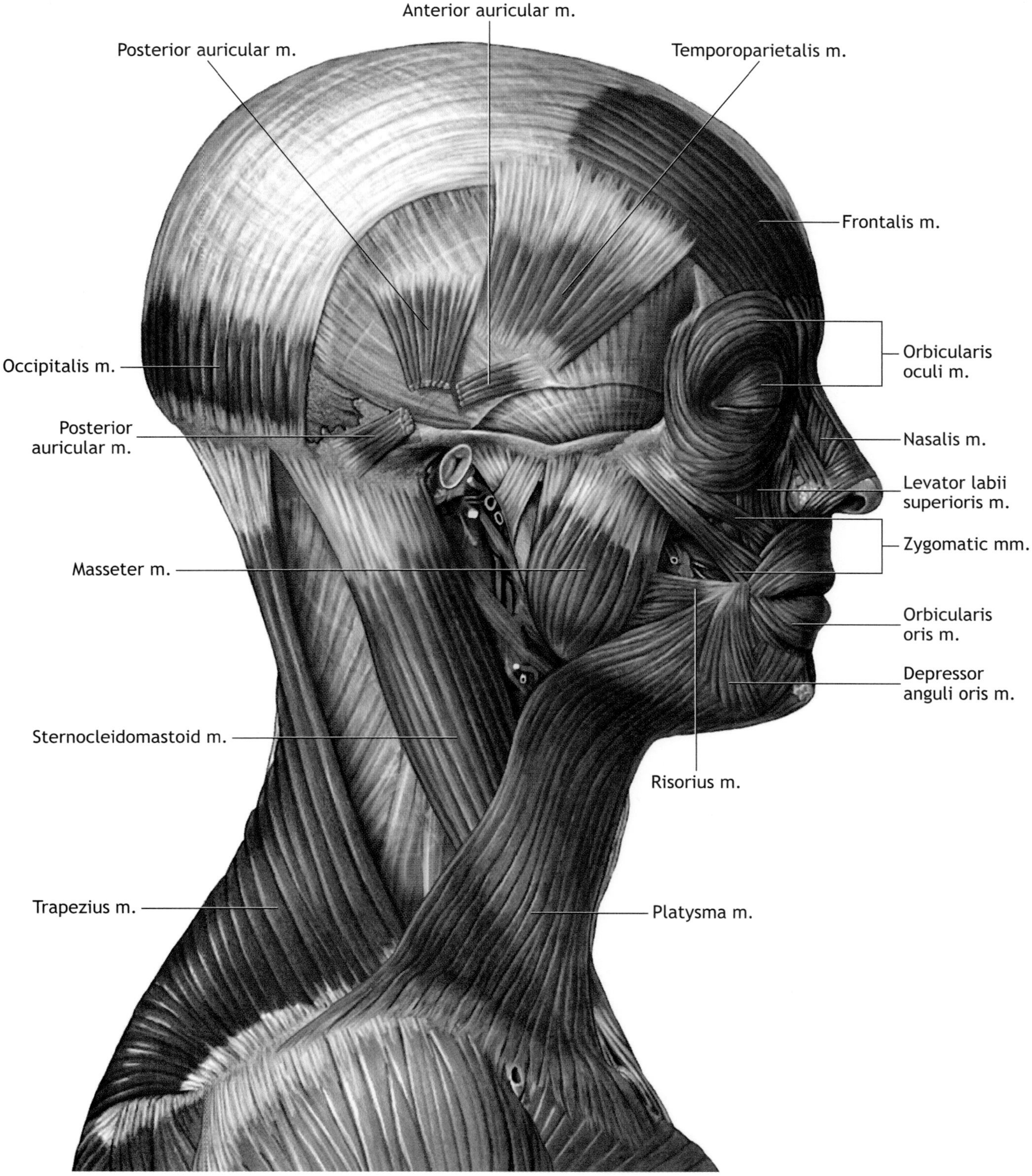
Anterior auricular m.
Posterior auricular m.
Temporoparietalis m.
Frontalis m.
Orbicularis oculi m.
Occipitalis m.
Posterior auricular m.
Nasalis m.
Levator labii superioris m.
Zygomatic mm.
Masseter m.
Orbicularis oris m.
Depressor anguli oris m.
Sternocleidomastoid m.
Risorius m.
Trapezius m.
Platysma m.

MUSCLES: FRONT VIEW

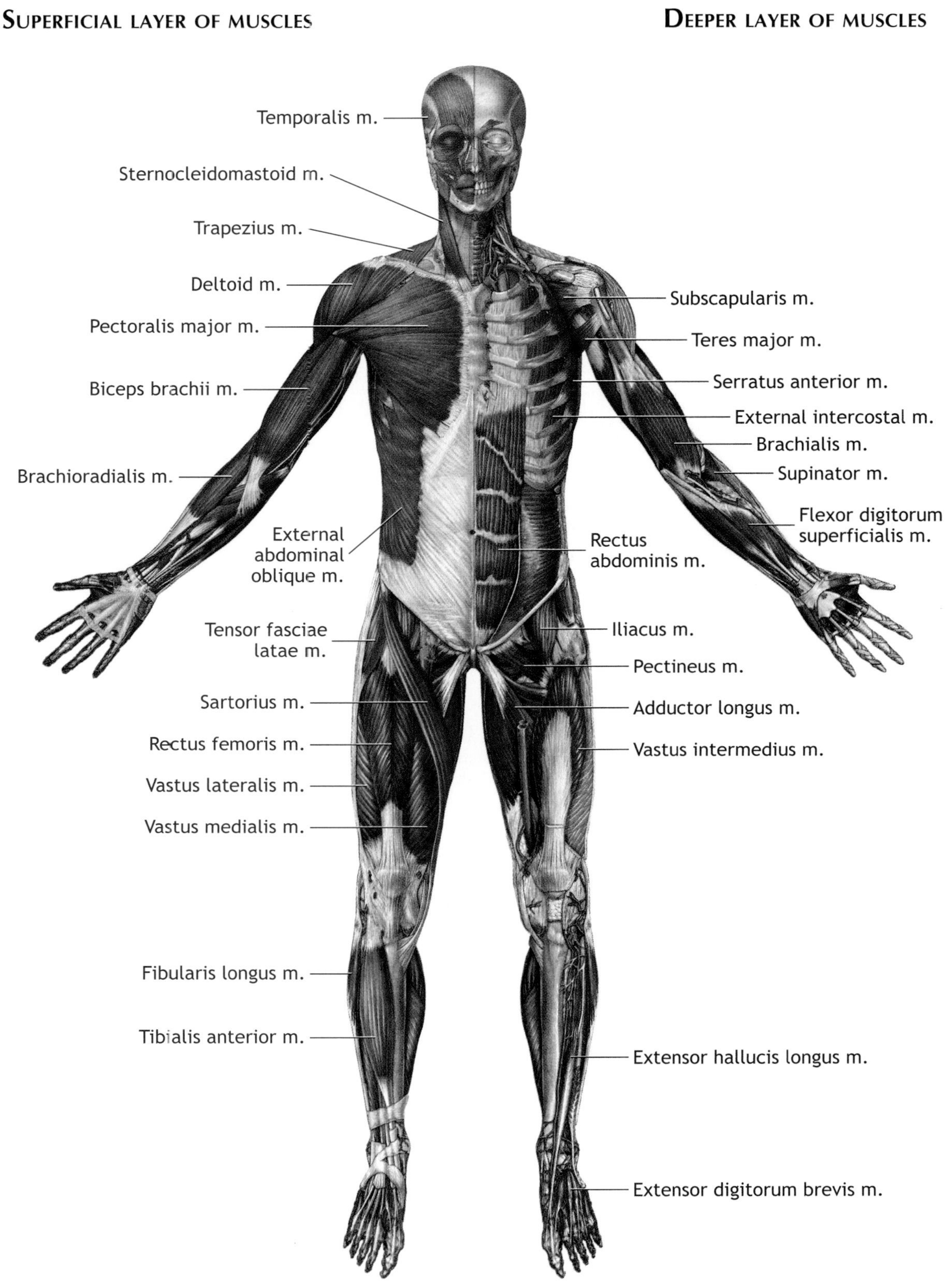
SUPERFICIAL LAYER OF MUSCLES
DEEPER LAYER OF MUSCLES
Temporalis m.
Sternocleidomastoid m.
Trapezius m.
Deltoid m.
Pectoralis major m.
Biceps brachii m.
Brachioradialis m.
External abdominal oblique m.
Tensor fasciae latae m.
Sartorius m.
Rectus femoris m.
Vastus lateralis m.
Vastus medialis m.
Fibularis longus m.
Tibialis anterior m.
Subscapularis m.
Teres major m.
Serratus anterior m.
External intercostal m.
Brachialis m.
Supinator m.
Flexor digitorum superficialis m.
Rectus abdominis m.
Iliacus m.
Pectineus m.
Adductor longus m.
Vastus intermedius m.
Extensor hallucis longus m.
Extensor digitorum brevis m.

Muscles: back view

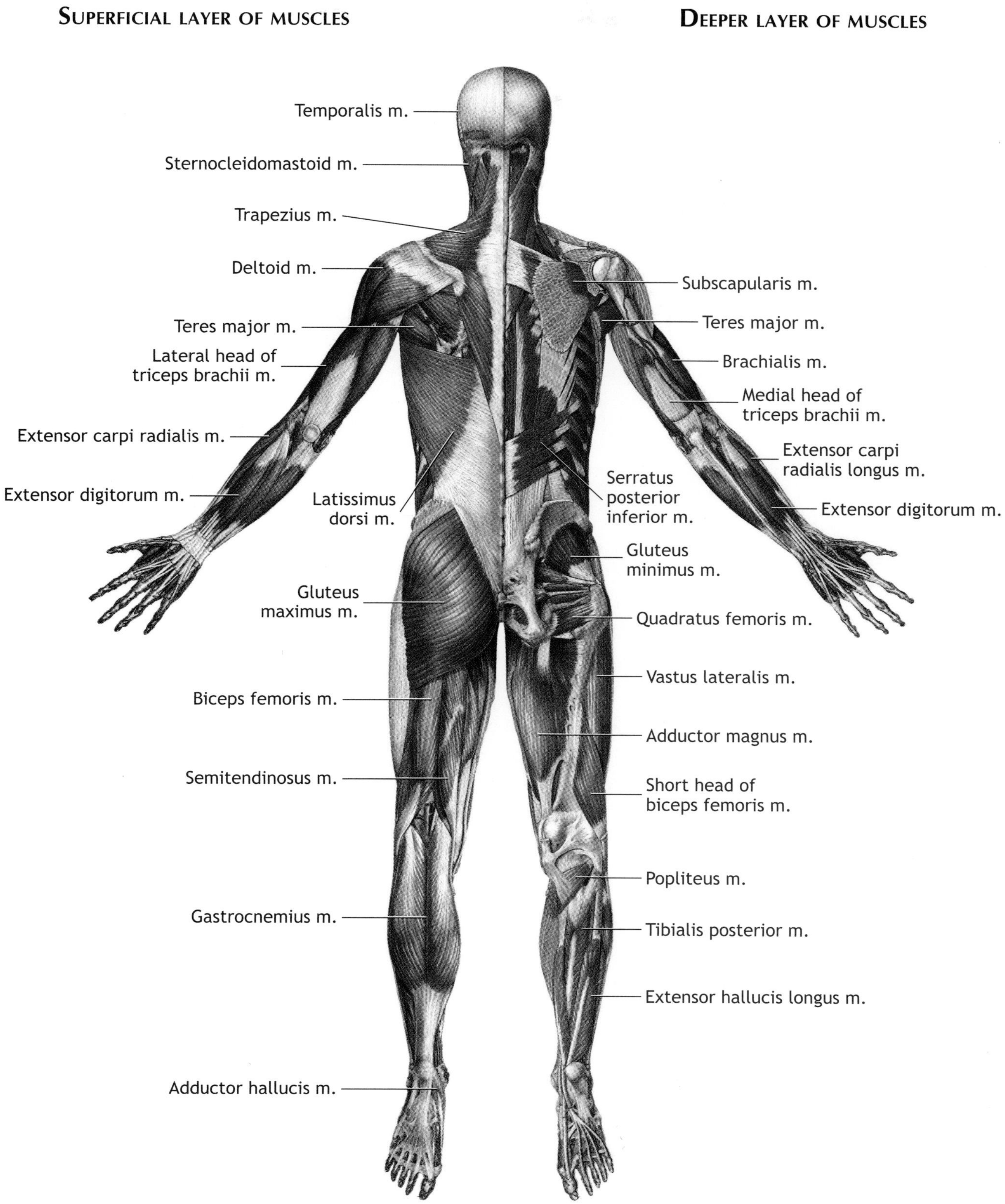
Superficial layer of muscles
Deeper layer of muscles
Temporalis m.
Sternocleidomastoid m.
Trapezius m.
Deltoid m.
Teres major m.
Lateral head of triceps brachii m.
Extensor carpi radialis m.
Extensor digitorum m.
Latissimus dorsi m.
Gluteus maximus m.
Biceps femoris m.
Semitendinosus m.
Gastrocnemius m.
Adductor hallucis m.
Subscapularis m.
Teres major m.
Brachialis m.
Medial head of triceps brachii m.
Extensor carpi radialis longus m.
Extensor digitorum m.
Serratus posterior inferior m.
Gluteus minimus m.
Quadratus femoris m.
Vastus lateralis m.
Adductor magnus m.
Short head of biceps femoris m.
Popliteus m.
Tibialis posterior m.
Extensor hallucis longus m.

Muscles of the Back and Spine

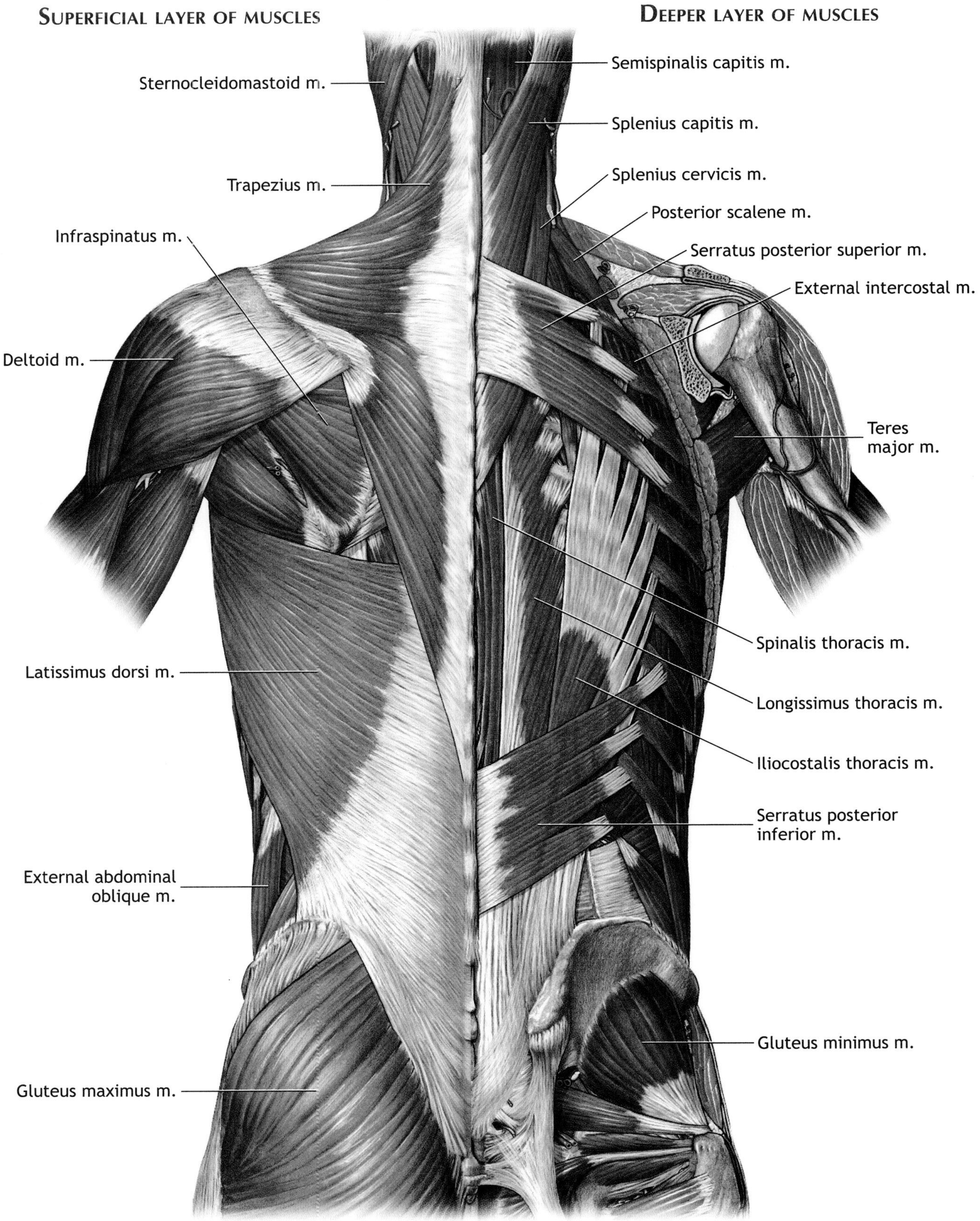
Superficial layer of muscles
Deeper layer of muscles
Sternocleidomastoid m.
Trapezius m.
Infraspinatus m.
Deltoid m.
Latissimus dorsi m.
External abdominal oblique m.
Gluteus maximus m.
Semispinalis capitis m.
Splenius capitis m.
Splenius cervicis m.
Posterior scalene m.
Serratus posterior superior m.
External intercostal m.
Teres major m.
Spinalis thoracis m.
Longissimus thoracis m.
Iliocostalis thoracis m.
Serratus posterior inferior m.
Gluteus minimus m.

Muscles of the Abdomen

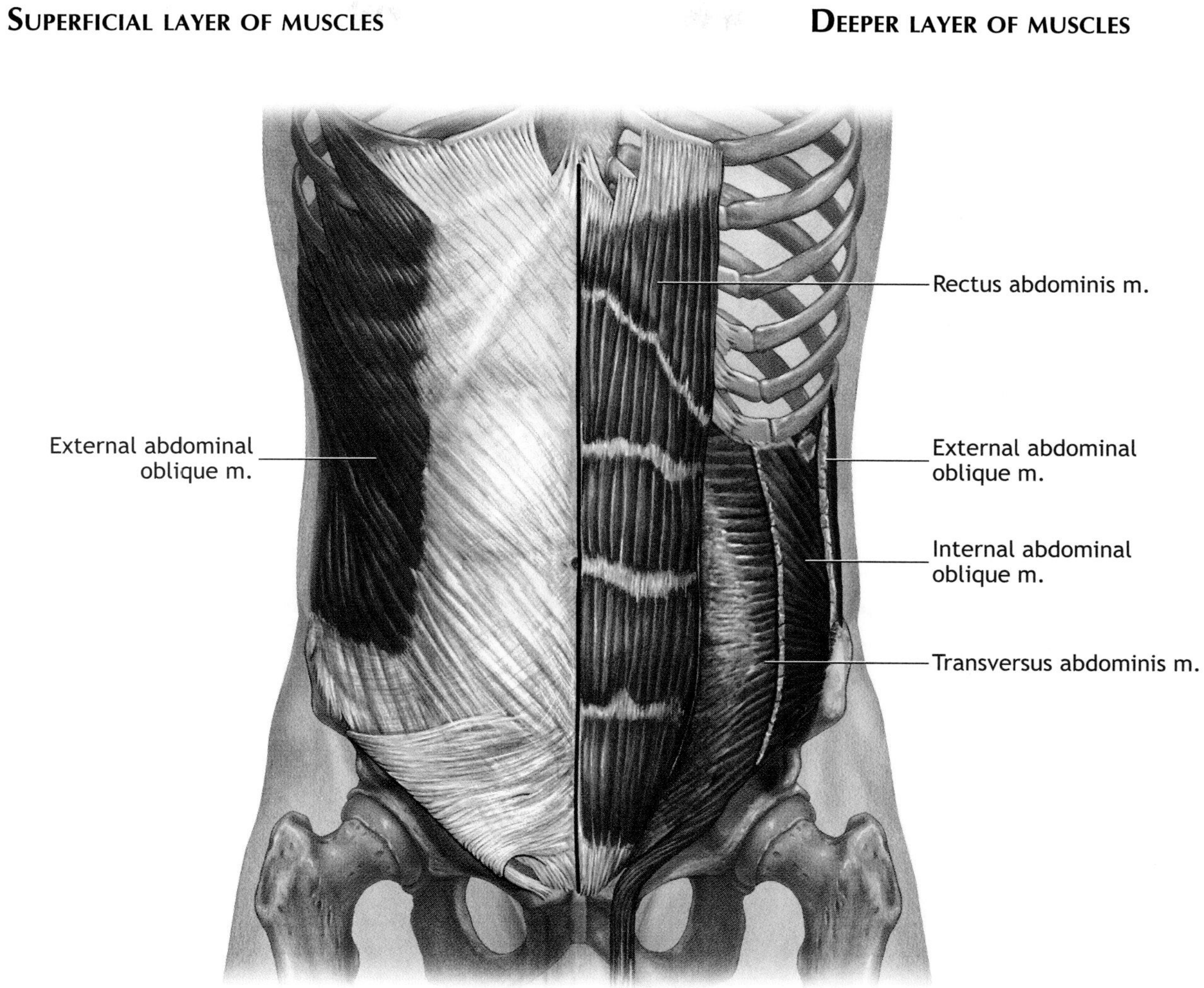

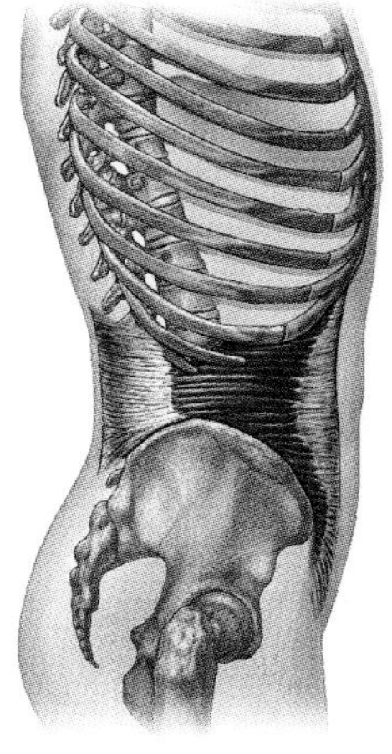

Transversus abdominis m.

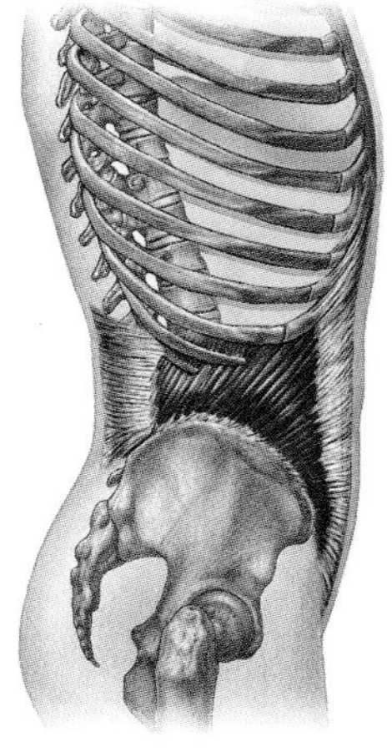

Internal abdominal oblique m.

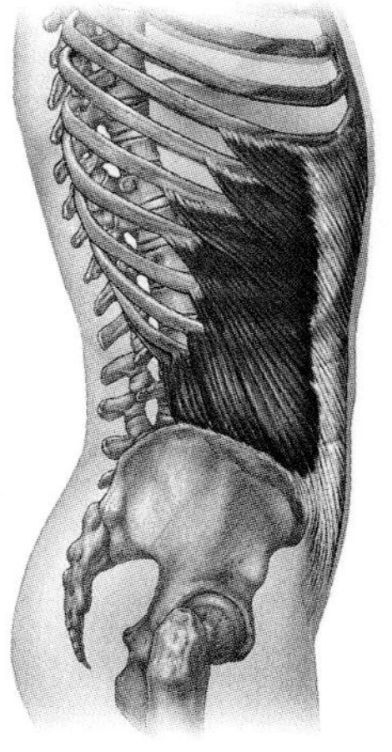

External abdominal oblique m.

Muscles of the Upper Limb

Front (anterior) view of the arm

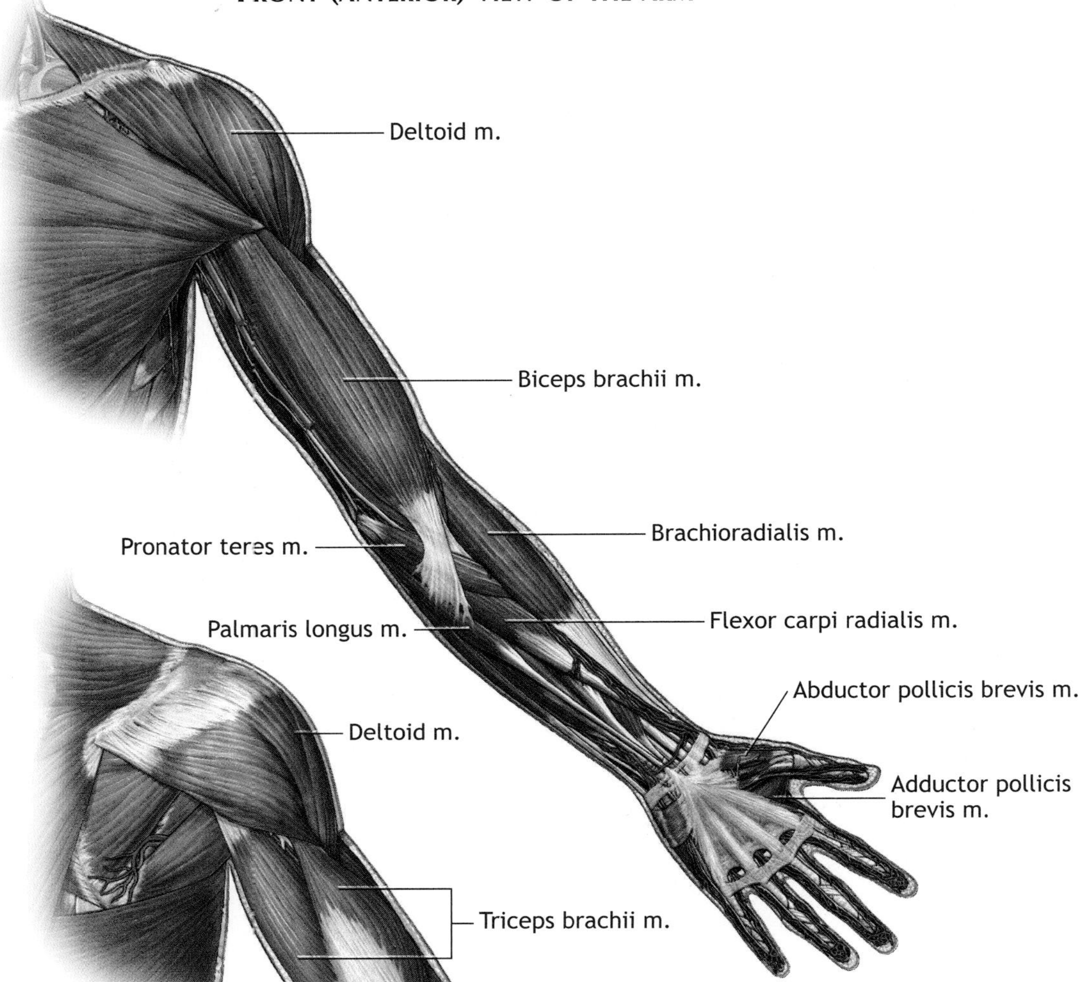

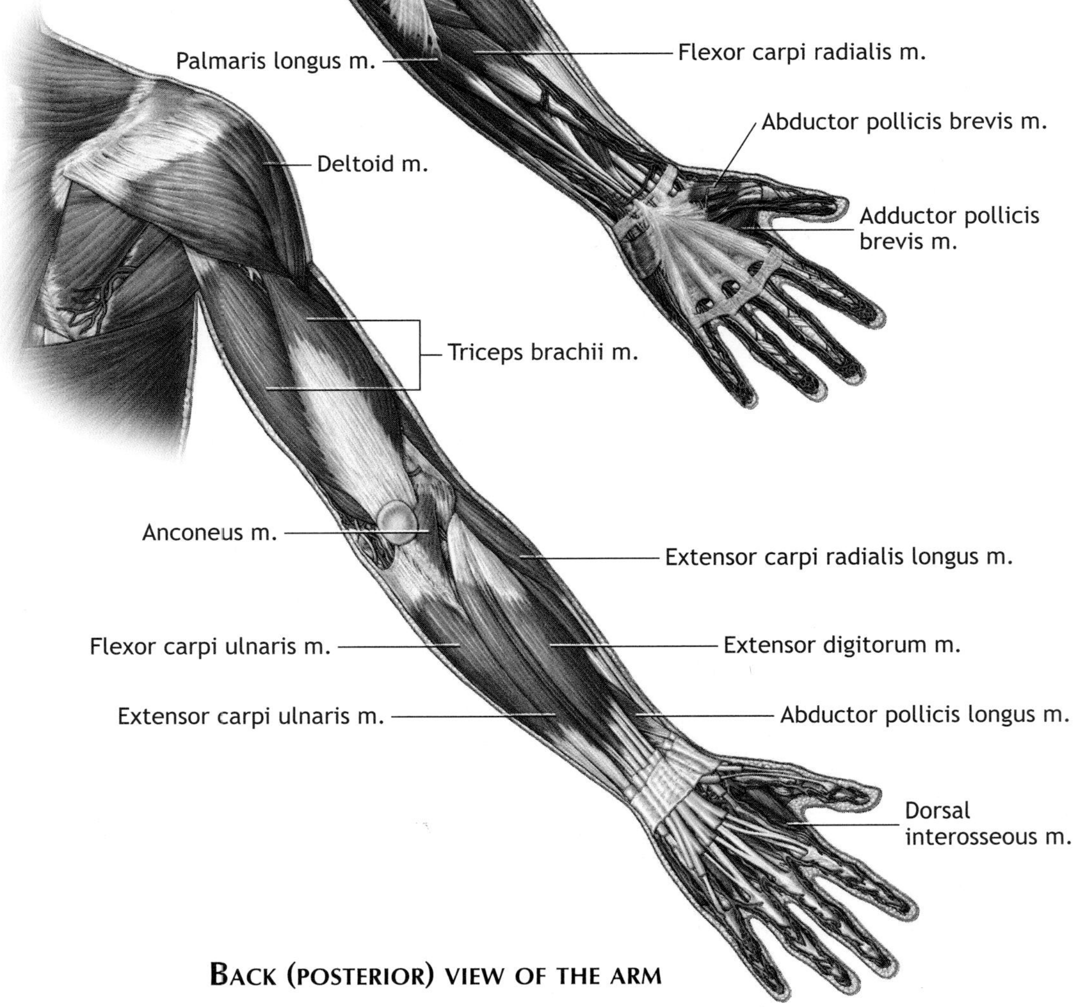

Back (posterior) view of the arm

Muscles of the lower limb

Front (anterior) view of the leg

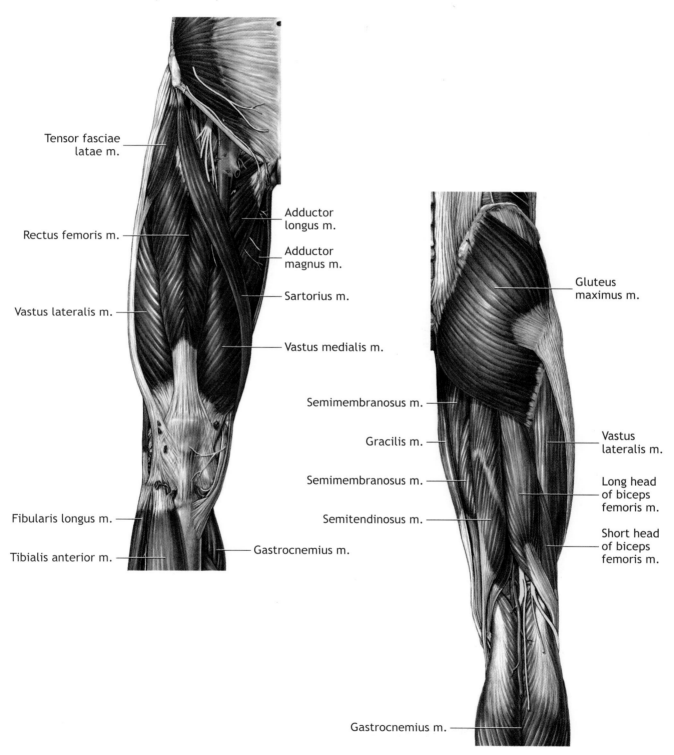

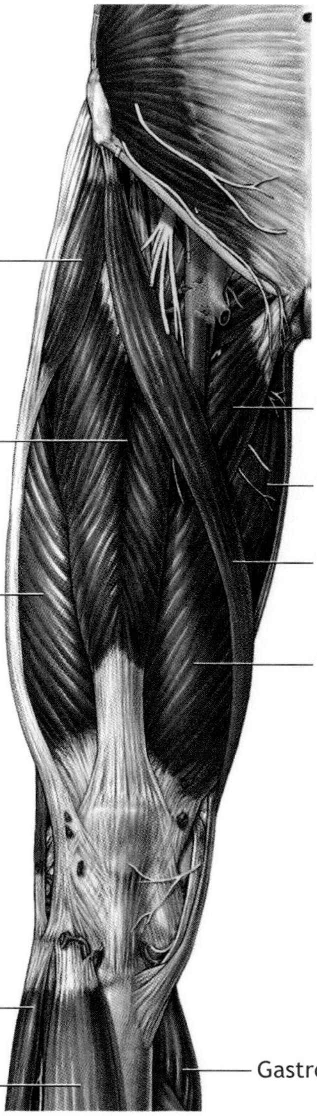

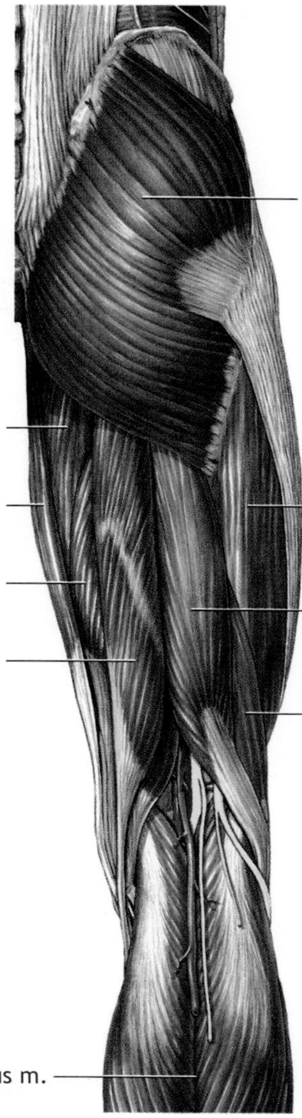

Back (posterior) view of the leg

ORGANS OF THE HEAD AND NECK

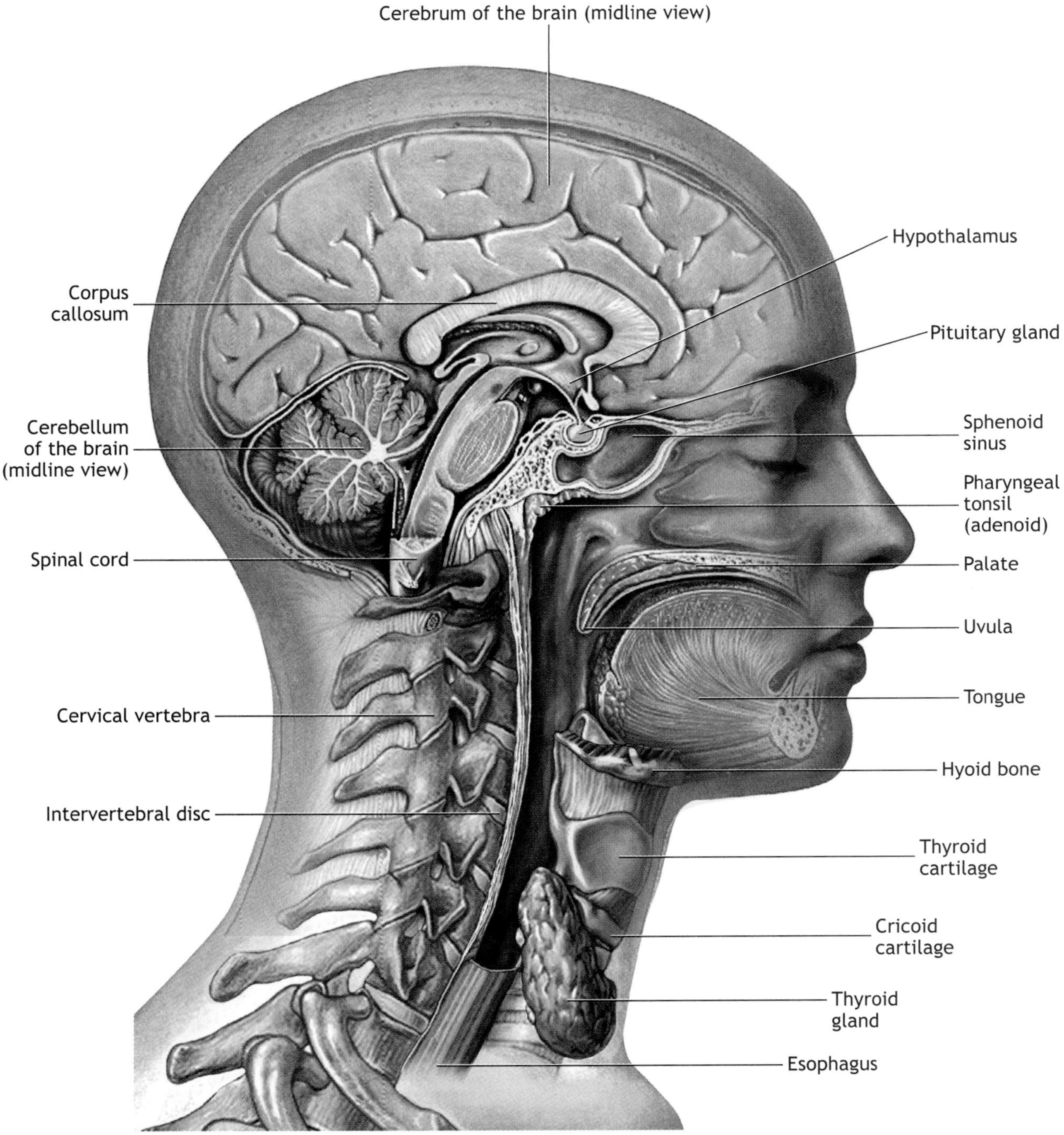
Cerebrum of the brain (midline view)
Hypothalamus
Corpus callosum
Pituitary gland
Cerebellum of the brain (midline view)
Sphenoid sinus
Pharyngeal tonsil (adenoid)
Spinal cord
Palate
Uvula
Tongue
Cervical vertebra
Hyoid bone
Intervertebral disc
Thyroid cartilage
Cricoid cartilage
Thyroid gland
Esophagus

Brain

Bottom (inferior) view of the brain

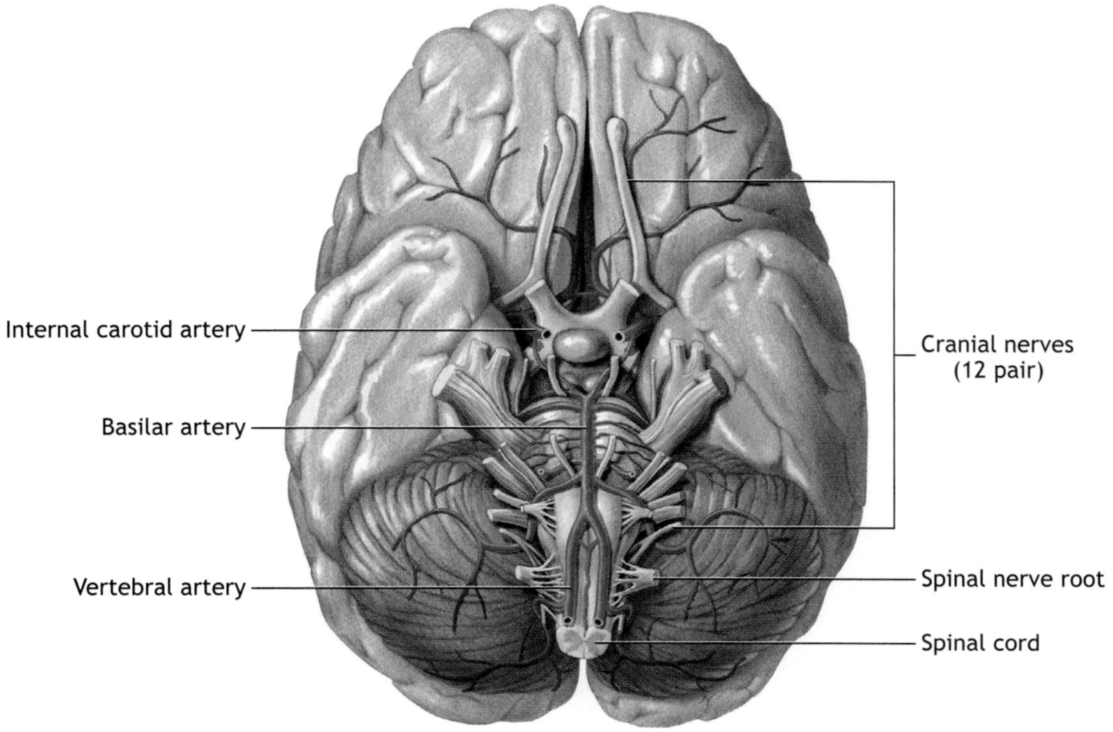

Side (left lateral) view of the brain

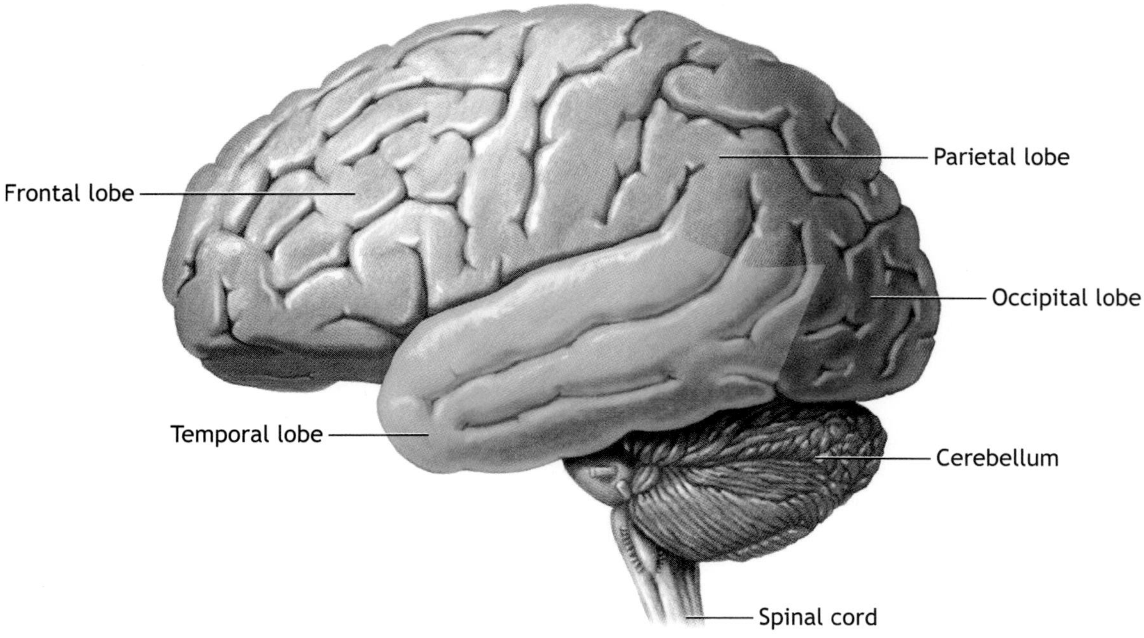

Eye

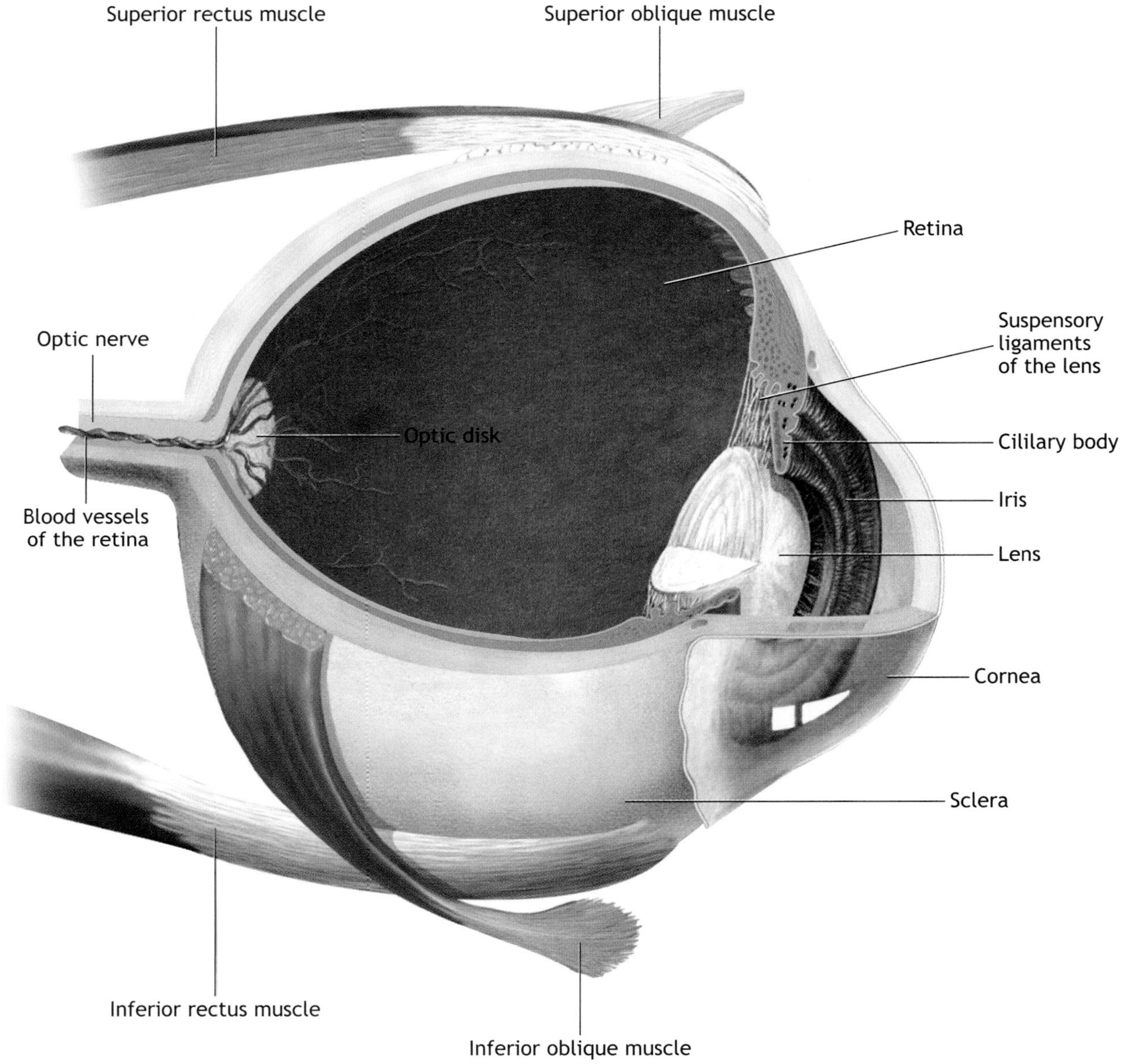
Superior rectus muscle
Superior oblique muscle
Retina
Suspensory ligaments of the lens
Optic nerve
Optic disk
Cililary body
Iris
Blood vessels of the retina
Lens
Cornea
Sclera
Inferior rectus muscle
Inferior oblique muscle

Organs of the Chest

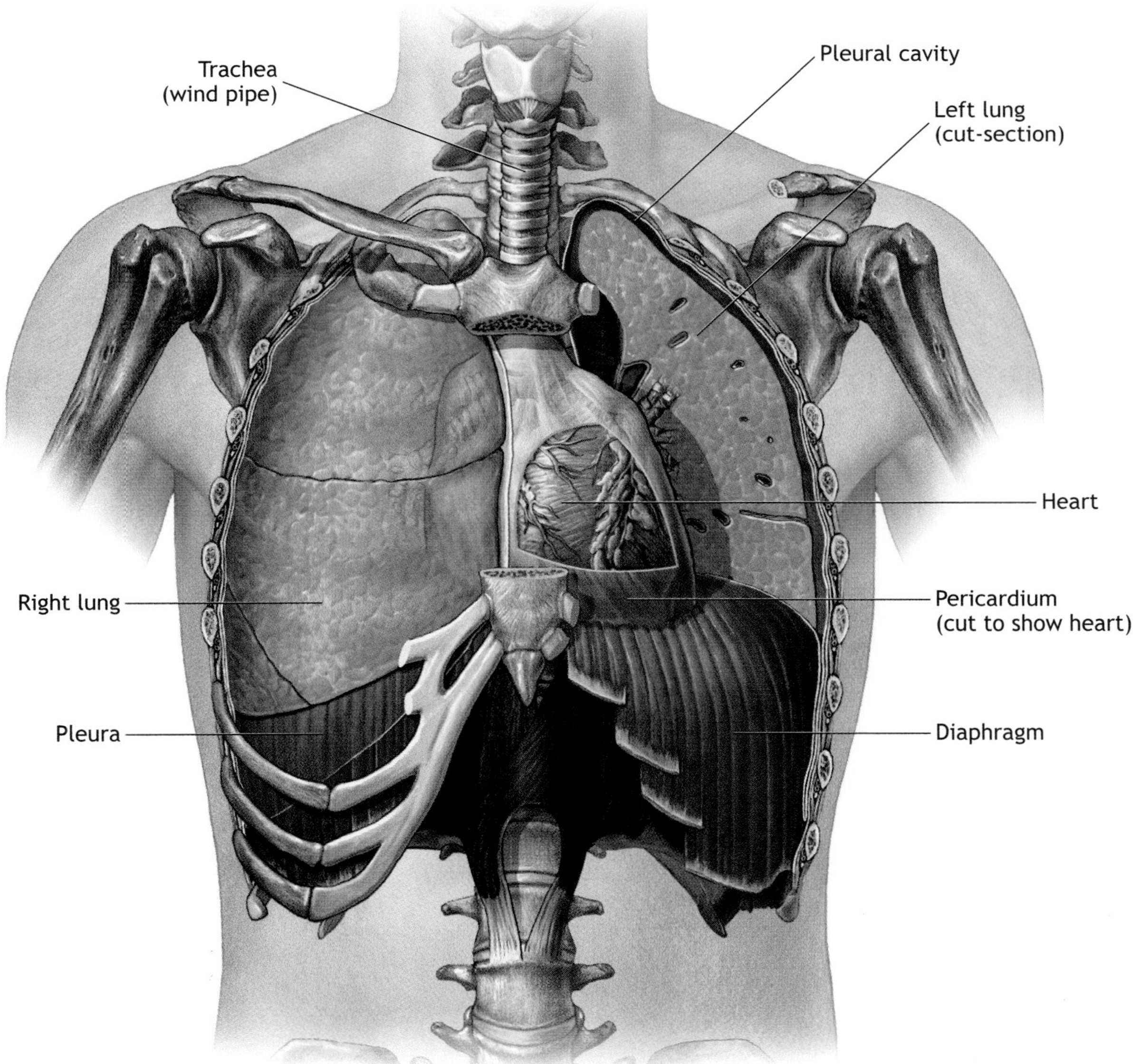

Heart and Great Vessels

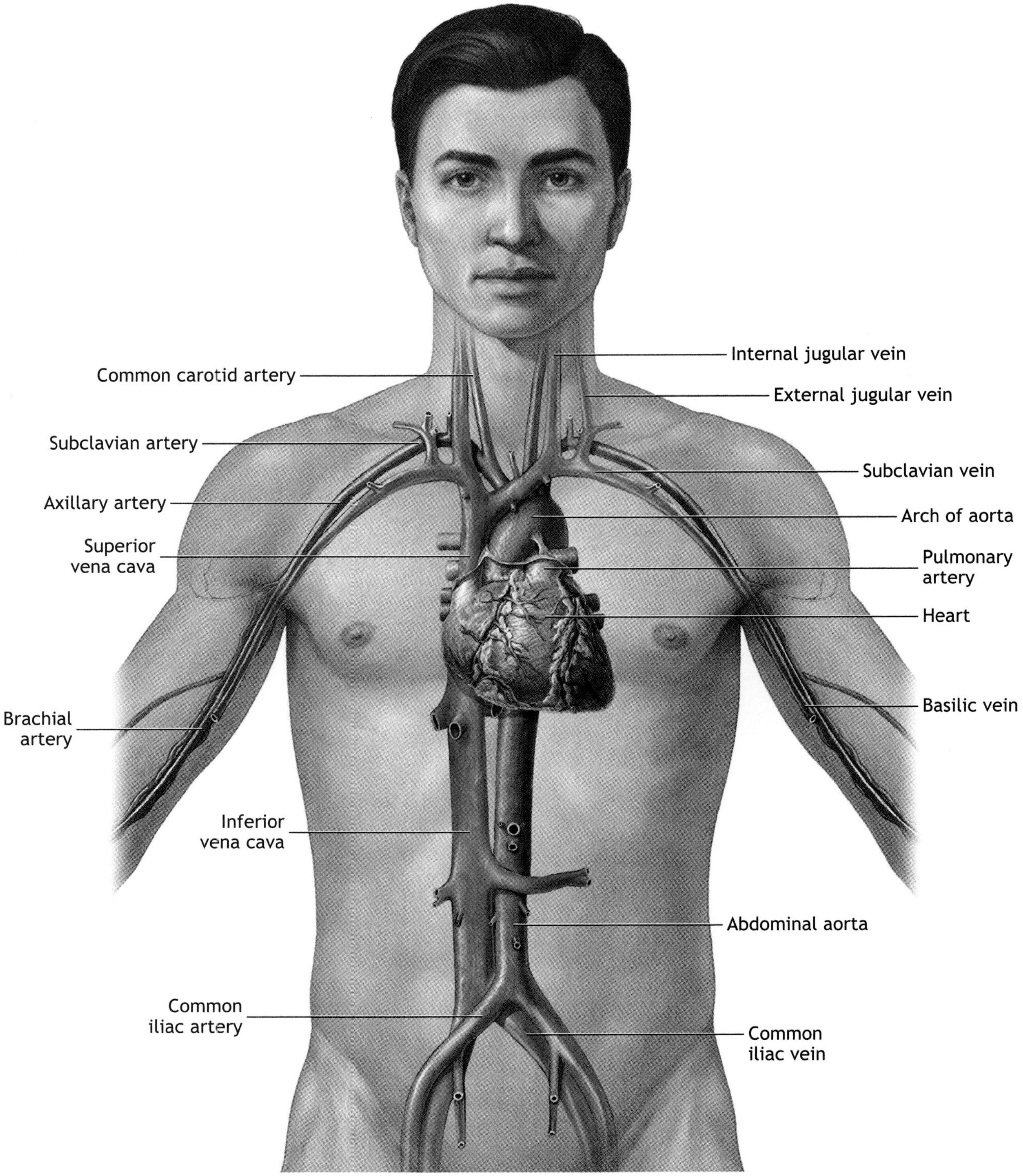
Common carotid artery
Subclavian artery
Axillary artery
Superior vena cava
Brachial artery
Inferior vena cava
Common iliac artery
Internal jugular vein
External jugular vein
Subclavian vein
Arch of aorta
Pulmonary artery
Heart
Basilic vein
Abdominal aorta
Common iliac vein

Valves of the Heart

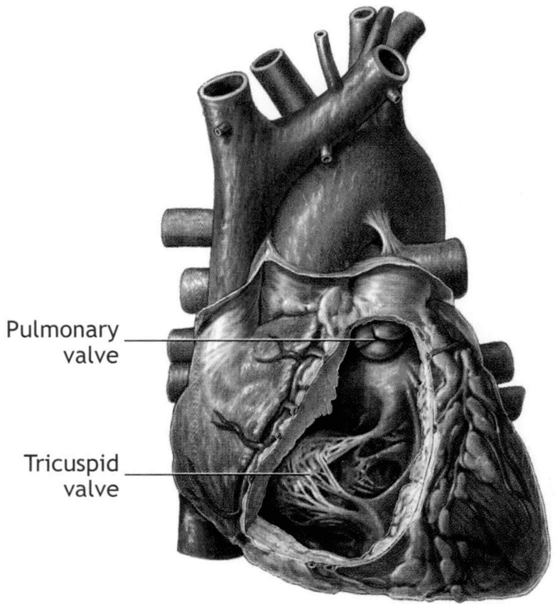

Right ventricle (cut-section)

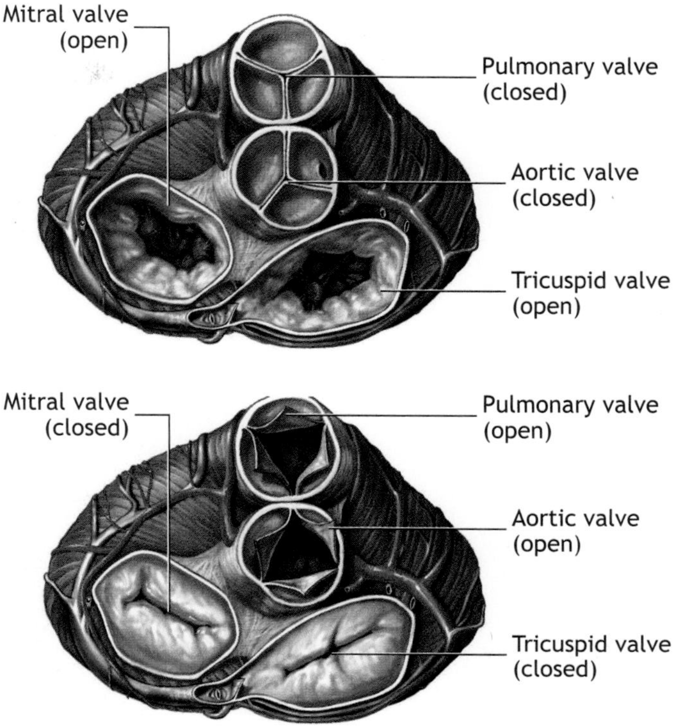

Top (superior) view of the heart

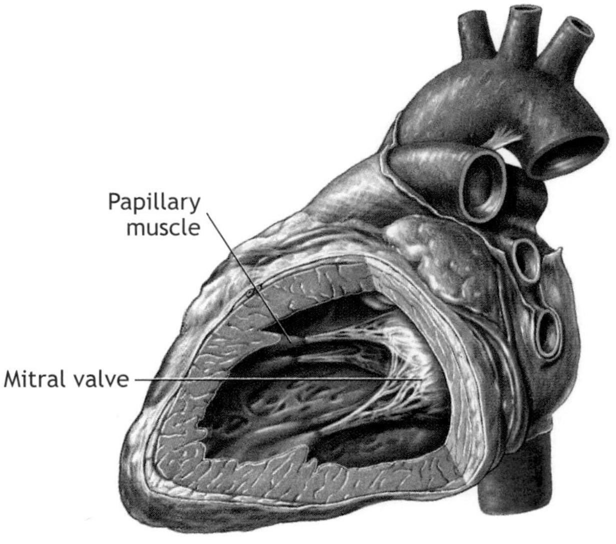

Left ventricle (cut-section)

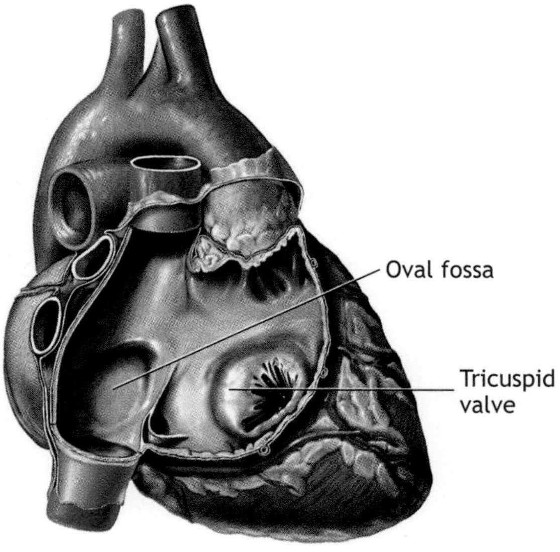

Right atrium (cut-section)

Organs of the abdomen

Digestive system

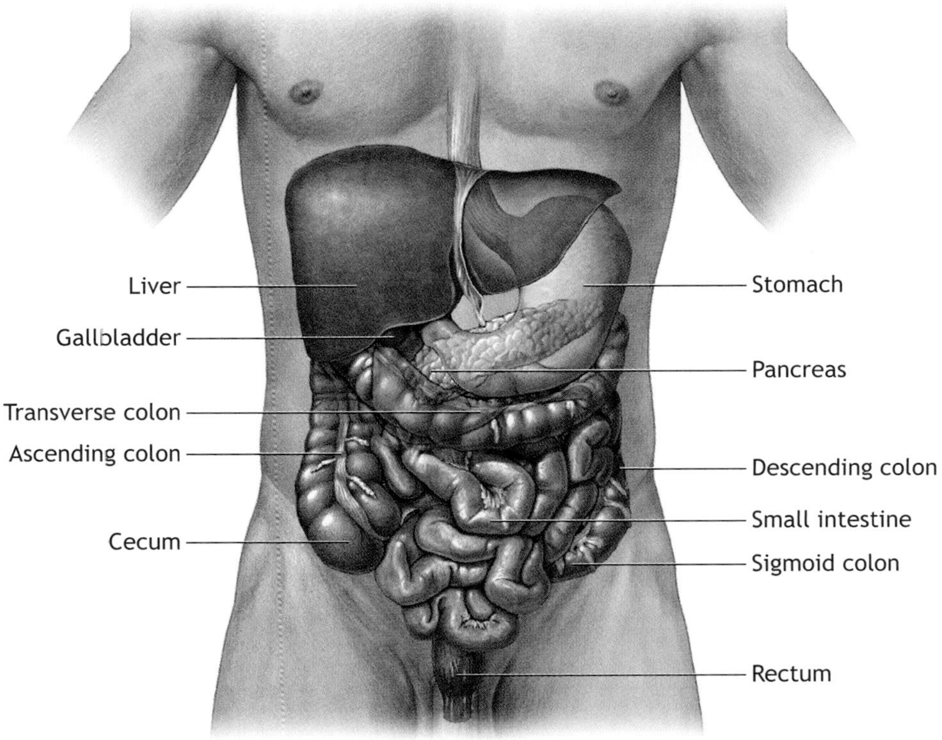

Cut-section layer

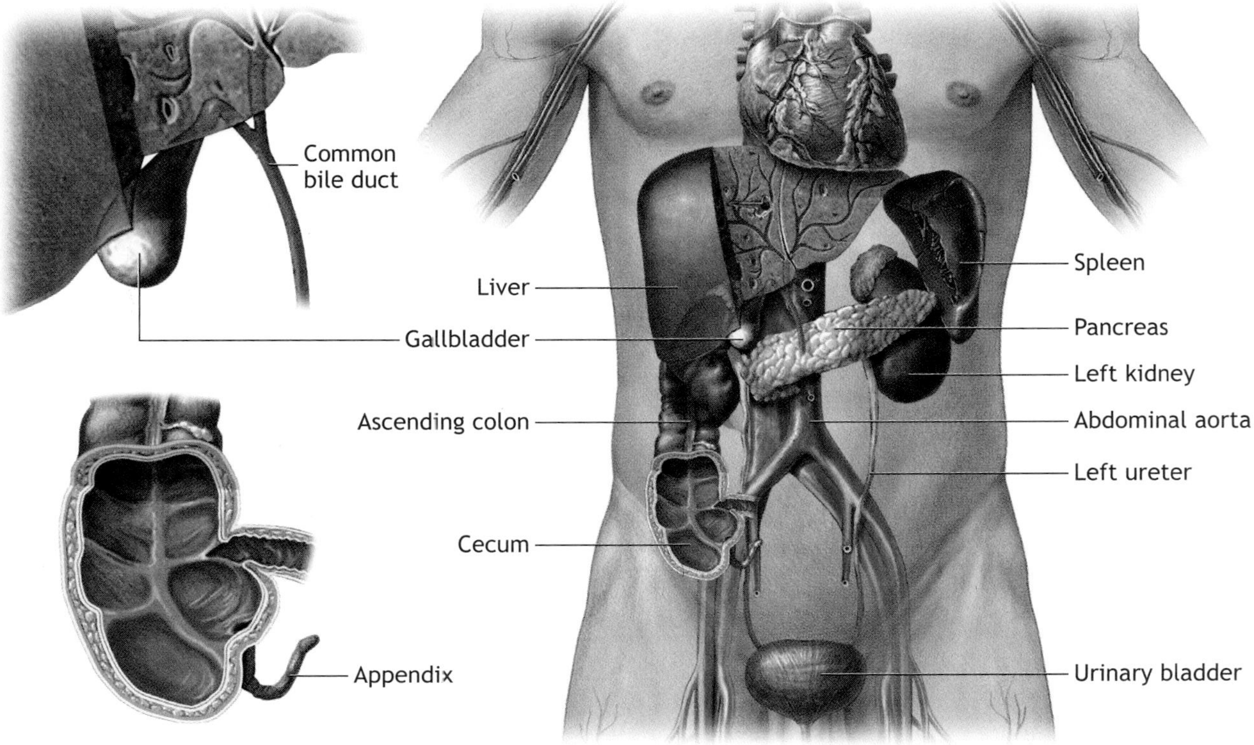

Lymphatic system

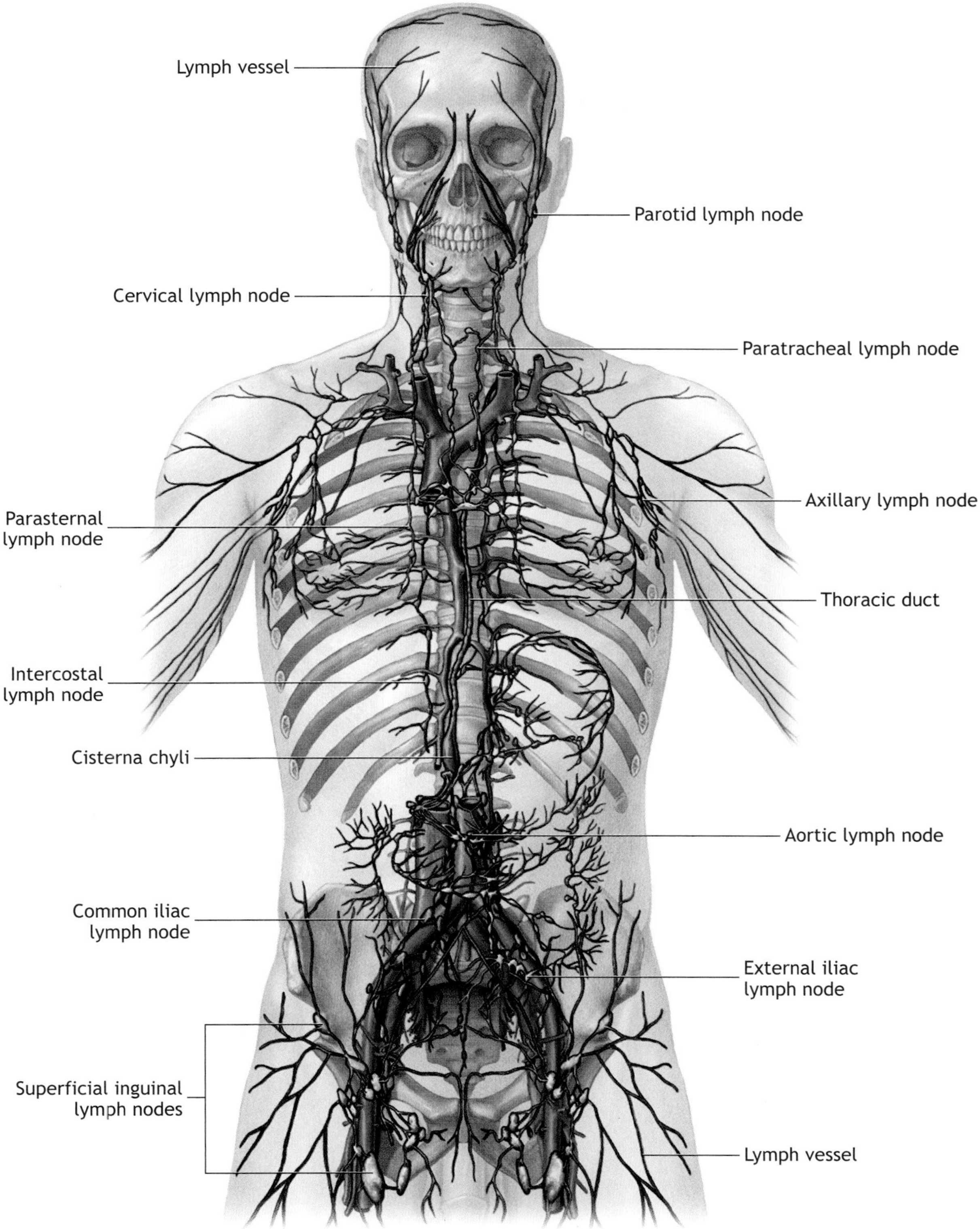
Lymph vessel
Parotid lymph node
Cervical lymph node
Paratracheal lymph node
Axillary lymph node
Parasternal lymph node
Thoracic duct
Intercostal lymph node
Cisterna chyli
Aortic lymph node
Common iliac lymph node
External iliac lymph node
Superficial inguinal lymph nodes
Lymph vessel

Urinary system

Cut-section view of the left kidney

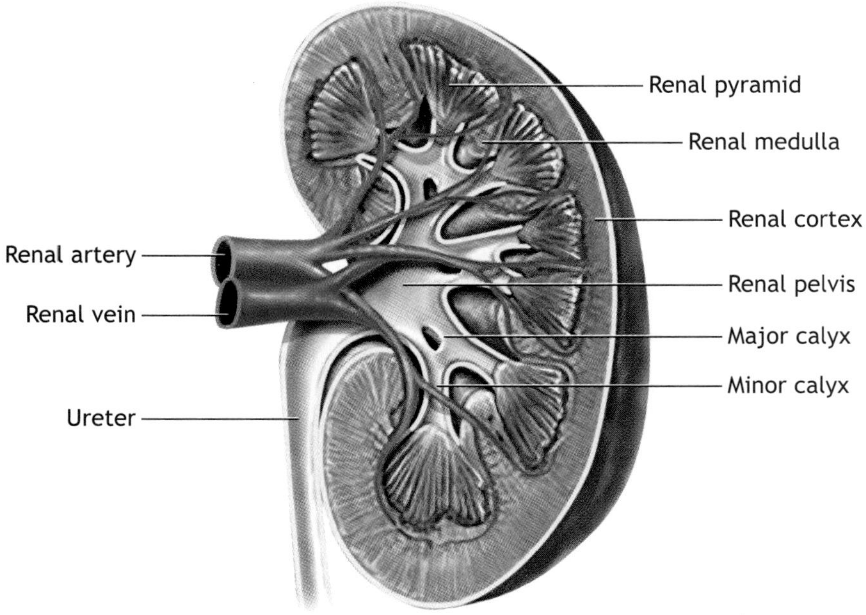

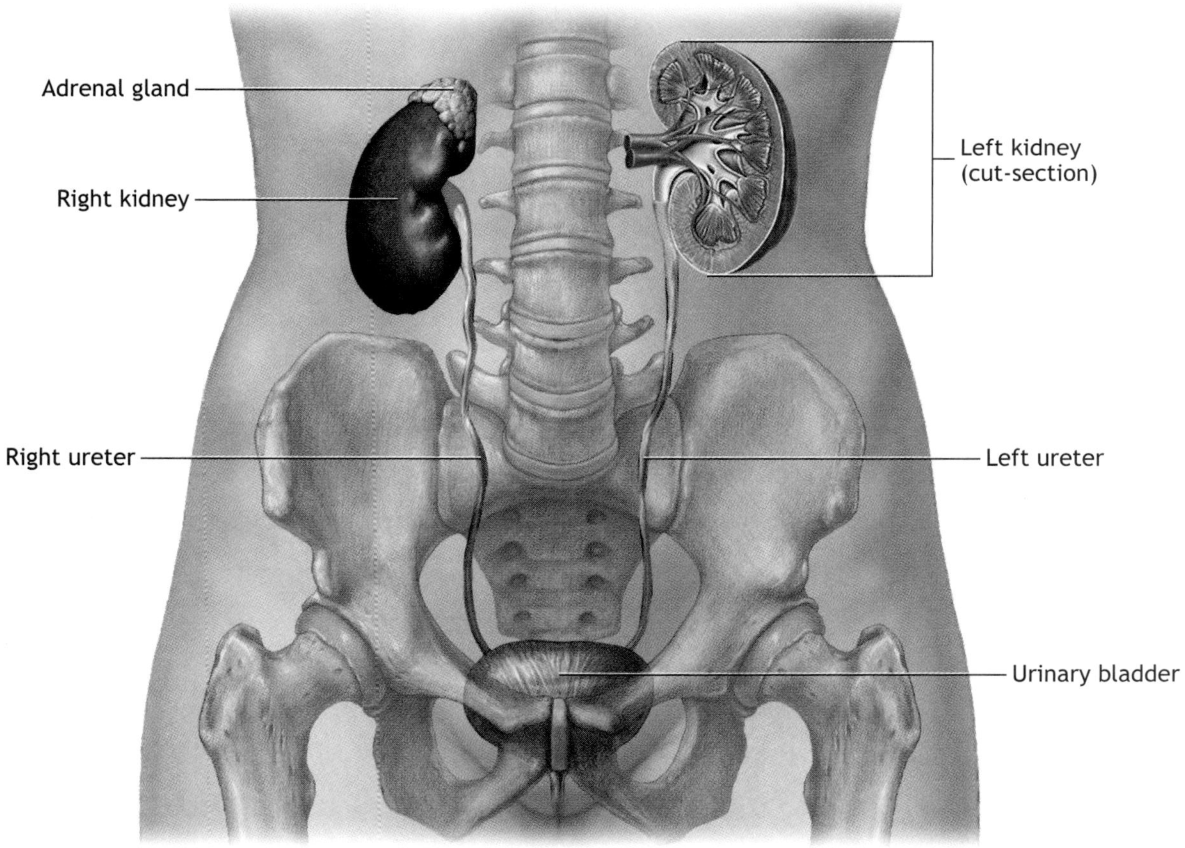

Reproductive system: male

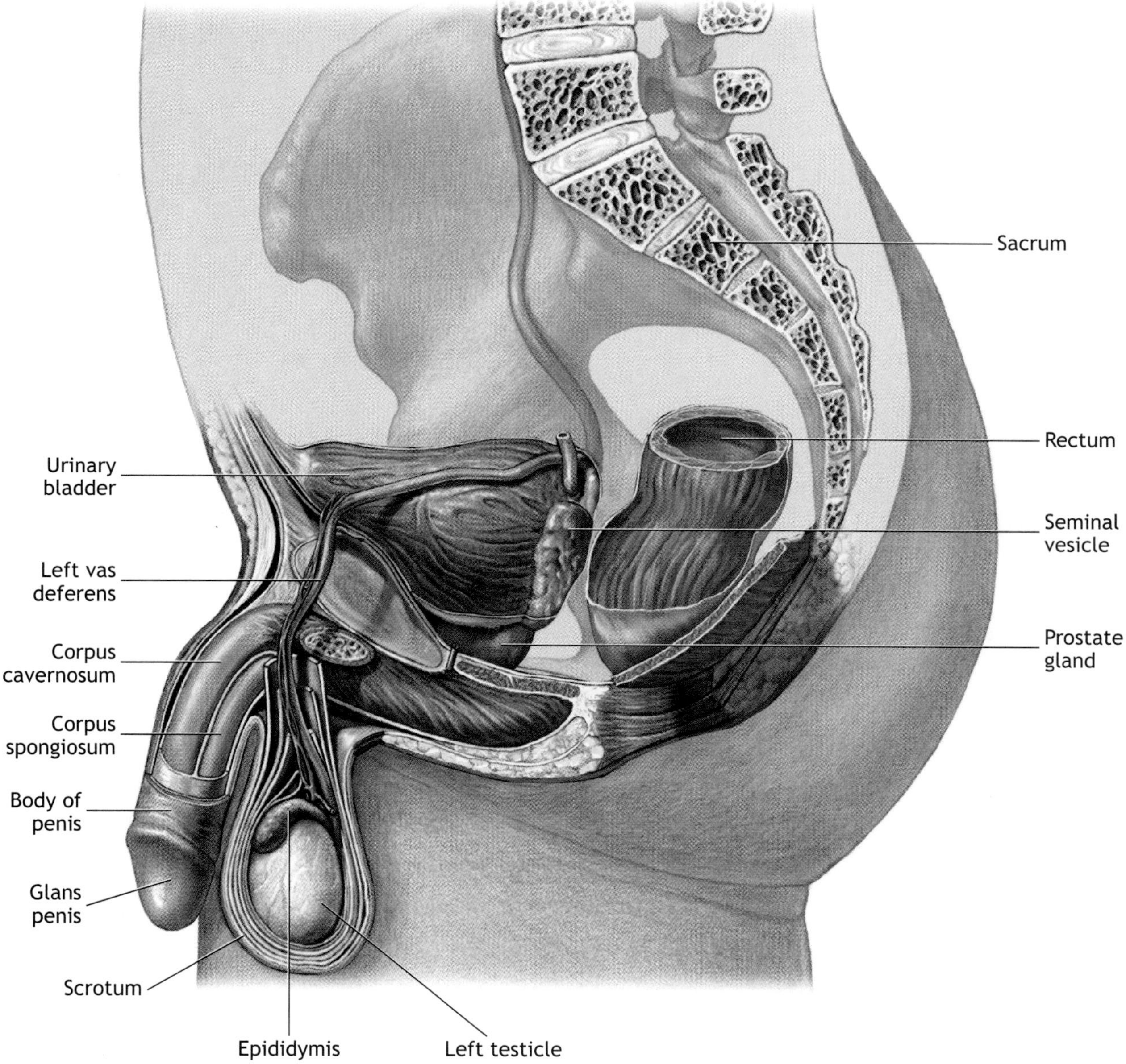

Reproductive system: female

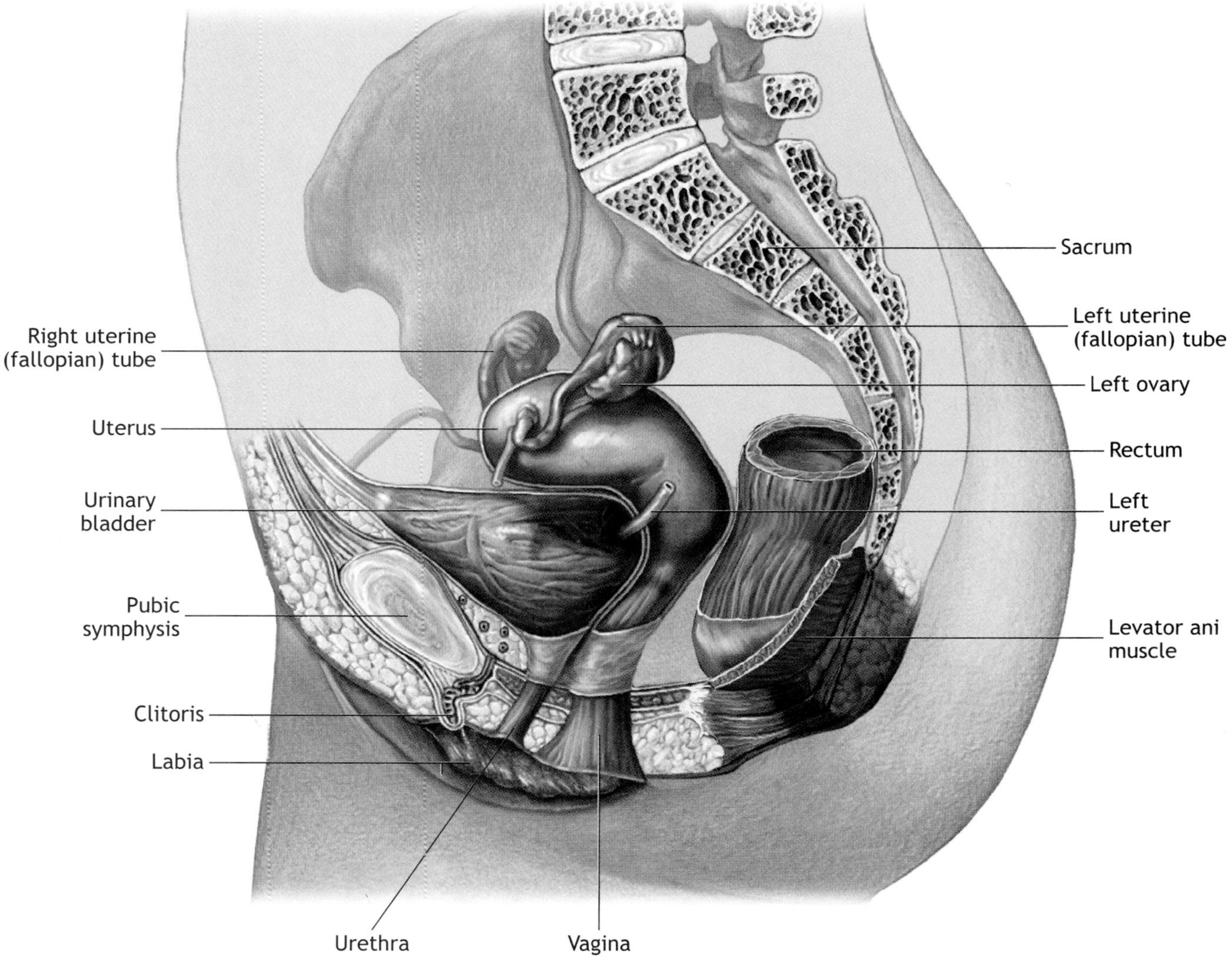

Pregnancy

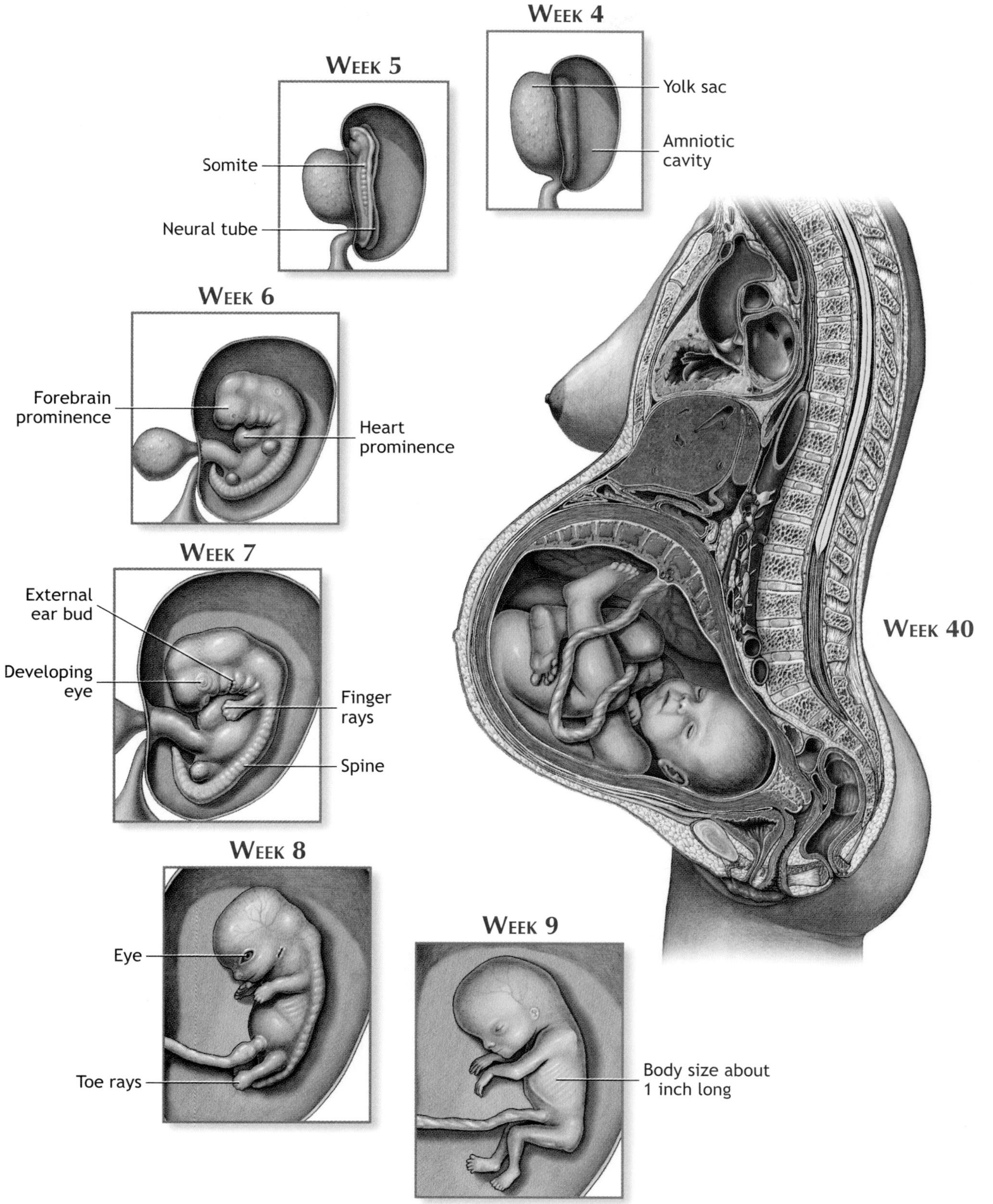
Week 4
Yolk sac
Amniotic cavity
Week 5
Somite
Neural tube
Week 6
Forebrain prominence
Heart prominence
Week 7
External ear bud
Developing eye
Finger rays
Spine
Week 8
Eye
Toe rays
Week 9
Body size about 1 inch long
Week 40

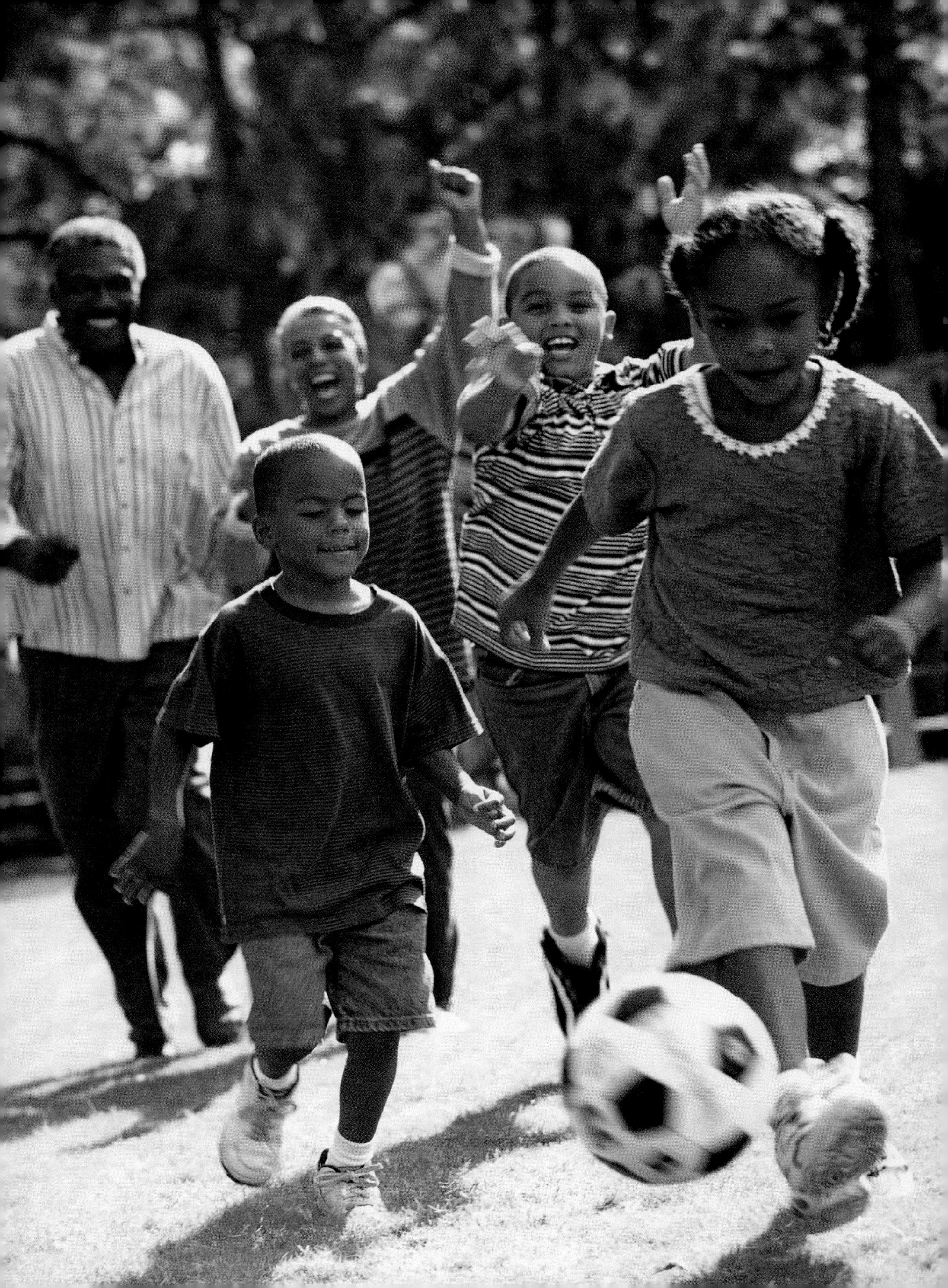

HEALTHY LIVING

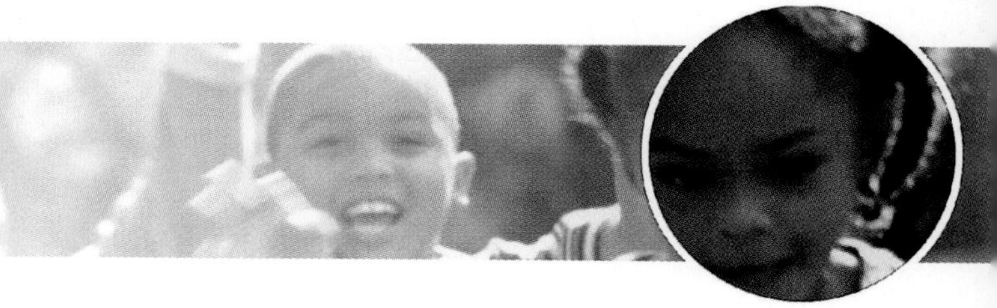

EXERCISE AND STAY ACTIVE

Physical fitness is essential to good health and is one of the best things you can do for your body, mind, and spirit. Exercise can greatly reduce your risk of many chronic diseases. It improves the way your body works and can make you look better, feel better, and even live longer.

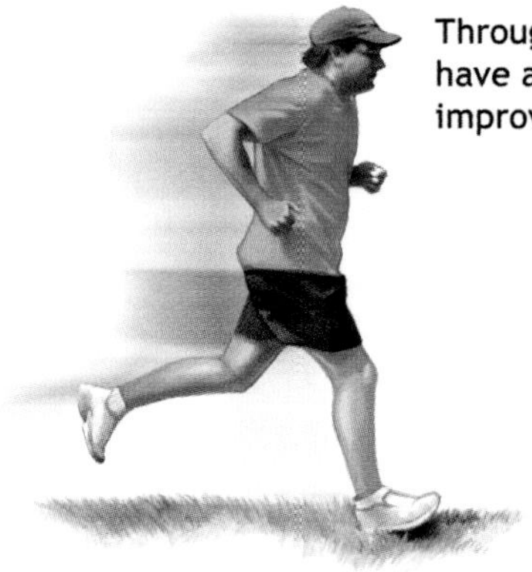

Through exercise, you have a powerful tool for improving your health

If you do not currently exercise, you may feel intimidated about starting. Exercise can be a tough adjustment to your lifestyle, but the rewards are great, and the obstacles become easier to overcome as you continue. Besides, you are giving yourself the best gift in the world: improved strength, endurance, and the satisfaction of taking care of yourself.

THE BENEFITS OF BEING IN SHAPE

Almost as soon as you start, exercise makes your brain release "endorphins" – hormones that make you feel good. This can help you enjoy the exercise and may improve your mood for several hours after your workout. Another benefit is that your muscles, having worked hard, can relax more easily. This helps you feel relaxed all over.

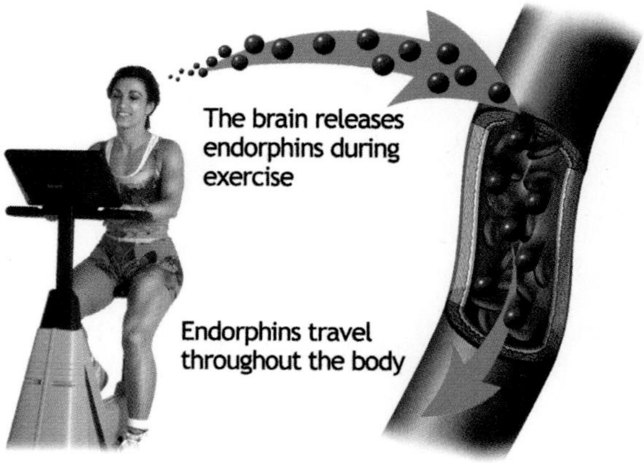
The brain releases endorphins during exercise
Endorphins travel throughout the body

In addition to the immediate rewards, your muscles will get stronger over time. Your heart will get stronger, too, and work more efficiently. Your bones will become denser, helping to prevent osteoporosis. Endurance increases, making most physical activities easier. And balance improves, lowering the risk of falls and fractures as you get older. You are also likely to experience less anxiety and depression and feel more self-assured.

PREVENT AND MANAGE CHRONIC DISEASES

Regular exercise can help PREVENT high blood pressure, high cholesterol, heart disease, type 2 diabetes, and possibly stroke from developing. You are also taking steps to reduce your risk of some forms of cancer, such as colon, breast, and prostate cancers.

If you already have certain chronic conditions, such as arthritis, osteoporosis, heart disease, Alzheimer's disease, and depression, exercise can help you manage them. Your blood pressure, cholesterol, and heart rate all may drop to healthier levels. Talk to your doctor about what is safe and best for you.

Lose weight

Exercise helps you shed extra pounds, particularly from fat. It helps tone muscles to increase your body's fitness. You're likely to experience less hunger. You will probably begin to burn more calories even while resting, making it easier to stay lean.

How much exercise is enough?

The U.S. Surgeon General recommends that everyone get a moderate amount of physical activity on most, if not all, days of the week. Physical activity is any activity that causes your body to work harder than normal.

- **For heart health** – To keep your heart healthy and maintain general fitness, you need to perform cardiovascular exercise (also called aerobic exercise). This type of exercise gets your heart beating fast over a sustained period of time. You benefit most when your heart beats between 50-75% of its maximum rate (your target zone) for at least 30 minutes total per day, at least 3 days per week. Your target heart zone is high enough to condition your heart without putting too much stress on it.
- **Losing weight** – If your goal is to lose weight, try to get 60 minutes of physical activity equivalent to brisk walking each day. This does NOT necessarily have to be aerobic exercise. The goal is to burn calories, and you can do that countless ways, such as using the stairs instead of the elevator, parking your car in the farthest parking space, or mowing the lawn or gardening. If you are doing an activity that takes more effort, like running, then 30 minutes a day should be sufficient. Or if you are doing something that takes about half the effort of brisk walking, like gardening, you'll have to do it twice as long – two hours.

Types of exercise

There are three major types of exercise, and each contributes something different to overall fitness. In general, a balanced program would include all three types.

- **Cardiovascular training** – also called aerobic training, this type of exercise keeps the heart pumping for an extended period of time. It strengthens your heart and blood vessels, improves cholesterol, and helps you lose weight. Examples include brisk walking, swimming, and cycling.
- **Flexibility training** – these exercises help your muscles stretch farther in a given direction. Flexibility training helps prevent cramps, stiffness, and injuries, and can give you a wider range of motion. These exercises also emphasize proper breathing, balance, and alignment. Some forms of flexibility training, such as yoga and tai chi, include meditation and breathing techniques that can reduce stress.

Three major types of exercise

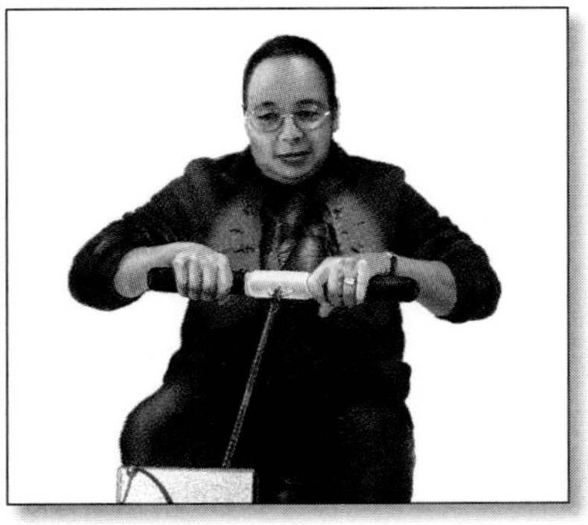

Cardiovascular training

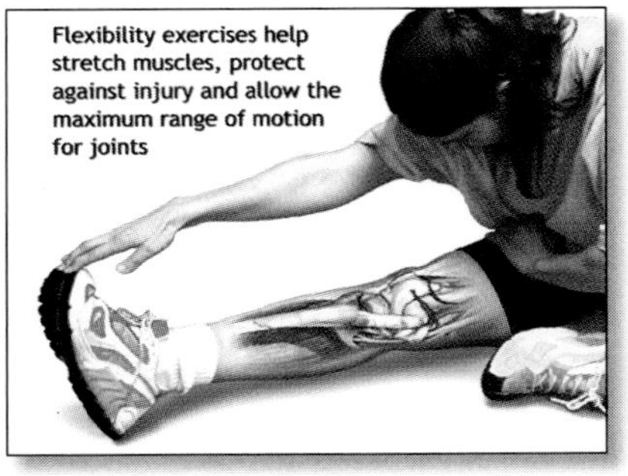

Flexibility exercises help stretch muscles, protect against injury and allow the maximum range of motion for joints

Flexibility training

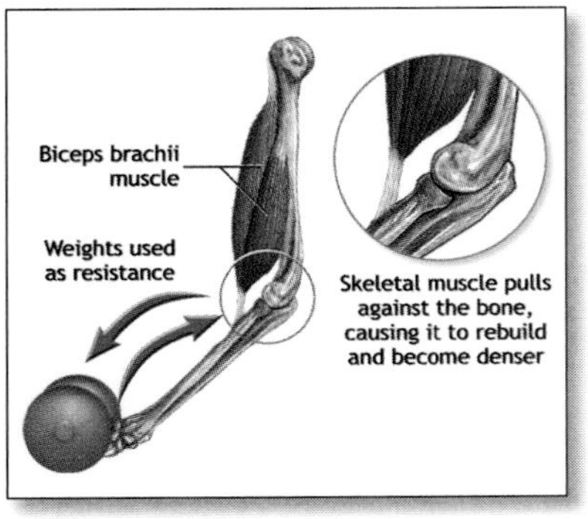

Weight training

- **Weight training** – also called strength or resistance training, these exercises build up your muscles and help maintain bone density. Strength training involves performing repetitions ("reps") that move specific muscles in the same pattern repeatedly against a resisting force. Aim for 10 to 20 minutes of strength training 2 to 3 times per week.

Stay safe

If you do not currently exercise, speak to your doctor before you begin, especially if you have any existing medical conditions or health risks.

Avoid injury by varying your workout, warming up and stretching, and cooling down adequately.

Drink plenty of water before, during, and after exercise. This is important no matter what the temperature is outside.

What motivates you?

For many people, the hardest part of exercising is getting out the door. Just about everyone who exercises struggles with this once in a while – getting motivated each day can be really tough! We asked people what gets them going, and below is a sample of their responses:

"Exercise helps me sleep better, which in turn gives me more energy the next day. I hate feeling tired at work."

"I enjoy spending time by myself first thing in the morning."

"I have family members who've had heart attacks, and I am doing what I can to keep that from happening to me."

"I want to be healthy as I get older. I don't want to lose my ability to stay active."

"There are several people I exercise with, and I enjoy their company. "

"I feel the results immediately – I feel like I have more energy."

Make the time for exercise to be a part of your regular routine, no matter what your age.

> **Tip**
>
> Having trouble doing your exercise all at once? That's no problem. Spread it out throughout the day in 10-minute chunks of activity. Doing this 3 to 6 times per day can still strengthen your heart and burn calories.

Eat for health

Despite the hype around whatever the latest and greatest diet is to make you thin, healthy, and happy, there are several principles that continue to stand the test of time:

- Control portions.
- Choose healthy fats and avoid unhealthy ones.
- Eat lots of fruits and vegetables.
- Get lots of fiber by having wholesome, unprocessed foods like whole grains.
- Select lean protein.

Although our desire for weight loss is what often draws us to particular diets, eating for health is not just about looking better. Unhealthy eating, together with other bad lifestyle habits, is estimated to cause 80% of all cases of heart disease and 90% of type 2 diabetes. Blood pressure, cholesterol, and our risk for cancer are also affected.

> **Watch your calories**
>
> Americans eat much larger portions compared to people in other countries. Even our candy bars are super-sized compared to every other nation. It's not hard to understand how 2 out of 3 Americans are overweight or obese.

To learn more about calories, see *Manage Your Weight*. For information on reading food labels, see *High Cholesterol*.

Good fat/bad fat

You want to limit *saturated fats* and *trans fatty acids* at the same time that you increase *monounsaturated fats* and *omega-3 fatty acids.* Eat foods like olive oil, fish, avocados, and nuts (especially walnuts and almonds). Cut back red meat, butter, ice cream, margarine, fried foods, and highly processed foods (like commercial baked goods). Not only does this switch help to protect your heart and maintain better sugar levels in your blood, you feel less hungry with some degree of healthy fat still in your diet.

Fruits and vegetables

It's not just an old-wives tale that lots of fruits and vegetables are good for you. Try to eat 5 to 9 half-cup servings of fruits and vegetables each day (equivalent to a medium apple, for example). These foods are low in calories and are jam-packed with flavonoids, carotenoids, and other antioxidants to help protect your eyes, skin, and heart. They may even help protect you from getting cancer. A general rule of thumb is the richer the color – like dark green or orange – the healthier the fruit or vegetable. For example, choose romaine over iceberg lettuce, or better yet spinach. Try cooked tomatoes to help protect your prostate. Eat plenty of berries (along with your carrots!) to prevent eye damage.

Eating grains in their most natural, wholesome form provides you with the most fiber possible. Fiber has many benefits, including:

- Controlling weight because you feel full sooner
- Regulating your bowels and relieving constipation by bulking up your stool
- Preventing diabetes and heart disease by improving blood sugar and lowering cholesterol
- Treating or preventing several bowel conditions, like diverticulosis, irritable bowel syndrome, hemorrhoids, and possibly colon cancer

Some of the best sources of fiber include:

- Oat bran, barley (although pearl barley has less), and wheat bran
- Nuts and seeds
- Beans, peas, and lentils
- Certain fruits and vegetables

Try to get 25 to 35 grams of fiber each day. A great way to start is to make oatmeal a part of your breakfast each morning. Try adding cinnamon and a touch of non-fat or low-fat yogurt, rather than butter or maple syrup. Make sure that you drink plenty of water with the high-fiber foods and throughout the day. Otherwise, the fiber may worsen (or bring on) constipation, bloating, and gas.

You probably see lots of references to the difference between soluble and insoluble fiber. Don't worry too much about this. The main point is to get as much fiber as possible. If you incorporate the foods mentioned, you will get plenty of both types.

The protein story

Despite the attention and interest that many high-protein diets draw (not to mention the many stories of successful weight loss you hear through the grapevine), they have NOT been researched adequately to show whether they will help you lose weight and keep it off over the long term. Remember, animal sources of protein are not only high in protein but also high in saturated fat. In addition, too much protein can cause kidney, bone, and liver problems. Animal sources of protein, for example, decrease calcium levels in your blood, potentially contributing to bone disorders like osteoporosis.

Luckily, the solution is rather simple:

- You DO NOT need protein at every meal.

- Choose beans, fish, soy, and poultry over red meat.
- Eat lean cuts of meat, when you do have red meat.

Manage your weight

People come in different shapes and sizes. While differences are normal, more than 60% of American adults weigh more than they should. In addition, about 25% of American children are overweight.

Experts agree that being too heavy is bad for your health. Having too much fat puts strain on the heart and can lead to serious health problems, including:

- Type 2 diabetes
- Heart disease, high cholesterol, and high blood pressure
- Sleep apnea
- Varicose veins
- Breast, endometrial, prostate, and colon cancers
- Arthritis
- Gallstones

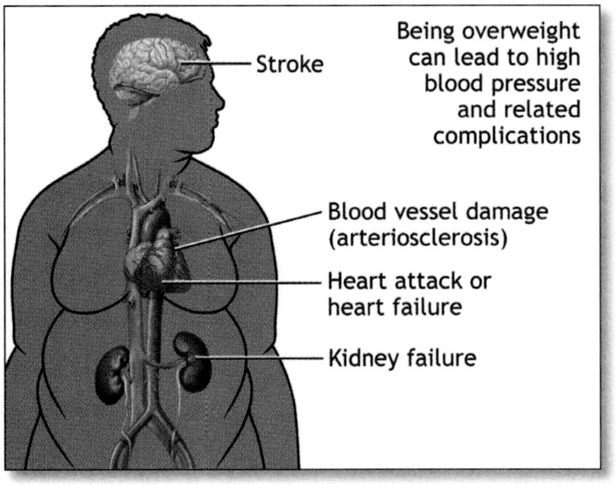

Next to smoking, obesity is the most common preventable cause of death in the United States.

Clearly, losing weight can have many potential health benefits. If you are overweight and have decided to shed some extra pounds, congratulations! You have already taken an important step toward improving your health and feeling better. If you've tried to lose weight before, don't view past efforts as failure. Instead, learn better weight-loss strategies, try again, and make this time different!

What is a healthy weight for you?

Doctors use a few different methods to determine whether you are overweight. One of these is called body mass index (BMI), a number calculated from your height and weight. (See the chart, next page.)

- **Adults:** A healthy BMI generally falls between 18.5 and 25. If your BMI is over 25, you are probably overweight. If it is 30 or higher, you are considered obese.
- **Elderly:** In the elderly it is often better to have a BMI between 25 and 27.
- **Children:** Talk to your child's doctor about what an appropriate weight is for his or her age.

For many people, efforts to lose weight mean intensive dieting, obsessive calorie counting, self-deprivation, and hunger. This approach to dieting usually fails because you suffer through it. For the most part, people who lose weight and manage to keep it off do so by adopting healthy habits that stay with them for the rest of their lives.

Take it slow and steady

Start with realistic, achievable goals. Don't expect to become "thin" overnight. Experts agree that slow, steady weight loss is healthier than a quick fix or remaining overweight. You should try to lose no more than one to two pounds per week.

While this can be frustrating, slow and steady weight loss is the only way to avoid "yo-yo dieting," where you lose a great deal of weight, only to regain it within a few months or years.

There are no miracles in weight loss; go for steady progress toward a healthier life.

Slow and steady weight loss is the only way to avoid "yo-yo" dieting, where you lose a lot of weight quickly only to regain it back

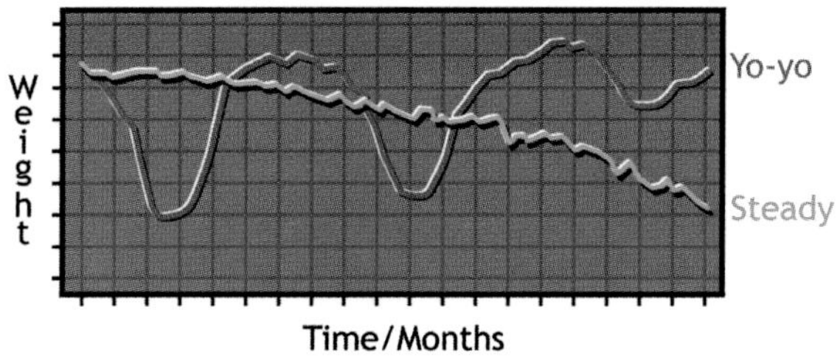

Body mass index chart

Find your height along the top and your weight along the side to determine your BMI.

Color key: Underweight | Healthy weight | Overweight | Obese | Extremely obese

	60″	62″	64″	66″	68″	70″	72″	74″	76″
100 lbs.	19.6	18.3							
110	21.5	20.2	18.9	17.8					
120	23.5	22	20.6	19.4	18.3				
130	25.4	23.8	22.4	21	19.8	18.7	17.7		
140	27.4	25.7	24.1	22.6	21.3	20.1	19	18.01	
150	29.4	27.5	25.8	24.3	22.9	21.6	20.4	19.3	18.3
160	31.3	29.3	27.5	25.9	24.4	23	21.7	20.6	19.5
170	33.3	31.2	29.2	27.5	25.9	24.4	23.1	21.9	20.7
180	35.2	33	31	29.1	27.4	25.9	24.5	23.2	22
190	37.2	34.8	32.7	30.7	28.9	27.3	25.8	24.4	23.2
200	39.1	36.7	34.4	32.3	30.5	28.8	27.2	25.7	24.4
210	41.1	38.5	36.1	34	32	30.2	28.5	27	25.6
220		40.3	37.8	35.6	33.5	31.6	29.9	28.3	26.8
230			39.6	37.2	35	33.1	31.3	29.6	28.1
240			41.3	38.8	36.6	34.5	32.6	30.9	29.3
250				40.4	38.1	35.9	34	32.2	30.5
260					39.6	37.4	35.3	33.5	31.7
270					41.1	38.8	36.7	34.7	32.9
280						40.3	38.1	36	34.2
290							39.4	37.3	35.4
300							40.8	38.6	36.6
310								39.9	37.8
320								41.2	39
330									40.3

The role of calories

The most common cause of weight gain is fairly simple: your energy input (the calories you eat) is greater than your energy output (the calories you burn).

Calories are the basic unit of energy within food. When you eat, your body converts calories into energy. Your body uses what it can and stores the rest in the form of fat.

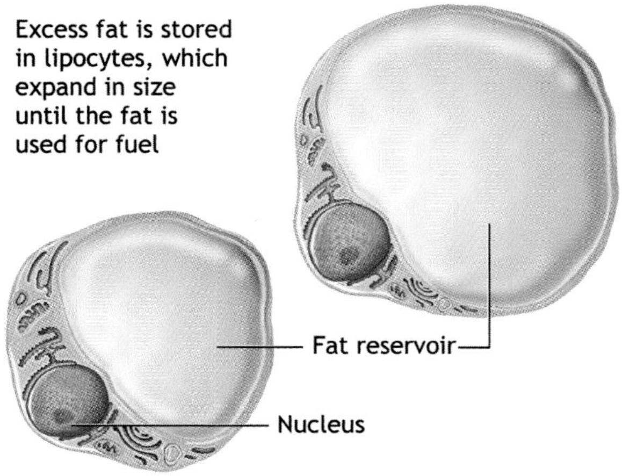

Thus, you should eat a **low-calorie diet** if you want to lose weight.

A calorie is a calorie, whether it comes from a brownie or raw broccoli. The important factors are the number of calories, nutrients, fat, and other ingredients in a typical **serving**.

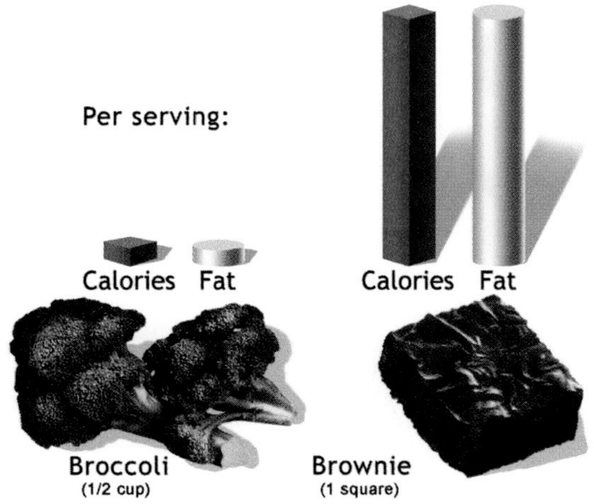

Food	Serving size	Calories	Fat (grams)
Broccoli	1/2 cup	12	0.2
Brownie	1 square	160	3

Some diets involve **calorie counting** – figuring out the number of calories in each food item you eat, then adding up the total at the end of the day. This method shows how quickly calories add up and where most of your calories come from. This can be valuable information, particularly when you first start your weight loss program.

Counting calories, however, quickly becomes tedious, and it does not necessarily train you to eat a healthy balance of foods. It is easy to become obsessed with the numbers and forget that the point is to eat healthily and vary your foods.

Healthy weight loss:

- Occurs slowly
- Promotes long-term healthy habits
- Fits into your lifestyle
- Includes physical activity
- Reduces calories but maintains a balance of nutrients

Eat less, or eat healthy?

Obviously, you can reduce calories simply by eating less. Although in theory this method should help you lose weight, it is not the healthiest or most successful.

First of all, you are not eating a balanced, nutritious diet, nor are you lowering your risk for chronic conditions like diabetes and heart disease. Furthermore, people who simply try to eat less, rather than changing food types, tend to get hungrier faster and snack more in between meals.

Instead, replace unhealthy and fattening foods with healthier alternatives – eat the same amount of food as before but **eat lower-calorie foods with a better balance of nutrients**.

Hints for eating nutritious foods

- Choose fresh fruits and vegetables over canned or processed foods.
- Lower your fat intake by eating a plant-based diet. Animal products tend to be higher in saturated fat and calories than most plant products.
- Choose products (like breads and pasta) with whole grains over those with white flour. These have more fiber, are more likely to fill you up, and are more nutritious. The fiber may even help lower your cholesterol.
- Allow yourself an occasional treat, so you don't feel deprived. It can be easier to change your habits if you know you can still have your favorite dessert or snack once in awhile.
- Eat fish instead of meat. Fish is a healthy, lean protein. Also, it contains a type of fat called "omega-3," which may help protect the heart.

Fish is great for people trying to lose weight:

- lean, low-calorie meat
- great source of protein
- contains omega 3

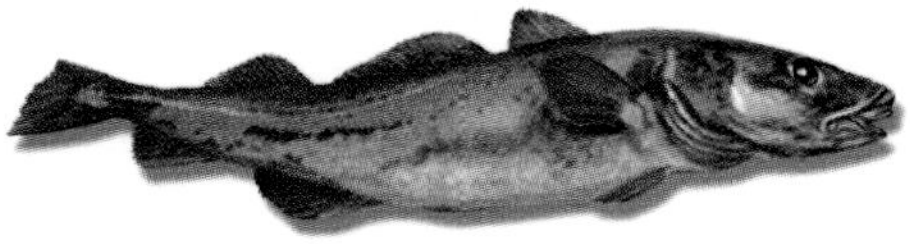

Some healthy food habits

- **Always eat regular meals, including breakfast** – Skipping meals delivers a double whammy to your weight loss efforts. When you skip meals, your body goes into "starvation mode," signaling your body to conserve as much energy as possible – this builds up body fat. Skipping meals is also likely to make you very hungry for your next meal, which could cause you to eat more. Try to eat meals and snacks at about the same time every day.
- **Eat only in the dining room or at the kitchen table** – this will keep you more disciplined about eating. Keep food out of sight so you won't be tempted to eat between meals.
- **Start with small portions** – You can always get more later, but your compulsion to "clean your plate" may encourage you to eat more than you should. Keep in mind that if you are used to eating large meals, your stomach will signal hunger until its size reduces. This takes weeks to months of eating smaller meals. It will be tougher to stick to smaller meals at the beginning, but that won't last.
- **Eat your vegetables first** – This will help you fill your stomach with relatively few calories and lots of fiber. You may be less hungry for the more fattening foods.
- **Slow down** – It takes time for your body to recognize you have eaten and for the feeling of hunger to go away. Eating too quickly may cause you to eat more food over the same period of time. Savor it.
- **Substitute healthy foods for unhealthy ones** – Instead of snacking on potato chips, try carrot sticks, fresh fruit, or yogurt. Sample different kinds of food for variety.
- **Drink plenty of water** – This will help you feel full sooner.

Finally, don't forget to take a walk after dinner! Exercise is vital to losing weight. See the article, *Exercise and Stay Active.*

If this isn't the first time that you've tried to lose weight, you are not alone. For most people, weight loss takes multiple attempts before getting it right. Losing weight is a significant undertaking; long-term success is a huge accomplishment and a lifetime commitment.

It may help to think about how far you have already come. You do not have to measure that by the number of pounds you have lost.

For example, think about how much farther or faster you can walk, jog or cycle compared to before you started. If good health is your goal (and it should be), you can measure success in many ways.

Eating right and exercising are the keys to a healthy life for everyone. Too few people – even thin people – respect their bodies enough to follow through with these important lifestyle habits. When you stick to achieving your weight loss goals, you will have accomplished more than many other people, and you will have something to be truly proud of!

> **KEY POINT**
>
> There is no magic drug, supplement, or other "quick fix". The key to successful weight loss is slow and steady change in diet and more physical activity.

DRINK RESPONSIBLY

Despite much media and popular attention around the idea that small, regular amounts of alcohol might be good for you, there are many health risks from drinking alcohol. It is important to understand these risks and know if you are a responsible drinker or not.

First and foremost, NEVER drink and drive. Alcohol is the leading cause of motor vehicle accidents in the United States. It slows reaction times and impairs your judgment.

Ongoing use of alcohol can:

- Damage your liver and possibly lead to cirrhosis.
- Increase your risk of cancer of the esophagus, throat, larynx, and mouth.
- Impair your ability to absorb certain essential nutrients from the stomach and small intestines.
- Diminish sexual function, even if it increases your sexual desire.
- Cause serious damage to a fetus if you are pregnant like failure to grow, reduced IQ, and malformed facial features. Alcohol should NOT be consumed if you are pregnant or trying to become pregnant.

How do you know if you have a drinking problem? Ask yourself the following:

- Have you ever thought that you needed to cut back on the amount of alcohol you drink?
- Has a spouse, friend, or coworker ever asked you to drink less?
- Do you ever feel guilty about the amount that you drink?
- Do you ever drink early in the day to nurse a hangover?

If you answer "yes" to 2 or more of these questions, you almost certainly have a drinking problem that requires attention. Talk to your doctor about helpful programs. Even if you answer "yes" to only 1 of these questions, talk to your doctor about such programs. Be honest with yourself; you have NOTHING to lose and EVERYTHING to gain.

Assuming that you don't have a drinking problem, how do you drink responsibly?

- ONLY drink if you are of legal age to do so.
- If you are out drinking, designate a driver or plan an alternative way home, like a taxi or a bus.
- DO NOT drink on an empty stomach. Snack before and during alcohol consumption.
- Drink slowly and only in moderation – preferably, no more than one drink per day for women and no more than two drinks per day for men.
- If you take medication, including over-the-counter medication, check with your pharmacist before drinking alcohol.

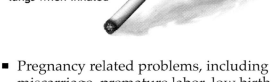

Finally, getting back to the potential health benefits of alcohol, it is important to know that these disappear when women drink more than 1 to 1 ½ alcoholic beverages per day and men more than 2 per day.

QUIT SMOKING

Over 38 million people in the United States have successfully quit smoking. Yet, there are still around 50 million Americans who smoke. The majority say they would like to quit.

And, while the number of cigarette smokers in the United States has dropped over recent years, the number of **smokeless tobacco** users has steadily risen. This trend is likely related to the false belief that smokeless tobacco is safe. It is NOT. Smokeless tobacco carries many of the same health risks as cigarettes. Some people who want to stop smoking, but who still crave the nicotine, turn to smokeless tobacco wrongly thinking that they are doing something good for themselves.

There are many reasons to quit using tobacco. Knowing these serious health risks can help motivate you to quit. When used over a long period, tobacco and its various chemical components (like tar, nicotine, and thousands of others) can increase your risk of:

- Coronary artery disease, including angina and heart attacks
- High blood pressure, blood clots, aneurysms, and strokes
- Cancer (especially in the lung, mouth, larynx, esophagus, bladder, kidney, pancreas, and cervix)
- Chronic lung disease – emphysema, chronic bronchitis

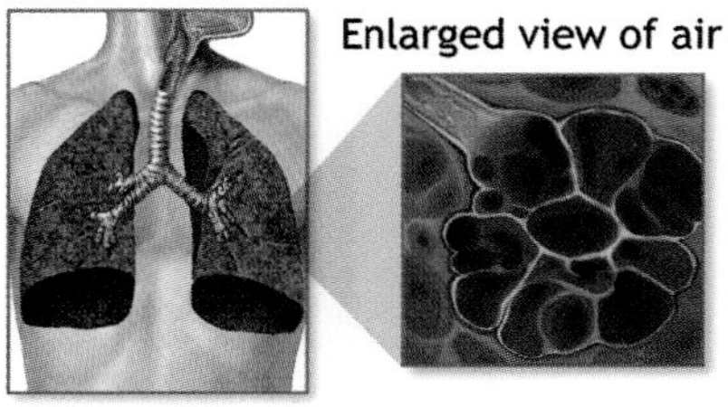

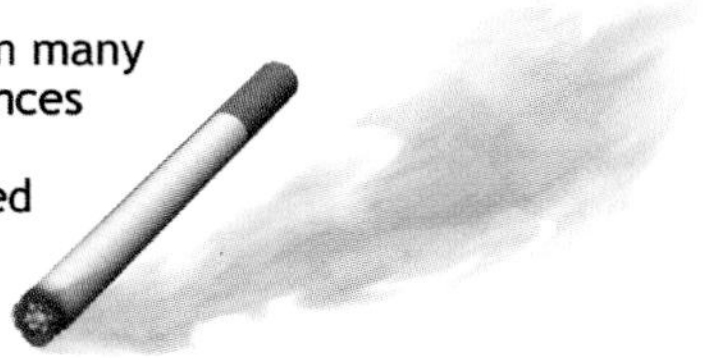

Cigarettes contain many hazardous substances that damage the lungs when inhaled

- Pregnancy related problems, including miscarriage, premature labor, low birth weight, and risk for SIDS (sudden infant death syndrome)
- Delayed wound healing
- Tooth and gum diseases; decreased senses of taste and smell

If you use smokeless tobacco long term, you have many of these same risks, plus a 50 times greater risk for oral cancer.

Even if you don't smoke yourself, but you are exposed regularly to secondhand smoke, you have a higher risk of:

- Lung cancer
- In infants and children, more respiratory infections (such as bronchitis and pneumonia), asthma, and poor lung function as the lungs mature
- Sudden and severe reactions, including eye, nose, throat, and lower respiratory tract symptoms

TIME TO QUIT

There are a lot of ways to quit smoking, and many resources to help you. Family members, friends, and coworkers may be supportive or encouraging, but the desire and commitment to quit must be your own.

Most people who have been able to successfully quit smoking made at least one unsuccessful attempt in the past. Try not to view past attempts to quit as failures, but rather as learning experiences.

Feel ready to quit? Here are some tips:

- Make a list of the reasons why you want to quit. Include both short- and long-term benefits.
- Ask your health care provider for help. Find out whether prescription medications (such as Zyban) might be useful for you. Find out about nicotine patches (Nicorette), gum, and sprays.
- Ask your family, friends, and coworkers for support.
- Set a quit date.
- Get rid of all of your cigarettes by that date. Throw them out if you have to!
- Quit completely – cold turkey.
- Exercise – It relieves the urge to smoke.
- Learn self-hypnosis from a qualified practitioner. This helps some people.
- Make a plan about what you will do, instead of smoking, when stressed or other times you have the urge for tobacco. Be as specific as possible.
- Avoid smoke-filled settings and situations in which you are more likely to smoke.

Like any addiction, quitting tobacco is difficult, particularly if you are acting alone. If you join smoking cessation programs, you have a much better chance of success. Such programs are offered by hospitals, health departments, community centers, and work sites.

If you aren't successful the first time, simply look at what occurred or what didn't work, develop new strategies, and try again. Many attempts are often necessary to finally "beat the habit."

When to contact a medical professional

Call your doctor if you are a smoker and:

- You want an individual health risk profile
- You want to learn about methods to stop tobacco use
- You are pregnant, planning a pregnancy in the future, or using birth control pills
- You have symptoms of specific diseases associated with tobacco use (even if you are a nonsmoker exposed to secondhand smoke)

Other resources include local chapters of the American Lung Association and the American Cancer Society. Both organizations have a wide range of resource materials and comprehensive smoking cessation programs.

Prevent osteoporosis

Osteoporosis literally means "porous bone." It is a condition in which your bones gradually lose density or strength and begin to deteriorate.

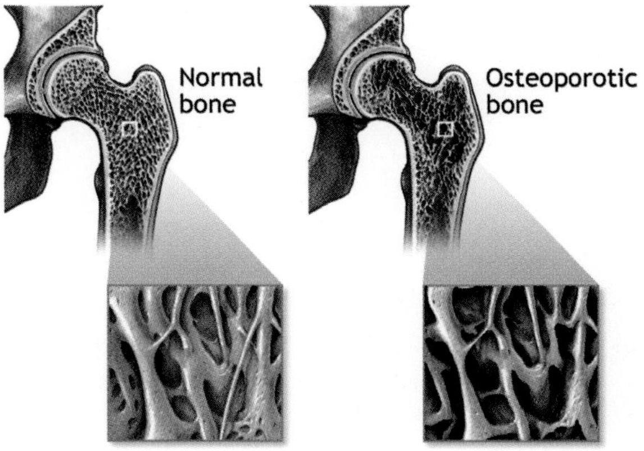

When you have osteoporosis, your bones become brittle and you are more likely to fracture your hip, spine, wrist, or other location. As many as 10 million Americans have osteoporosis and 18 million more have low bone mass (called **osteopenia**). When you have early signs of bone loss, this is a warning that osteoporosis is likely to develop unless you make some changes to prevent it.

The older you are, the more likely you are to get osteoporosis, although it can happen at any age. The loss of bone mass actually begins as early as childhood and adolescence, even though the effects are not usually seen for years.

The majority of those with this bone disorder are women beyond menopause, but men and younger women are also affected.

The good news is that there are lots of steps you can take to prevent further bone loss if it has already started. These same steps also protect your bones if they are still perfectly healthy. Most Americans can avoid osteoporosis altogether by eating a well-balanced diet, exercising regularly, and living a healthy lifestyle. It is never too late to make the following changes. But the younger you are when you get started on these changes, the better.

Change your diet

First and foremost, make sure that you get plenty of calcium, magnesium, and vitamin D in your diet. Most Americans consume less than half the amount of calcium recommended to build and maintain healthy bones. The recommended amounts of calcium are:

- **Children**: 800 to 1200 mg/day
- **Adolescent girls**: 1200 to 1500 mg/day
- **Premenopausal women** (19 to 50 years old): 1000 mg/day
- **Older adults** (51 to 70 years old): 1200 to 1500 mg/day

Good dietary sources of calcium include low-fat dairy products (such as milk, yogurt, and cheese), dark green, leafy vegetables (such as broccoli, collard greens, and spinach), sardines and salmon, tofu, and almonds. Since most people have difficulty getting enough calcium from their diet alone, supplements are important. There are a variety of supplements available, so your doctor can help you choose the most appropriate one for you. Calcium citrate tends to be the most easily absorbed and digested form.

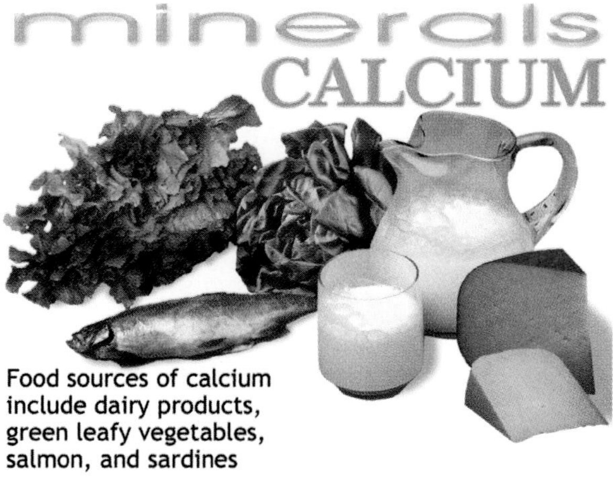

Food sources of calcium include dairy products, green leafy vegetables, salmon, and sardines

Vitamin D plays a major role in calcium absorption and bone health. Vitamin D supplements or exposure to the sun (about 20 minutes a day), in combination with calcium, can help heal bone fractures and decrease the risk of future bone breaks.

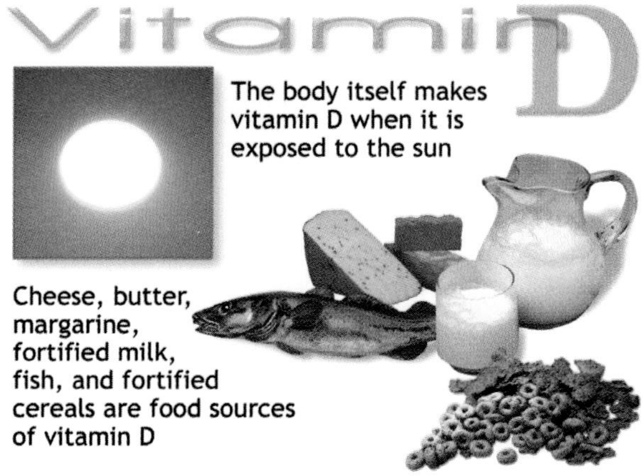

The body itself makes vitamin D when it is exposed to the sun

Cheese, butter, margarine, fortified milk, fish, and fortified cereals are food sources of vitamin D

The recommended amounts of vitamin D are:

- **Before age 50**: 200 IU/day
- **Age 51 to 70 years old**: 400 IU/day
- **71 years and older**: 600 IU/day

If you have already had a bone fracture, you may need 800 IU, especially during the winter months.

Exercise

Exercise early in life boosts bone mass, while exercise later in life helps you maintain your existing amount of bone. Exercise also increases strength, coordination, flexibility, and balance – all important tools to help prevent falls that cause fractures, especially in the elderly.

A combination of exercises may be best: weight-bearing endurance activity (such as walking), strength-training (such as weight-lifting), and flexibility and coordination exercises (such as tai chi or yoga). Together these activities prevent bone loss and increase muscle and bone mass, even if you already have osteoporosis.

Medications

Several medications can help prevent and treat osteoporosis. Talk to your doctor about the possibilities, which include estrogen, bisphosphonates, and raloxifene.

- **Estrogen** can treat and prevent bone loss. However, the risks may outweigh the benefits. Estrogen can greatly increase your risk for endometrial cancer, unless taken with progesterone. New information has proven that estrogen plus progesterone (commonly called hormone replacement therapy) increases your chances of breast cancer and, possibly, stroke and heart disease. Together with your doctor, you should weigh the pros of estrogen to help keep your bones strong against the cons of endometrial and breast cancer risks. Keep in mind that there are lots of other options available today to strengthen your bones without relying on hormones.
- **Bisphosphonates (alendronate and risedronate)** boost bone density, slow or stop bone loss, and reduce your risk of fractures. Side effects include abdominal pain, heartburn, nausea, and irritation of the esophagus. You can help reduce the likelihood of these effects by taking this medication first thing in the morning before eating anything else. Take with 8oz.

Tips to prevent falls

As we age, we become more likely to fall. This is related to poor eyesight, disorientation, lapses in judgment, and being on medications that cause dizziness or confusion. At the same time, our bones become weaker and more brittle as we grow older. Therefore, the biggest risk from a fall is fracturing your hip or other body part.

Most falls happen at home, especially in bathrooms and on stairways. Here are some ways to prevent falls:

- Place a nonskid surface on the bottom of your bathtub and shower.
- Don't use bath oils. They are slippery.
- Place a handrail near your toilet and in your tub.
- Use handrails when walking up and down stairs.
- Eliminate throw rugs and exposed electrical cords around the house.
- Keep rooms well lit.
- Get regular eye exams.

Also, consider wearing a personal emergency response system that dials directly to a medical emergency center in case you do fall and can't get up.

of water and stand upright for at least 30 minutes after taking the pill.

- **Selective Estrogen Receptor Modifiers (raloxifen)** has estrogen-like effects on bone (prevents bone loss) but does not seem to increase the risk for breast cancer. Side effects can include hot flashes and blood clotting.

Dental care for adults

Tooth decay and gum disease are largely caused by plaque, a sticky combination of bacteria and food.

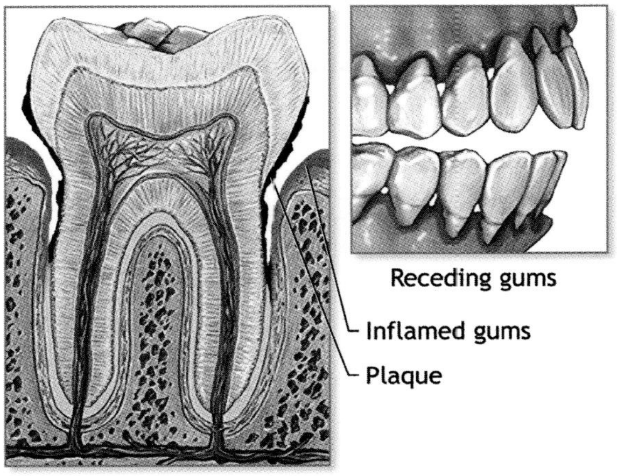

Plaque begins to accumulate on teeth within 20 minutes after eating. If this plaque is not removed thoroughly each day, tooth decay will flourish. Over time, plaque will harden into tartar.

Plaque and tartar lead to a number of problems:

- **Cavities** – holes that damage the structure of teeth
- **Gingivitis** – swollen, inflamed, bleeding gums
- **Periodontitis** – destruction of the ligaments and bone that support the teeth, often leading to tooth loss
- **Bad breath** (halitosis)
- Abscesses, pain, inability to use teeth
- A variety of health problems outside the mouth, from preterm labor to heart disease

Healthy teeth are clean and have few cavities. Healthy gums are pink and firm.

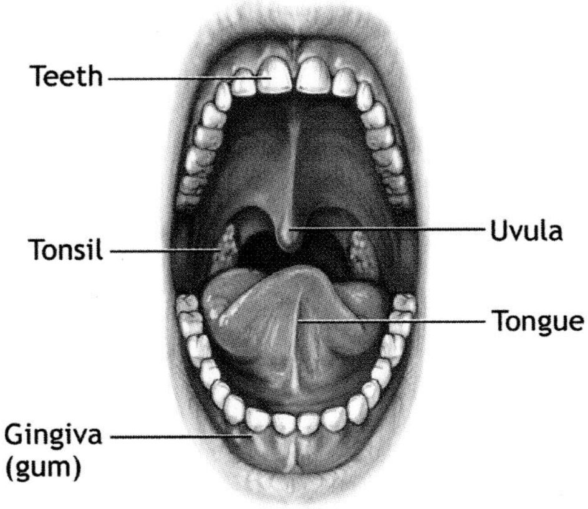

To maintain healthy teeth and gums, follow these steps:

- Brush your teeth at least twice daily, preferably after every meal and at bedtime.
- Floss at least once per day.
- Schedule an appoint with a dentist for a routine cleaning and examination. Many dentists recommend having the teeth professionally cleaned every 6 months.
- Keep dentures, retainers, and other appliances clean. This includes regular brushing and may include soaking them in a cleansing solution.

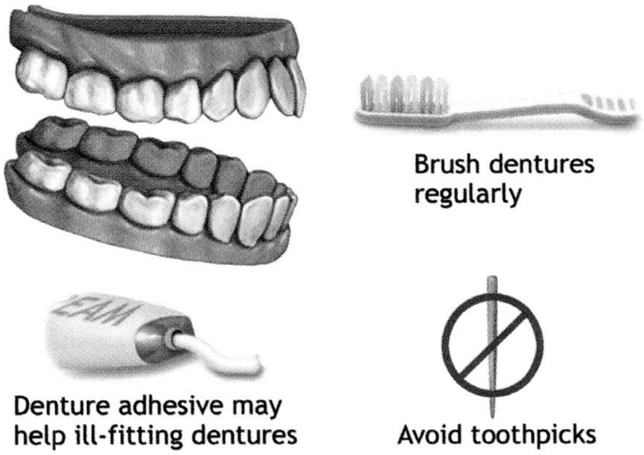

Ask your dentist:

- What toothbrush you should use, and where your problem areas are located.
- How to properly floss your teeth. Overly vigorous or improper flossing may injure the gums.
- Whether you should use any special appliances or tools, such as water irrigation or electric toothbrushes. These may sometimes help supplement (but not replace) brushing and flossing.
- Whether you could benefit from particular toothpastes or mouth rinses. In some cases, over-the counter pastes and rinses may be doing you more harm than good, depending on your condition.

Dental care for children

Healthy teeth and gums are essential to your child's overall good health. If the child's teeth develop diseases or become injured, or don't develop properly, this can result in poor nutrition, painful and dangerous infections, problems with speech development, and problems with self image.

Caring for an infant's teeth

Even though newborns and infants do not have teeth, it is important to take care of their mouth and gums. Follow these tips:

- Use a damp washcloth to wipe your infant's gums after each meal.
- DO NOT put your infant or young child to bed with a bottle of milk, juice, or sugar water. Use only water for bedtime bottles.
- Begin using a soft toothbrush instead of a washcloth to clean your child's teeth as soon as his first tooth shows (usually between 5-8 months of age).
- Ask your pediatrician if your infant needs fluoride added to his diet.

The first trip to the dentist

- Your child's first visit to the dentist should be between the time the first tooth appears (5-8 months) and the time when all the primary teeth are visible (before 2 1/2 years).
- Many dentists recommend a "trial" visit to expose the child to the sights, sounds, smells, and feel of the office before the actual examination.
- Children who are accustomed to having their gums wiped and teeth brushed every day will be more comfortable going to the dentist.

Caring for a child's teeth

- The child's teeth and gums should be brushed at least twice each day and especially before bed.

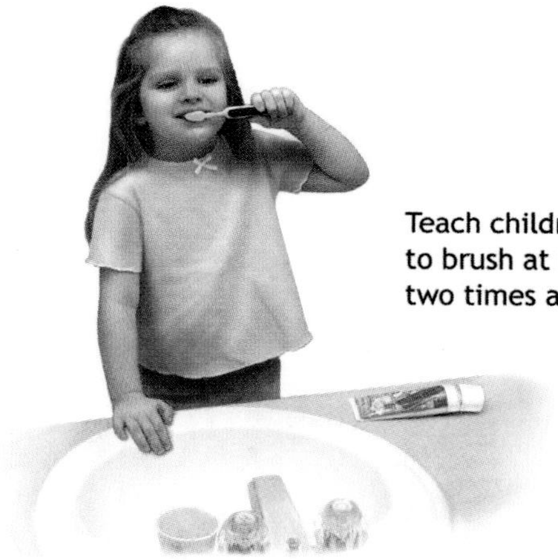

Teach children to brush at least two times a day

- Take your child to a dentist every 6 months. Let the dentist know if your child thumbsucks or breathes through the mouth.
- When your child gets permanent teeth, he or she should begin flossing each evening before bed.
- When the child reaches the teens, braces or extractions may be needed to prevent long-term problems.
- If your child loses an adult (permanent) tooth during a fall or other injury, see *Broken or Knocked Out Tooth* for first aid

instructions. If you act quickly, you can often save the tooth.

- Teach your child how to play safe and what to do if a tooth is broken or knocked out.

Practice Safe Sex

Safe sex means taking precautions during sex that can keep you from getting a sexually transmitted disease (STD), or from giving an STD to your partner. These diseases include genital herpes, genital warts, HIV, chlamydia, gonorrhea, syphilis, hepatitis B and C, and others.

Most of the diseases are transferred by direct contact with a sore on the genitals or mouth. However, some organisms can be transferred in body fluids without causing a visible sore. They can be transferred to another person during oral, vaginal, or anal intercourse.

Abstinence is an absolute answer to preventing STDs. However, abstinence is not always a practical or desirable option.

Next to abstinence, the least risky approach is to have a monogamous sexual relationship with someone that you know is free of any STD. Ideally, before having sex with a new partner, each of you should get screened for STDs, especially HIV and hepatitis B, and share the test results with one another.

Use condoms to avoid contact with semen, vaginal fluids, or blood. Both male and female condoms dramatically reduce the chance you will get or spread an STD. However, condoms must be used properly:

- The condom should be in place from the beginning to end of sexual activity and should be used every time you have sex.
- Lubricants may help reduce the chance a condom will break. Use only water-based lubricants, because oil-based or petroleum-type lubricants can cause latex to weaken and tear. Do not use codoms nonoxynl-9 lubricant. (These help prevent pregnancy, but may increase HIV transmission.)
- Use latex condoms for vaginal, anal, and oral intercourse.
- Keep in mind that STDs can still be spread, even if you use a condom, because a condom does not cover surrounding skin areas. But a condom definitely reduces your risk.

Here are additional safe-sex steps:

- **Know your partner.** Before having sex, first establish a committed relationship that allows trust and open communication. You should be able to discuss past sexual histories, any previous STDs or IV drug use. You should not feel coerced or forced into having sex.
- **Stay sober.** Alcohol and drugs impair your judgment, communication abilities, and ability to properly use condoms or lubricants.
- **Be responsible.** If you have an STD, like HIV or herpes, advise any prospective sexual partner. Allow him or her to decide what to do. If you mutually agree on engaging in sexual activity, use latex condoms and other measures to protect the partner.
- **If pregnant, take precautions.** If you have an STD, learn about the risk to the infant before becoming pregnant. Ask your provider how to prevent the fetus from becoming infected. HIV positive women should not breastfeed their infant.

In summary, safe sex requires prior planning and good communication between partners. Given that, couples can enjoy the pleasures of a sexual relationship while reducing the potential risks involved.

Birth control

There are many different birth control and family planning methods to help sexually active individuals and couples prevent pregnancy. The information below summarizes many of the pros and cons of each method.

Condoms

- A condom is a thin sheath placed on the penis or, in the case of the female condom, within the vagina prior to intercourse. Semen is collected inside the condom, which must be carefully kept in place and then removed after intercourse.
- Condoms are readily available in most drug and grocery stores. Some family planning clinics offer free condoms.
- Latex condoms help prevent HIV and other STDs.
- About 14 pregnancies occur over 1 year out of 100 couples using male condoms, and about 21 pregnancies occur over 1 year out of 100 couples using female condoms. They are more effective when spermicide is also used.

Spermicides

- Spermicides are chemical jellies, foams, creams, or suppositories that kill sperm.
- They can be purchased in most drug and grocery stores.
- This method used by itself is not very effective. About 26 pregnancies occur over 1 year out of 100 women using this method alone. Spermicides are generally combined with other methods (such as condoms or diaphragm) as extra protection.
- Warning: nonoxynol-9 can help prevent pregnancy, but also may increase the risk of transmitting HIV.

Diaphragm

- A diaphragm is a flexible rubber cup that is filled with spermicidal cream or jelly, and then placed into the vagina, over the cervix, before intercourse. It should be left in place for 6 to 8 hours after intercourse.
- Diaphragms must be prescribed by a woman's health care provider, who determines the correct type and size of diaphragm for the woman.
- About 5-20 pregnancies occur over 1 year in 100 women using this method, depending on proper use.
- A similar, smaller device is called a cervical cap.

Birth control pills

- Also called oral contraceptives or just the "pill", this method uses the hormones estrogen and progestin to prevent ovulation.
- A health care provider must prescribe birth control pills.
- The method is highly effective if the woman remembers to take her pill consistently each day.
- Women who experience unpleasant side effects on one type of pill are usually able to adjust to a different type.
- About 2 to 3 pregnancies occur over 1 year out of 100 women who never miss a pill.

The mini-pill

- The "mini-pill" is a type of birth control pill that contains only progestin, no estrogen.
- It is an alternative for women who are sensitive to estrogen or cannot take estrogen for other reasons.
- The effectiveness of progestin-only oral contraceptives is slightly less than that of the combination type. About 3 pregnancies occur over a 1 year period in 100 women using this method.

Progestin implants

- Implants, such as Norplant, are small rods implanted surgically beneath the skin, usually on the upper arm. The rods release a continuous dose of progestin to prevent ovulation.

- Implants work for 5 years. The initial cost is generally higher than some other methods, but the overall cost may be less over the 5-year period.
- Less than 1 pregnancy occurs over 1 year out of 100 women using this type of contraception.

Hormone injections

- Progestin injections, such as Depo-Provera, are given into the muscles of the upper arm or buttocks. This injection prevents ovulation.
- A single shot works for up to 90 days.
- Less than 1 pregnancy occurs over 1 year in 100 women using this method.

Skin patch

- The skin patch (Ortho Evra) is placed on your shoulder, buttocks, or other convenient location. It continually releases progestin and estrogen. Like other hormone methods, a prescription is required.
- The patch provides weekly protection. A new patch is applied each week for three weeks, followed by one week without a patch.
- About 1 pregnancy occurs over 1 year out of 100 women using this method.

Vaginal ring

- The vaginal ring (NuvaRing) is a flexible ring about 2 inches in diameter that is inserted into the vagina. It releases progestin and estrogen. Like other hormone methods, a prescription is required.
- The woman inserts it herself and it stays in the vagina for 3 weeks. Then, she takes it out for one week.
- About 1 pregnancy occurs over 1 year out of 100 women using this method.

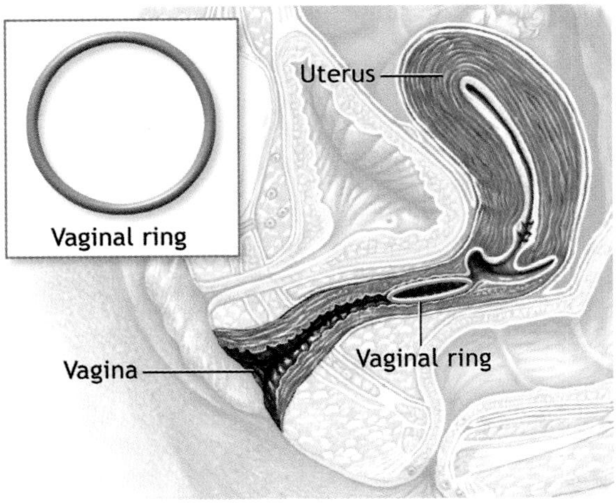

IUD

- The IUD is a small plastic or copper device placed inside the woman's uterus by her health care provider. IUDs may be left in place for up to ten years in some patients.
- The method should not be used by women who have a history of pelvic infection or ectopic pregnancy.
- 1 to 3 pregnancies occur per year out of 100 women using this method.

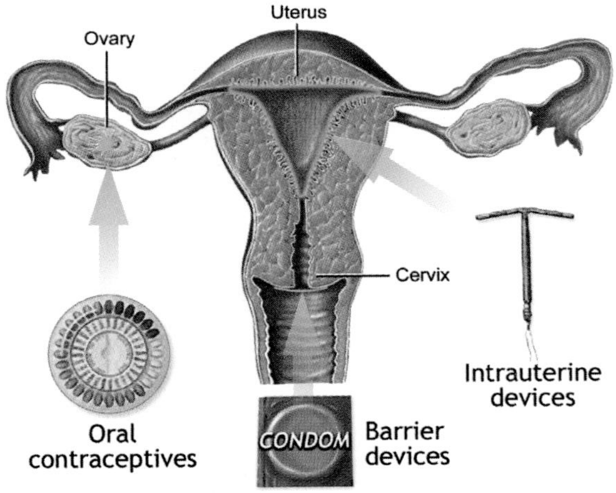

Methods of birth control include hormone contraceptives to prevent ovulation, and barrier or implantation devices, such as a condom or IUD.

Natural family planning

- This method involves observing a variety of body changes in the woman (such as cervical mucus changes, basal body temperature changes) and recording them on a calendar to determine when ovulation occurs. The couple abstains from unprotected sex for several days before and after the assumed day ovulation occurs.
- This method requires special education and training in recognizing the body's changes as well as a great deal of continuous and committed effort.
- About 15 to 20 pregnancies occur over 1 year out of 100 women using this method (for those who are properly trained).

Tubal ligation

- During tubal ligation, a woman's fallopian tubes are cut, sealed, or blocked by a special clip, preventing eggs and sperm from entering the tubes.
- The operation can sometimes be reversed if a woman later chooses to become pregnant. However, tubal ligations are best for women and couples who believe they never wish to have children in the future. Tubal ligations are best viewed as a permanent method.

Vasectomy

- A vasectomy is a simple, permanent procedure for men. The vas deferens (the tubes that carry sperm) are cut and sealed.
- Vasectomies can sometimes be reversed. However, vasectomies are best for men and couples who believe they never wish to have children in the future. Vasectomies are best viewed as a permanent method.

Emergency ("morning after" birth control

- The "morning after" pill consists of two doses of hormone pills taken as soon as possible within 72 hours after unprotected intercourse.
- The pill may prevent pregnancy by temporarily blocking eggs from being produced, by stopping fertilization, or keeping a fertilized egg from becoming implanted in the uterus.
- The morning after pill may be appropriate in cases of rape; having a condom break or slip off during sex; missing two or more birth control pills during a monthly cycle; and having unplanned sex.
- Call your provider for more information about the morning after pill.

Unreliable methods

- **Coitus interruptus** – withdrawal of the penis from the vagina prior to ejaculation. Some semen frequently escapes prior to full withdrawal, enough to cause a pregnancy.
- **Douching shortly after sex** – sperm can make their way beyond the cervix within 90 seconds after ejaculation, so this method is ineffective and unreliable.
- **Breastfeeding** – women who are breastfeeding CAN become pregnant.

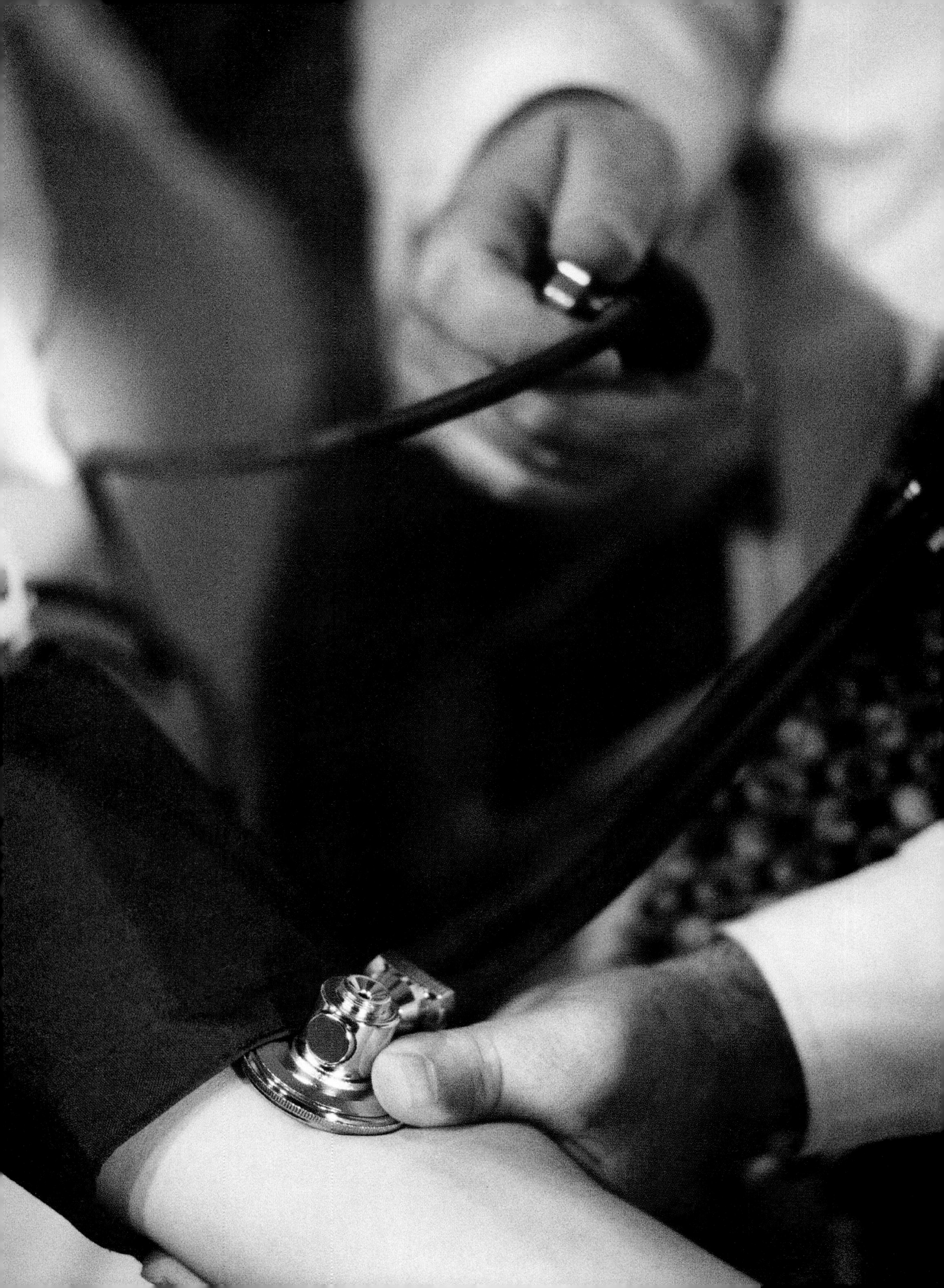

SCREENING AND CHECKUPS

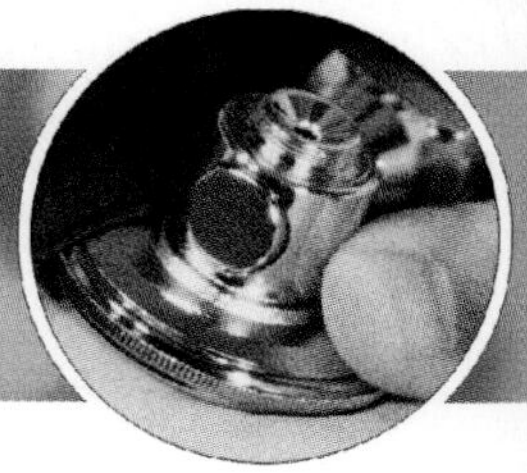

NORMAL VITAL SIGNS

Your blood pressure, pulse, breathing rate, and body temperature are referred to as "vital signs." These important measurements help a health care provider evaluate you during a physical exam. When your vital signs are not within a normal range, they may indicate a problem and point your provider in the direction of what might be causing any symptoms you have. Even when you are feeling fine and see your provider for a general checkup, he or she may find one of these numbers to be abnormal. If so, this could be a warning sign that something is wrong.

BLOOD PRESSURE

Blood pressure is usually measured while you are sitting down with your arm at the level of your heart. The blood pressure cuff is wrapped snugly around your upper arm so that the lower edge is 1 inch above your elbow. The cuff is inflated until heartbeat sounds can no longer be heard through the stethoscope, which is placed over an artery in your arm. As the air is let out of the cuff, the number where your heartbeat is first heard is your systolic blood pressure. The second number recorded, or diastolic blood pressure, is when the sound of your heartbeat disappears again.

You want your blood pressure reading to be **lower** than "120 over 80." Blood pressure varies depending on what you are doing, what you are feeling, what position you are in, your body temperature, any medications that you are taking, and other factors. For more information on blood pressure values, see the article on high blood pressure.

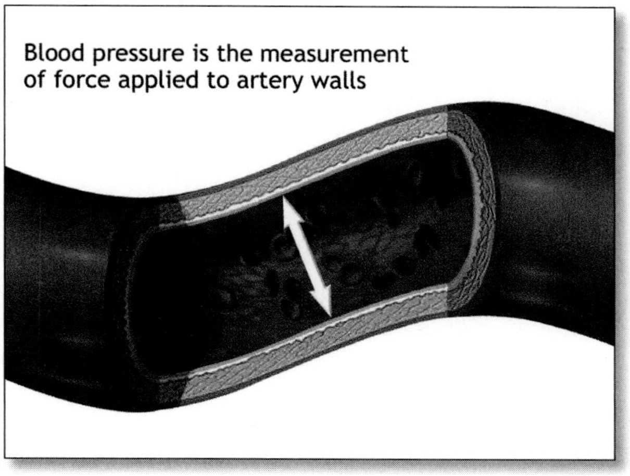

Blood pressure is the measurement of force applied to artery walls

A child's blood pressure is normally lower than an adult's, and depends on height, age, and sex. As an example, boys of average height are at risk for developing high blood pressure if they exceed the following levels:

Ages 3 to 5	108/67
Ages 6 to 9	113/74
Ages 10 to 12	119/77
Ages 13 to 15	127/79

Children should have their blood pressure at every well-child visit, beginning at age 3. They should never go 2 years without having their blood pressure checked. More frequent follow-up may be needed if a blood pressure reading is high or the child has risks for high blood pressure, like being overweight, having a strong family history, or having kidney or heart disease.

CAN BLOOD PRESSURE BE TOO LOW?

The answer depends on the individual. For some people, their blood pressure always runs on the low side – for example, between 80/50 and 95/75. However, if your blood pressure is notably lower than your usual readings (for example, 100/70 compared to your usual 130/80), this would be considered abnormal and a possible sign of an illness.

Blood pressure below 80/50 or your usual readings can be a sign that your brain and other organs are not getting enough blood. This means they are not getting enough oxygen and other nutrients. Low blood pressure may mean that you are dehydrated, bleeding somewhere (may be internal), or have an infection. It may also mean your heart is functioning poorly, which can be from bad congestive heart failure, a heart attack, or other problems.

The serious risk from low blood pressure is the possibility of going into shock. (For more information, see the article on shock.)

Pulse

Your pulse is checked in order to measure the number of times your heart beats each minute. This is also called your heart rate. Your pulse can be felt in many places throughout your body – wherever an artery is close to the surface of the skin. Your provider will usually check your pulse at the wrist or neck.

You can measure your own pulse. Place your index and middle fingers over the underside of the opposite wrist, below the base of your thumb. With your fingers flat, press firmly and count the beats you feel for 1 full minute (or for 15 seconds and multiply by 4).

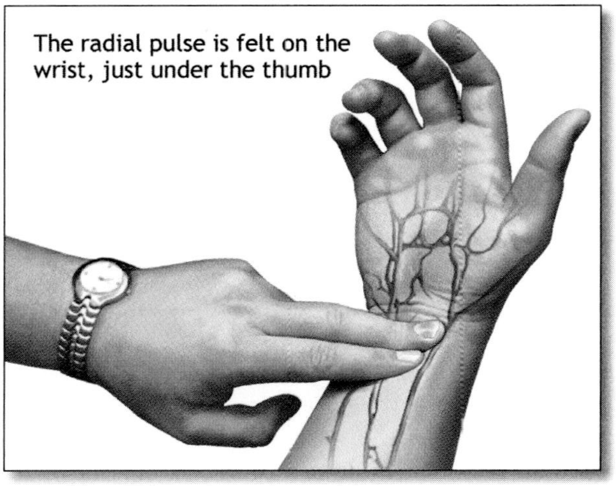

The radial pulse is felt on the wrist, just under the thumb

Normal heart rates are as follows:

Group	Beats per minute
Infants	80 - 160
Children 1 - 10	70 - 130
Adolescents	55 - 110
Adults	60 - 100
Well-trained athletes	40 - 60

If your heart rate is too fast, this may mean that you have an infection or are dehydrated. Your pulse rate normally goes up during exercise, but should return to normal soon afterward. A very fast or very slow heart rate may also be a sign of an abnormal heart rhythm. If your pulse is not normal when your vital signs are measured, your doctor may do an electrocardiogram (ECG) in the office to check your heart rhythm.

Breathing rate

Most adults take 8 - 16 breaths per minute. Infants can take as many as 44 breaths per minute or more. You probably won't be aware that a health care professional is measuring your breathing rate. They do this by observing you and checking the clock.

A fast breathing rate is known as hyperventilation. This can happen during exercise, but may also happen if you are anxious, have a problem with your lungs or heart, or for other medical reasons.

A slow breathing rate, called hypoventilation, leads to accumulation of carbon dioxide in your blood. Possible causes include diabetic coma and medications.

When someone stops breathing for a short period of time, this is called apnea. Infants who have apnea lasting 20 seconds or longer are at risk for Sudden Infant Death Syndrome (SIDS). Adults who have periods of apnea while sleeping need to be evaluated by a doctor.

Temperature

Your body temperature is a measurement of your body heat. The normal, safe range for this number depends on where your temperature is checked – under your tongue, under your armpit, or in your rectum. When speaking to a health care provider, report both the temperature and how you checked it. The normal range in children over 13 and adults is 97.8 to 99.1°F, with an average of 98.6°F. Infants and children tend to have slightly higher temperatures, up to a degree, depending on age.

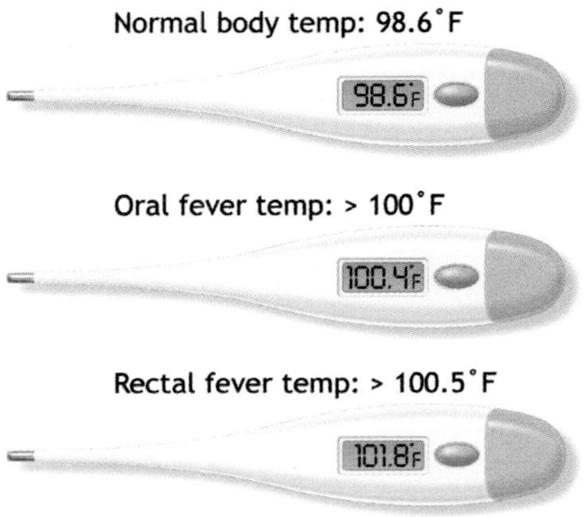

Your body temperature is checked to see if you have a fever. Fevers may be a sign of infection. Your temperature should not be measured for at least one hour after exercising or taking a hot bath. Similarly, wait for at least 20 to 30 minutes after eating, drinking a hot or cold liquid, or smoking.

Healthy men's screenings

The key to being (and staying) healthy is prevention. The *Healthy Men's Table* can serve as a guide for how often men need particular screening tests. The information assumes that you have no risk factors or signs of particular diseases. If you do, your doctor may want you to have certain tests performed earlier or more often. For example, if high cholesterol runs in your family, you may need this checked more often than every five years.

Different medical organizations may vary in their recommendations for tests included in this chart. The intent here is NOT for this chart to serve as medical advice. Always talk to your own doctor about what is best for you, and find out how often you should have routine physical exams.

Healthy women's screenings

The key to being (and staying) healthy is prevention. The *Healthy Women's Table* can serve as a guide for how often women need particular screening tests. The information assumes that you have no risk factors or signs of particular diseases. If you do, your doctor may want you to have certain tests performed earlier or more often. For example, if your mother or sister had breast cancer before menopause, your doctor will likely recommend starting mammograms at age 35.

Different medical organizations may vary in their recommendations for tests included in this chart. The intent here is NOT for this chart to serve as medical advice. Always talk to your own doctor about what is best for you, and find out how often you should have routine physical exams.

Breast self-exam

Breast cancer is easier to treat the earlier it is found. For that reason, some experts recommend that women over age 20 perform a monthly breast self-exam to look for new lumps and other changes. The self exam has limitations, however, and is NOT a substitute for regular breast examinations from your doctor or screening mammograms.

Healthy men's table

	Men ages 20 - 39	Men ages 40 - 49	Men ages 50 - 59	Men over 60
Testicular self-exam [1]	Every month for men with risk factors	Every month for men with risk factors	Every month for men with risk factors	Every month for men with risk factors
Prostate specific antigen [2]			Talk to your provider at regular physical	Talk to your provider at regular physical
Colorectal screening [3]			Frequency depends on tests performed	Frequency depends on tests performed
Blood pressure check [4]	At least every 2 years	At least every 2 years	At least every 2 years	At least every 2 years
Cholesterol test [5]	Every 5 years	Every 5 years	Every 5 years	Every 5 years
Body Mass Index [6]	Every physical	Every physical	Every physical	Every physical
Skin self-exam [7]	Every month	Every month	Every month	Every month
Eye exam [8]				Every year after age 65
Dental cleaning and exam	Every 6 months	Every 6 months	Every 6 months	Every 6 months

[1] Recommendation by the American Cancer Society. Risk factors include a family history of testicular cancer or history of cryptorchism. For instructions on how to perform this exam, see *Testicular Self-Exam*. This supplements, but does not replace, a periodic exam by your provider.

[2] Recommendation by the American Cancer Society. PSA may be measured starting at age 40 or 45 if you have risk factors for prostate cancer, like you are African American or you have a father or brother diagnosed at an early age.

[3] Recommendation by the American Cancer Society. Colorectal screening may include fecal occult blood test, flexible sigmoidoscopy, barium enema, and/or colonoscopy. If you have a strong family history of colon cancer or polyps, or if you have had inflammatory bowel disease or polyps yourself, colon cancer screening would be started at an earlier age and be performed more frequently.

[4] Recommendation by the American Heart Association and the United States Preventive Task Force.

[5] Recommendation by the American Heart Association and the National Cholesterol Education Panel (NCEP) of the NIH.

[6] Recommendation by the United States Preventive Task Force.

[7] Recommendation by the American Cancer Society. For instructions on how to perform the exam, see *Skin Self-Exam*. This supplements, but does not replace, a periodic exam by your provider.

[8] Recommendation by the United States Preventive Task Force.

Healthy Women's Table

	Women ages 20 - 39	Women ages 40 - 49	Women ages 50 - 59	Women over 60
Breast self-exam [1]	Every month (optional)	Every month (optional)	Every month (optional)	Every month (optional)
Mammogram [2]		Every year [3]	Every year	Every year
Pap smear and pelvic exam [4]	Every 1 to 2 years	Every 1 to 2 years	Every 1 to 2 years	Every 1 to 2 years [5]
Chlamydia screening [6]	Every physical up to age 25			
Bone density study [7]			Discuss with your provider [8]	At least once after age 65
Colorectal screening [9]			Frequency depends on tests chosen	Frequency depends on tests chosen
Blood pressure check [10]	At least every 2 years	At least every 2 years	At least every 2 years	At least every 2 years
Cholesterol test [11]	Every 5 years	Every 5 years	Every 5 years	Every 5 years
Body Mass Index [12]	Every physical	Every physical	Every physical	Every physical
Skin self-exam [13]	Every month	Every month	Every month	Every month
Eye exam [14]				Every year after age 65
Dental cleaning and exam	Every 6 months	Every 6 months	Every 6 months	Every 6 months

[1] Recommendation by the American Cancer Society. For instructions on how to do this self-exam, see *Breast Self-Exam*. This supplements, but does not replace, a periodic exam by your provider.

[2] Recommendation by the American Cancer Society. If you have a mother or sister with a history of breast cancer before menopause, your provider may start mammograms for you at age 35. Your provider may also consider other screening tests, like a breast ultrasound or MRI.

[3] The American Cancer Society recommends annual mammograms starting at age 40. However, some professional organizations may recommend every 2 years between the ages of 40 and 50, assuming no other risk factors.

[4] Recommendation by the American Cancer Society. You should begin to have Pap smears when you turn 21 or when you become sexually-active – whichever happens first. If you have a normal Pap smear for 3 years in a row and you are over age 30, you may be able to have them every 2 to 3 years instead of 1 to 2 years. Talk to your provider. Regardless of past results, you should have a Pap smear within a year of having a new sexual partner.

[5] After age 70, if you have had 3 or more normal Pap smears in a row and no abnormal Pap smears in the last 10 years, you may be able to stop having this screening test performed. Talk to your provider.

[6] Recommendation by the United States Preventive Task Force.

[7] Recommendation by the United States Preventive Task Force and the American College of Obstetricians and Gynecologists.

[8] Women who have had a fracture or who are at high risk for osteoporosis may benefit from early screening.

[9] Recommendation by the American Cancer Society. If you have a strong family history of colon cancer, polyps, or if you have had inflammatory bowel disease or polyps yourself, colon cancer screening would be started at an earlier age and be performed more frequently.

[10] Recommendation by the American Heart Association and the United States Preventive Task Force.

[11] Recommendation by the American Heart Association and the National Cholesterol Education Panel (NCEP) of the NIH.

[12] Recommendation by the United States Preventive Task Force.

[13] Recommendation by the American Cancer Society. For instructions on how to perform the exam, see *Skin Self-Exam*. This supplements, but does not replace, a periodic exam by your provider.

[14] Recommendation by the United States Preventive Task Force.

Talk to your health care provider about the pros and cons of performing self-exams. If you do perform monthly exams, do them 3-5 days after your period, when your breasts are the least tender and lumpy.

First, lie on your back. Place your right hand behind your head. With the middle fingers of your left hand, gently yet firmly press down using small motions to examine the entire right breast. Then, while sitting or standing, examine your armpit (commonly skipped) because breast tissue extends to that area. Gently squeeze the nipple, checking for discharge. Repeat the process on the left breast.

Use one of the patterns shown in the diagram to make sure that you are covering all of the breast tissue. You are feeling for any lump or thickness that stands out or feels new.

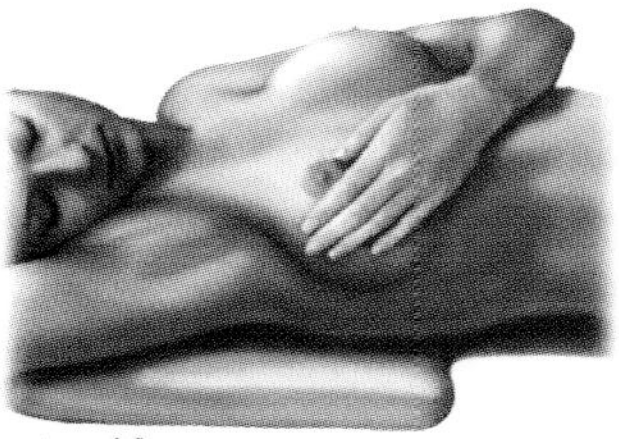

Breast self-exam: manual inspection (reclining)

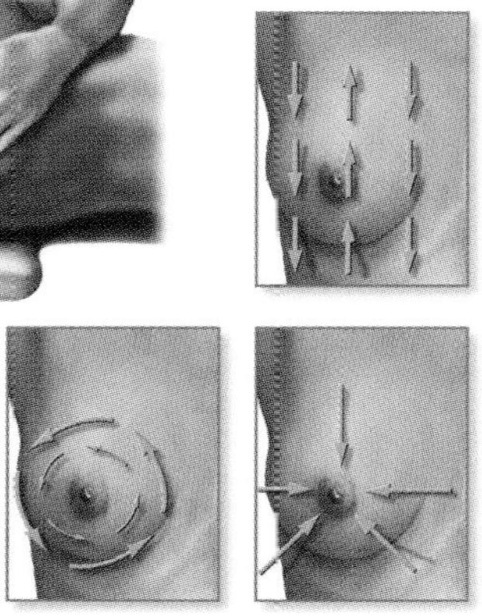

With fingertips close together, gently probe each breast in one of these three patterns

Although some women find it easiest to do the exam in the shower, when the skin is soft and wet, you are more likely to examine all of the breast tissue if you are lying down.

Next, stand in front of a mirror with your arms by your side. Look at your breasts directly AND in the mirror for changes in skin texture (such as dimpling, puckering, indentations, or skin that looks like an orange peel), shape, contour, or the nipple turning inward. Do the same with your arms raised above your head.

Discuss any changes you find right away with your doctor. It is helpful to know that all women have some lumps. If you do monthly exams, it is important do them at the same time in your monthly cycle. Know that the value of breast self-exams is controversial. The American Cancer Society considers them to be optional. Talk to your health care provider about what is right for you.

See also *Breast Lumps*.

Skin self-exam

Skin cancer is the most common form of cancer in the Unites States. For this reason, perform a skin self-exam once a month. This helps you detect skin cancer (or other skin abnormalities) and get treatment as early as possible.

Skin cancers can have many different appearances. They can be small, shiny, or waxy; scaly or rough; firm and red; crusty or bleeding; or have other features. Any suspicious mole, sore, or skin growth should be looked at by a doctor as soon as possible.

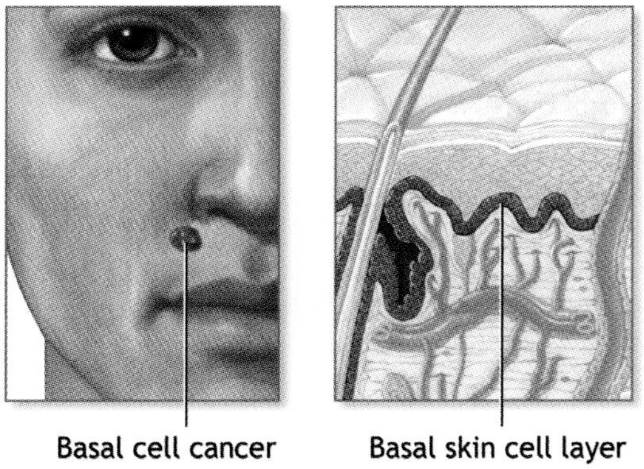

Basal cell carcinoma is a slow-growing skin tumor involving cancerous changes in the basal layer of the skin. It is the most common form of skin cancer in the United States.

How to do it

The easiest time to do the exam may be after you take a bath or shower. Women may wish to perform their skin self-exam at the same time that they perform amonthly breast self-exam.

Ideally, the room should have a full-length mirror and bright lights so that you can see your entire body well. It is important to examine all areas of your skin, including hard-to-see areas such as the genitals, buttocks, scalp, and back. (Have a partner, friend, or relative help.) Don't forget to check under your arms and below facial hair.

When you are performing the skin self-exam, look for:

- NEW skin markings (e.g., moles, blemishes, colorations, bumps)
- Moles that have CHANGED their size, texture, color, or shape
- Moles or lesions that won't heal or that continue to bleed
- Moles with ragged edges, differences in coloration, or lack of symmetry

How to prevent skin cancer

Minimizing sun exposure is the best way to prevent skin damage, including many types of skin cancer:

- Protect your skin from the sun when you can – wear protective clothing such as hats, long-sleeved shirts, long skirts, or pants.
- Try to avoid exposure during midday, when the sun is most intense.
- Use sunscreen with an SPF of at least 15. Apply sunscreen at least one-half hour before sun exposure, and reapply frequently.
- Apply sunscreen during winter months as well.

Testicular self-exam

A lump on the testicle may be the first sign of testicular cancer. Starting in puberty, men at risk for testicular cancer should examine their testicles for lumps on a monthly basis. This includes men with a family history of testicular cancer, men who have had a previous testicular tumor, or men with an undescended testicle. Most cases of testicular cancer occur when men are between ages 15 and 40, although it can happen at older or younger ages.

How to do it

Perform this test during or after a shower. This way, the scrotal skin is warm and relaxed. The test is best done while standing.

1. Gently feel your scrotal sac to locate a testicle.
2. Firmly yet gently roll the testicle between the thumb and fingers of both hands to examine the entire surface.
3. Repeat the procedure with the other testicle.

Each testicle should feel firm but not rock hard. One testicle may, or may not, be lower or slightly larger than the other. Normal testicles contain blood vessels and other structures that can make the exam confusing. Performing the self-exam monthly allows you to become familiar with your normal anatomy. Then, if you notice any changes from the previous exam, this alerts you to contact your doctor. Always ask you doctor if you have any doubts or questions.

When to contact a medical professional

If you find a small hard lump (like a pea), have an enlarged testicle, or notice any other concerning differences from your last self-exam, see your doctor as soon as you can.

Also consult your doctor if:

- You can't find one or both testicles – the testicles may not have descended properly in the scrotum
- There is a soft collection of thin tubes above the testicle – it may be a collection of dilated veins (varicocele)
- There is pain or swelling in the scrotum – it may be an infection or a fluid-filled sac (hydrocele) causing blockage of blood flow to the area

Pregnancy checkups

The best time to start prenatal care is *before* getting pregnant. Schedule a visit if you are trying to conceive or you are not using birth control. To lower the risk of having a baby with neural tube defects, take folic acid. Start taking folic acid when you stop birth control, or better yet, first become sexually active.

Once you know you're pregnant, see your provider regularly as your pregnancy progresses.

Here's what to expect during the first prenatal visit. After a blood or urine test confirms your pregnancy, your health care provider will give you a complete medical exam. She'll also take a detailed medical history and assess any pregnancy risks. She'll need honest answers about the following:

- Do you drink alcohol? If so, how often and how much?
- Do you smoke? Does someone near you smoke?
- Do you take any over-the-counter medications or supplements?
- Any prescription drugs or illegal drugs?
- What regular exercise do you get?
- What chemicals or hazardous substances are you exposed to?

Having a clear, complete picture of your medical history and lifestyle helps her provide the best care possible for you and your baby, so it's important not to leave out any details – even embarrassing ones.

Next, she'll give you a blood test to determine your **Rh factor**. Though it's rare, having a different Rh factor than your fetus can cause Rh disease, which may lead to serious illness or even death for your baby. This is easily prevented if Rh incompatibility is spotted early.

Your provider will check your blood for signs of exposure to syphilis, rubella, hepa-

Rh incompatibility

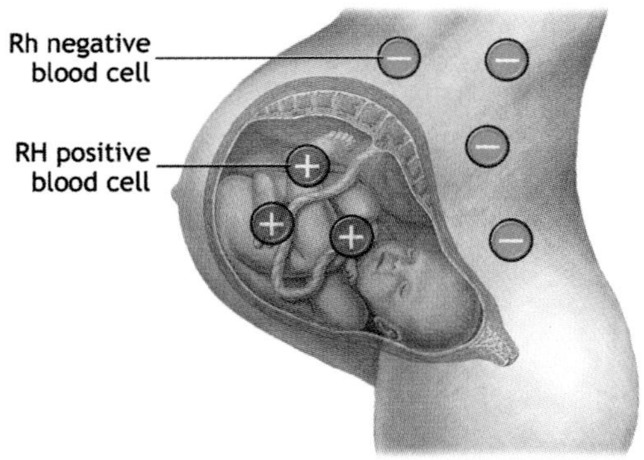

Rh incompatibility occurs when the mother's blood type is Rh negative and her fetus' blood type is Rh positive.

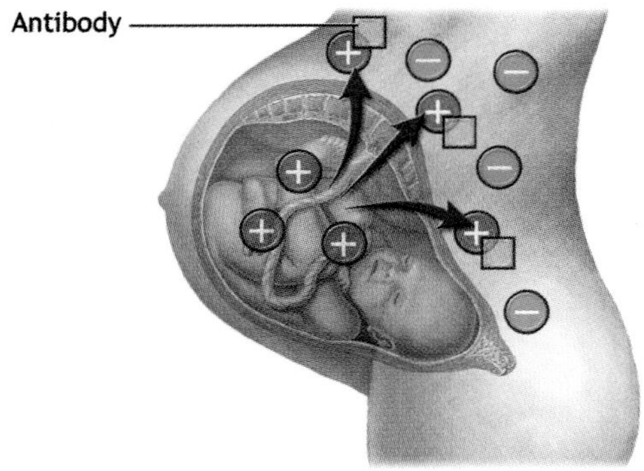

If some of the fetus' blood passes into the mother's blood stream, her body will produce antibodies in response.

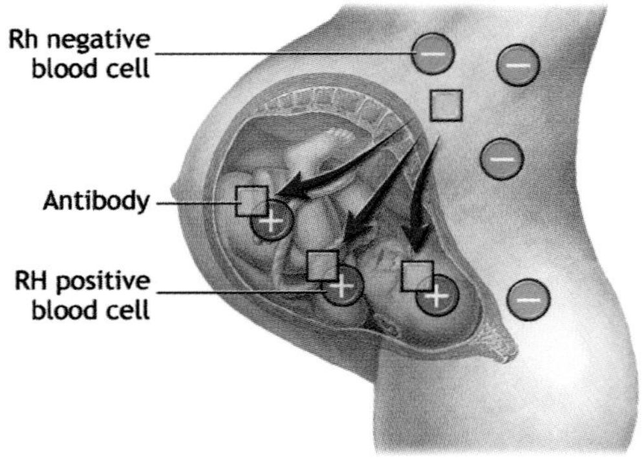

These antibodies could pass back through the placenta and harm the fetus' red blood cells, causing mild to serious anemia in the fetus.

titis B, and possibly HIV. Other lab work includes urine tests for infection or diabetes, and a cervical culture to check for sexually transmitted diseases, such as gonorrhea and chlamydia.

Your health care provider will also talk about nutrition during pregnancy. In addition to warning you away from alcohol, mercury, tobacco, and certain herbs, she may advise you to consume more iron, folic acid, vitamin B6, zinc, or other nutrients. Because it can be hard to get enough of certain nutrients, she will likely recommend that you take a daily prenatal vitamin.

A note about calcium: Calcium requirements DO NOT go up during pregnancy, but the consequences of calcium deficiency are greater. The March of Dimes estimates that only about 6% of American women of childbearing age get enough calcium from their foods and supplements. Women aged 19 to 50, pregnant or not, need at least 1,000 mg per day. Most Americans get only 700 mg.

If you are otherwise healthy and your pregnancy seems uncomplicated, you can count on going to your provider once every month or two during the first two trimesters. Sometime during the third trimester, the visits accelerate to every two weeks and then every week by the end. The actual schedule varies depending upon your provider, and if you are in a high- or low-risk category.

Pregnancy is a uniquely special time. Take the opportunity to learn about you and your baby, and to start caring for your child even before the baby is born.

IF YOU ARE PREGNANT – WATCH FOR THESE COMPLICATIONS

Most women only experience the normal discomforts that take place during pregnancy. However, sometimes there can be complications that need immediate medical attention.

If you experience any of the symptoms listed below, contact your health care provider immediately, or go to the hospital or emergency room.

- Vaginal bleeding, change in vaginal discharge, or leakage of fluid from the vagina
- Severe, persistent, frequent headaches
- Pain or burning with urination, or decrease in urination
- Persistent nausea or vomiting
- Sharp pelvic pain or severe cramping
- Frequent dizzy spells or fainting
- Visual disturbances such as blurred vision, white lights or flashes, dots in front of the eyes
- Sudden swelling in hands, feet, and face
- Falling or hitting your abdomen
- Noticeable decrease or absence of fetal movement
- High fever with chills, over 100.4° Fahrenheit orally
- Contractions more often than four an hour if you are less than 37 weeks
- Low back pain that comes and goes but never goes away
- Any other problem that feels unusual

Immunizations (vaccines)

Our bodies are designed to protect us from diseases. When you are exposed to an illness, your immune system actually learns from the experience. The next time your body is exposed to the same illness, your immune system often recognizes the culprit and sets out to destroy it.

Immunization exposes you to a very small, very safe amount of the most important diseases you are likely to encounter at some point in your life. This mild exposure helps your immune system recognize and attack the disease efficiently. If you are exposed to the full-blown disease later in life, you will either not become infected or have a much less serious infection. This is a natural way to deal with infectious diseases.

Immunizing children

Babies get so many shots these days! Many parents are concerned that the sheer number of vaccines might overwhelm, weaken, or use up a baby's immature immune system. But a baby's immune system is built to make antibodies to as many as 10,000 foreign proteins. If a baby were to receive all 11 available vaccines at once, this would engage only a tiny fraction of the immune system.

Mercury

A small amount of mercury (called thimerosal) is a preservative in some multi-dose vaccines. Despite concerns, thimerosal-containing vaccines have NOT been shown to cause autism or ADHD. Nevertheless, all of the routine vaccines are also available without added thimerosal.

Immunization schedule

The recommended immunization schedule is updated at least every 12 months by organizations such as the American Academy of Pediatrics. Consult your provider about specific immunizations for you or your child. The current recommendations are available at www.cdc.gov/nip. **At every doctor visit, ask about the next recommended immunizations.**

Tips for parents

Immunizations must be given as an injection (shot). The following tips can help make the experience easier for your child:

- Tell older children that the shot is needed to keep them safe and healthy. Knowing what to expect ahead of time may reassure the child.
- Explain to the child that it is OK to cry, but suggest that the child try to be brave. Explain that you do not like injections either, but *you* try to be brave, too. Praise the child after the injection is over, whether or not he or she cries.
- Distract the child at the moment of the injection. For example, point out a picture on the wall, have them count or say their "ABCs", or tell them something funny.
- Try to be calm. The child will notice if you cringe before the shot!
- Plan something fun to do afterward. A trip to the park, eating out, or other entertainment after the shot can make the next one less scary.

Immunizations for adults

Immunizations are not only for children. Each year the CDC posts recommended adult immunizations on their website. Go there to learn about tetanus booster shots, the flu shot, hepatitis A and B vaccines, the pneumococcal vaccine, MMR, and immunizations for chickenpox and meningitis.

Travelers

The CDC website (www.cdc.gov) gives travelers detailed information on immunizations and other precautions. Many immunizations should be obtained at least a month before travel.

Well-child visits

Childhood is a time of rapid growth and change. Regular well-child visits are important. They are most frequent during the first year and a half.

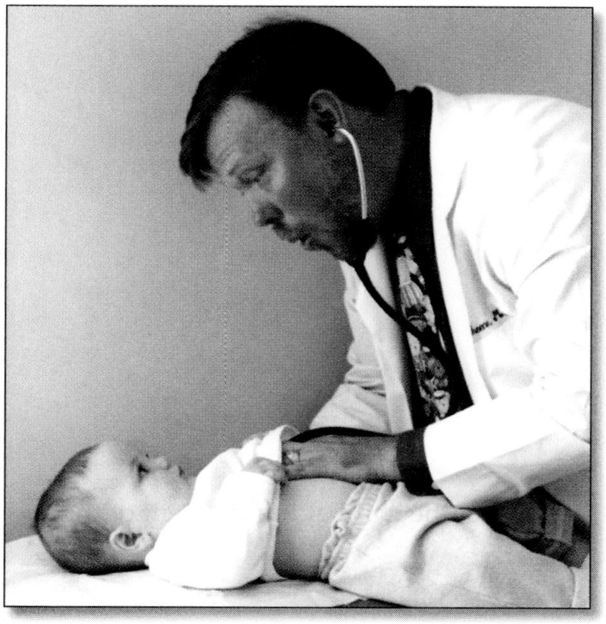

Each visit includes a complete physical exam. This will assess the child's growth and development and help identify problems early. Height, weight, and other factors are recorded. Hearing, vision, and other tests will be a part of some visits. These assessments are important for raising healthy children.

Well-child visits are also a time for communication. You'll be told about normal development, nutrition, sleep, safety, infectious diseases that are "going around," and other important topics for parents.

Make the most of these visits by writing down your most important questions and concerns to bring with you.

You might also want to bring this book with you to the visits, and ask your doctor or nurse to mark your child's growth on the included charts. This can be a great springboard for discussion. Ask your doctor about the BMI curve, which is the most important curve for identifying and preventing obesity.

Remember...

Make the most of well-child visits. Always bring your most pressing questions.

There are several schedules for routine well-child visits. The American Academy of Pediatrics schedule is given below.

Preventive health care schedule

A visit with a pediatrician *before* the baby is born is important for first-time parents, those with high-risk pregnancies, and any other parent who wishes to discuss common issues such as feeding and circumcision.

After the baby is born, the next visit should be 2-3 days after bringing the baby home (for breast-fed babies) or when the baby is 2-4 days old (for all babies discharged from a hospital before 2 days old).

Thereafter, visits should occur at the following points:

By 1 month	2 years
2 months	3 years
4 months	4 years
6 months	5 years
9 months	6 years
1 year	8 years
15 months	10 years
18 months	Each year after until age 21

Of course, visits and phone calls to a health care provider should be made any time a baby or child seems ill or whenever the parent is concerned about a baby's health or development.

BMI growth curve

Childhood obesity is a public health emergency. Well-child visits can help prevent your child from becoming obese. Ask your doctor about the BMI growth curve.

Growth charts

Growth charts help parents and their doctors evaluate a child's physical development. The charts help gauge a child's height, weight, head circumference, and other factors relative to other children of the same age and gender.

Bring this book with you (or a photocopy of the charts) to doctor visits to make a record of your child's growth. Ask your doctor to mark your child's measurements on each chart. If you have more than one child, you might use different symbols on the graph for each, such as X's for one and O's for another.

The pattern of your children's growth can tell you quite a bit about their health now and their health risks for the future. Your doctor should explain what the "percentiles" mean. Anytime your child falls into less than the 5th percentile or greater than the 95th percentile, it should be looked into more carefully. The child may be healthy, but should be checked for potential nutrition or health problems.

Here are a few things to watch out for.

Head circumference

Most children whose head circumference is above the 95th percentile or below the 5th percentile are healthy. But there is an increased chance that some of these children might have developmental problems. They should be checked to be sure.

Length

A child may be less than the 5th percentile for length and still be at the perfect length for him or her. However, the child should be checked to be sure the child is not short due to an illness, a genetic problem, or poor nutrition.

Weight-for-length

This chart is the best to use for infant and toddlers to see if they are getting the right amount to eat. If they are less than the 5th percentile on this chart, they may be undernourished. If they are above the 95th percentile, they may be overweight. Be sure to talk about either of these with your doctor.

Body mass index

For kids age 2 and above, this is the most important growth chart. The Body Mass Index chart combines height, weight, and age to give one score. Children under the 5th percentile may be undernourished. Children above the 85th percentile are at high risk for becoming overweight children and obese adults. Children above the 95th percentile are already overweight. High BMI also means a higher risk of high blood pressure, high cholesterol, and diabetes in children.

Birth to 36 Months: Length and Weight

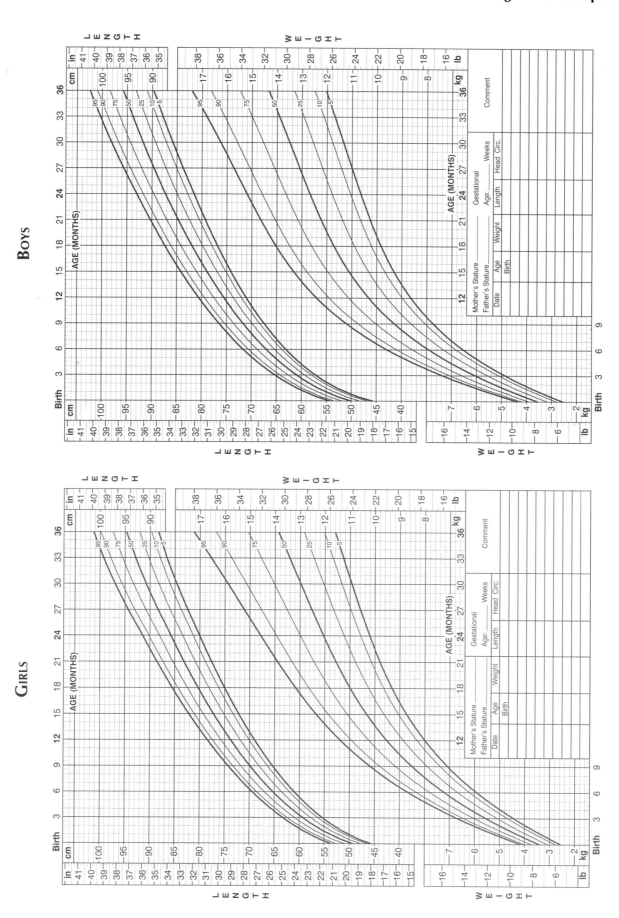

Girls

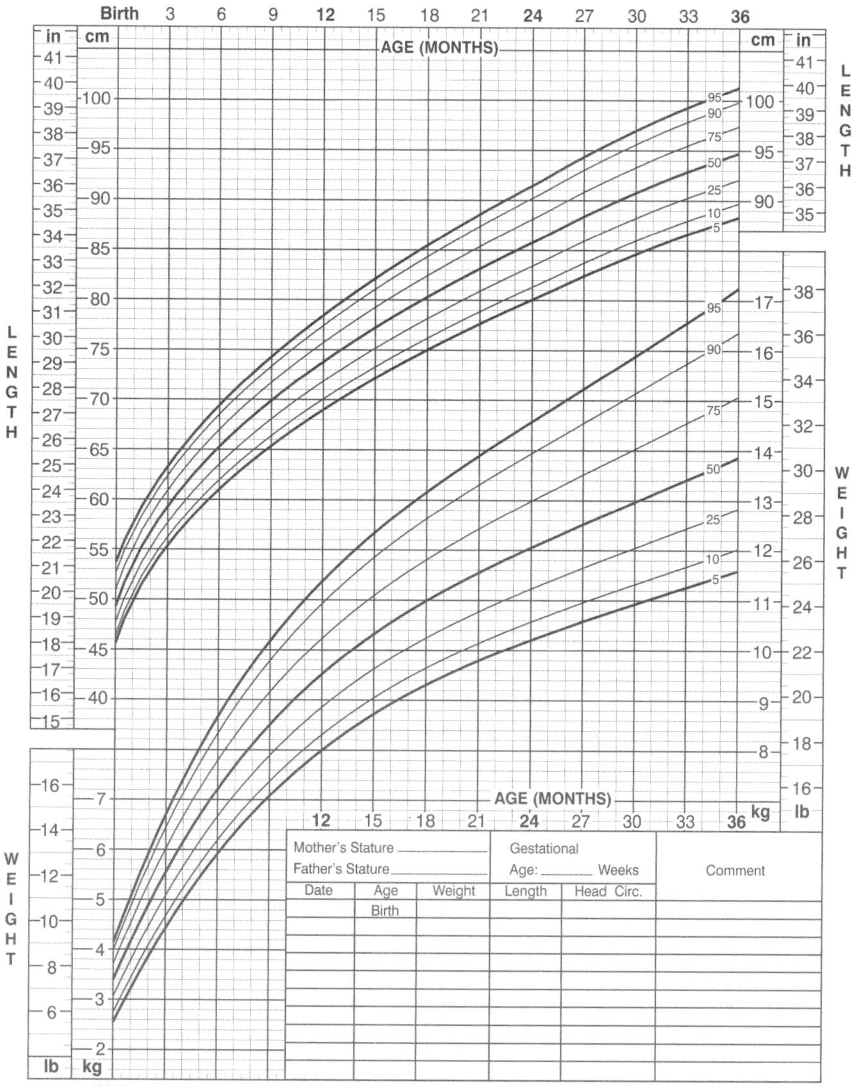

Boys

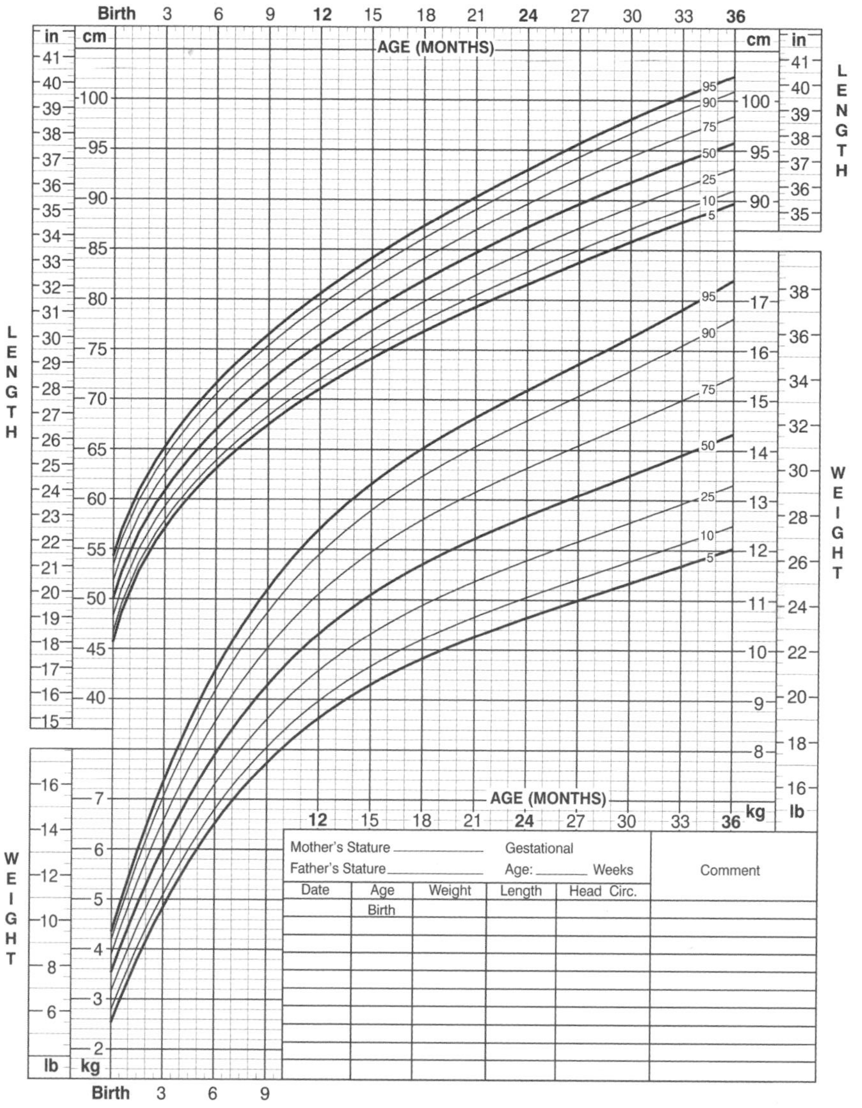

2 TO 20 YEARS OLD: HEIGHT AND WEIGHT

BOYS

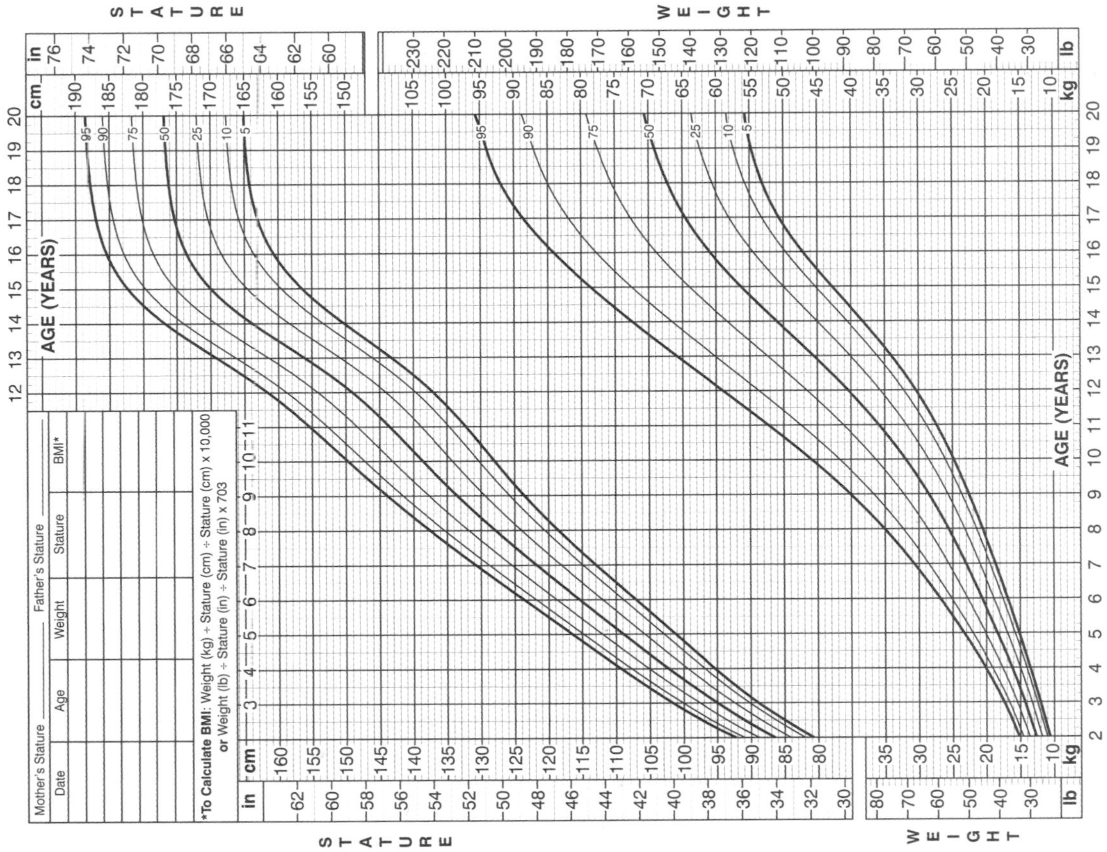

GIRLS

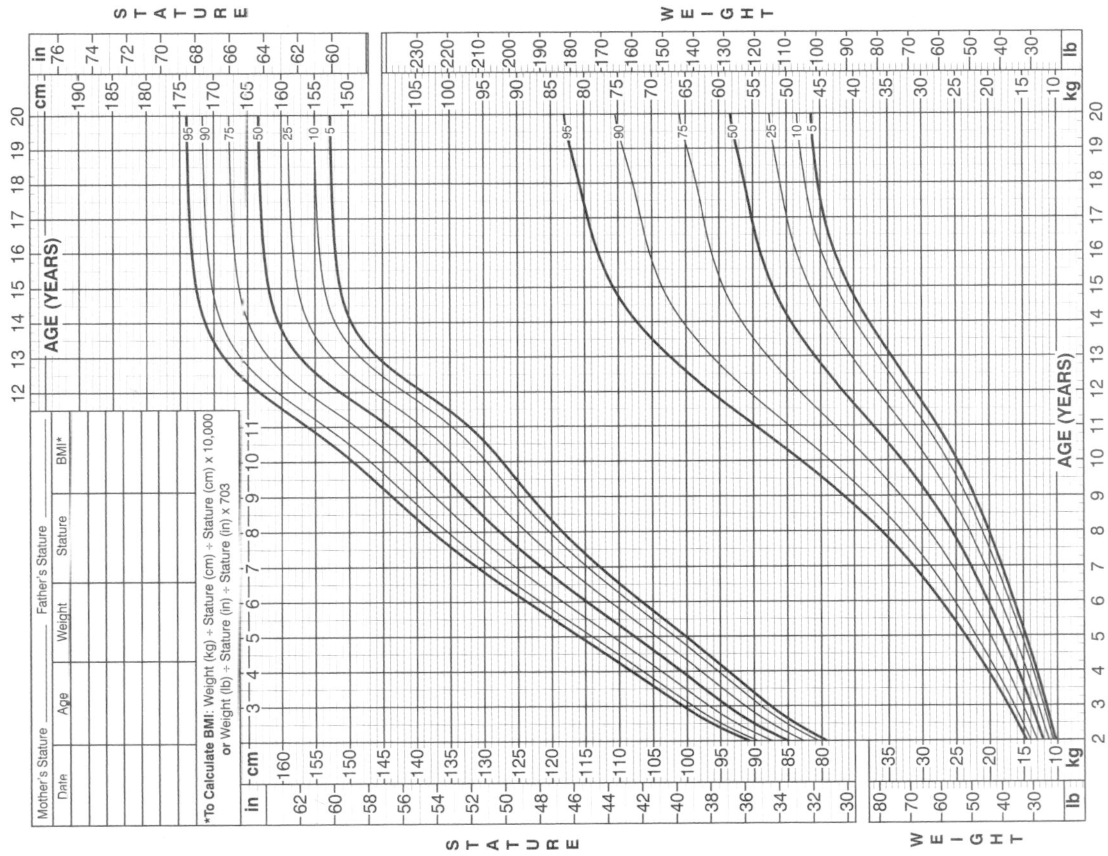

2 TO 20 YEARS OLD: BODY MASS INDEX

GIRLS

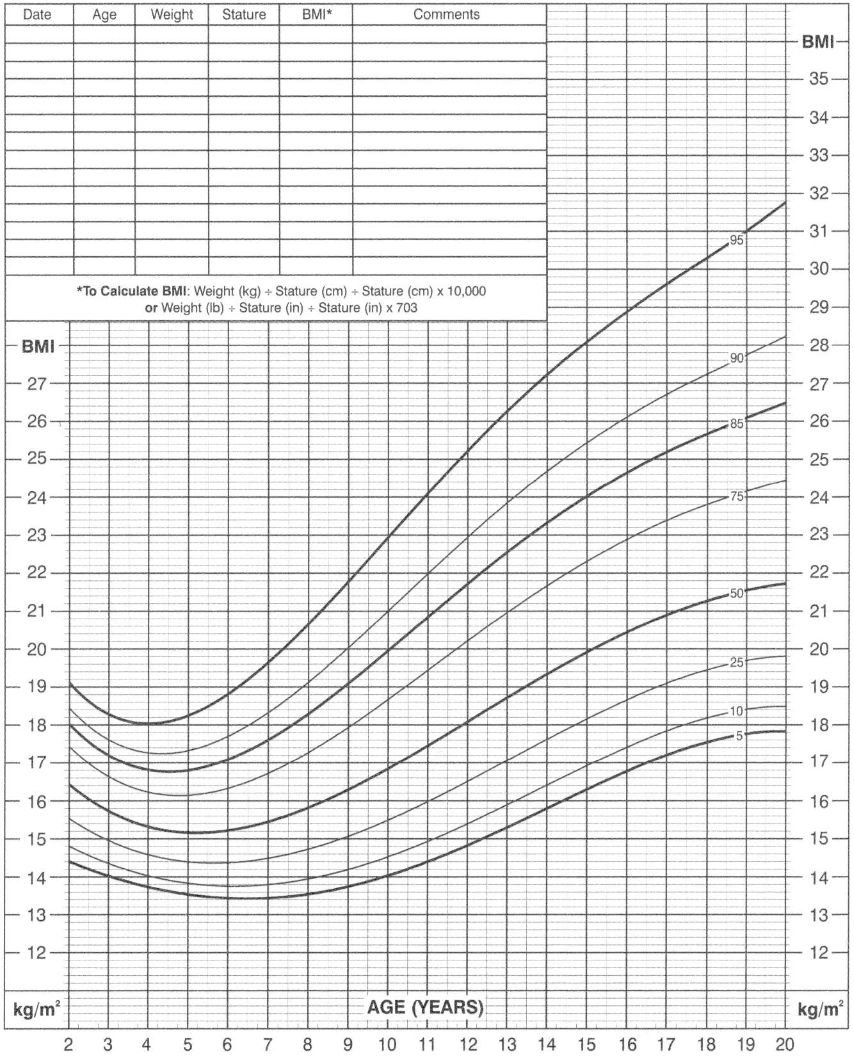

BOYS

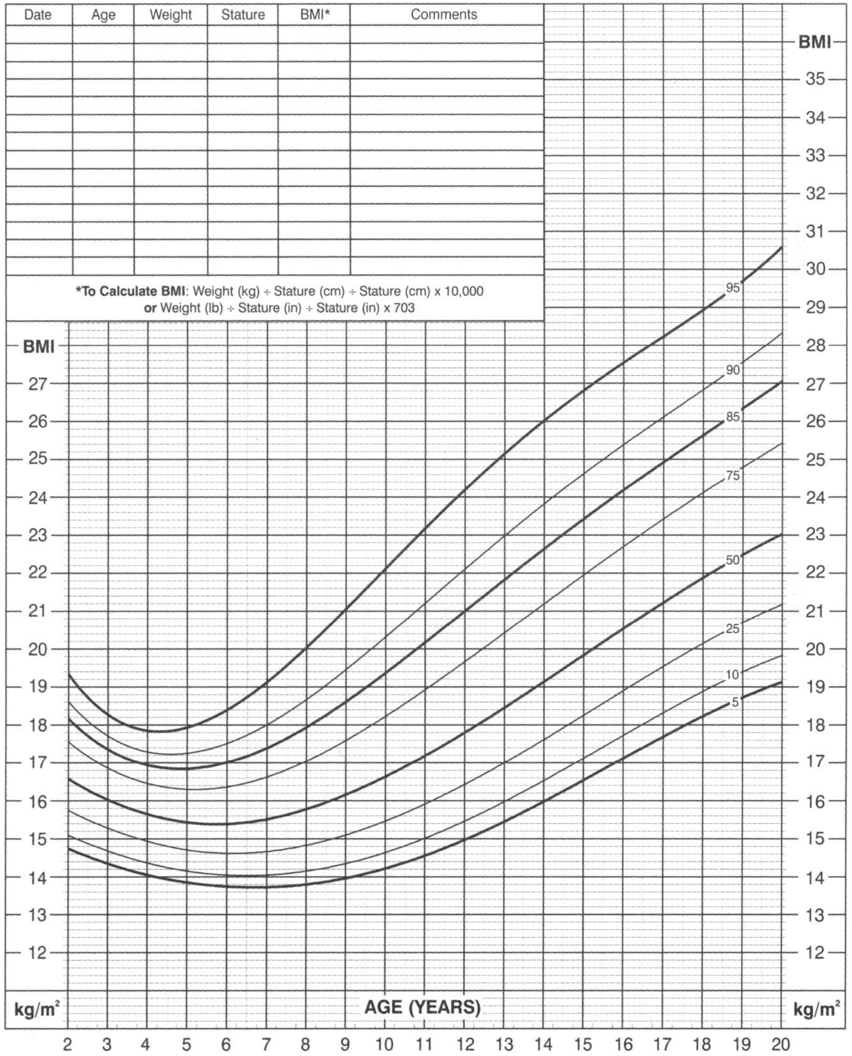

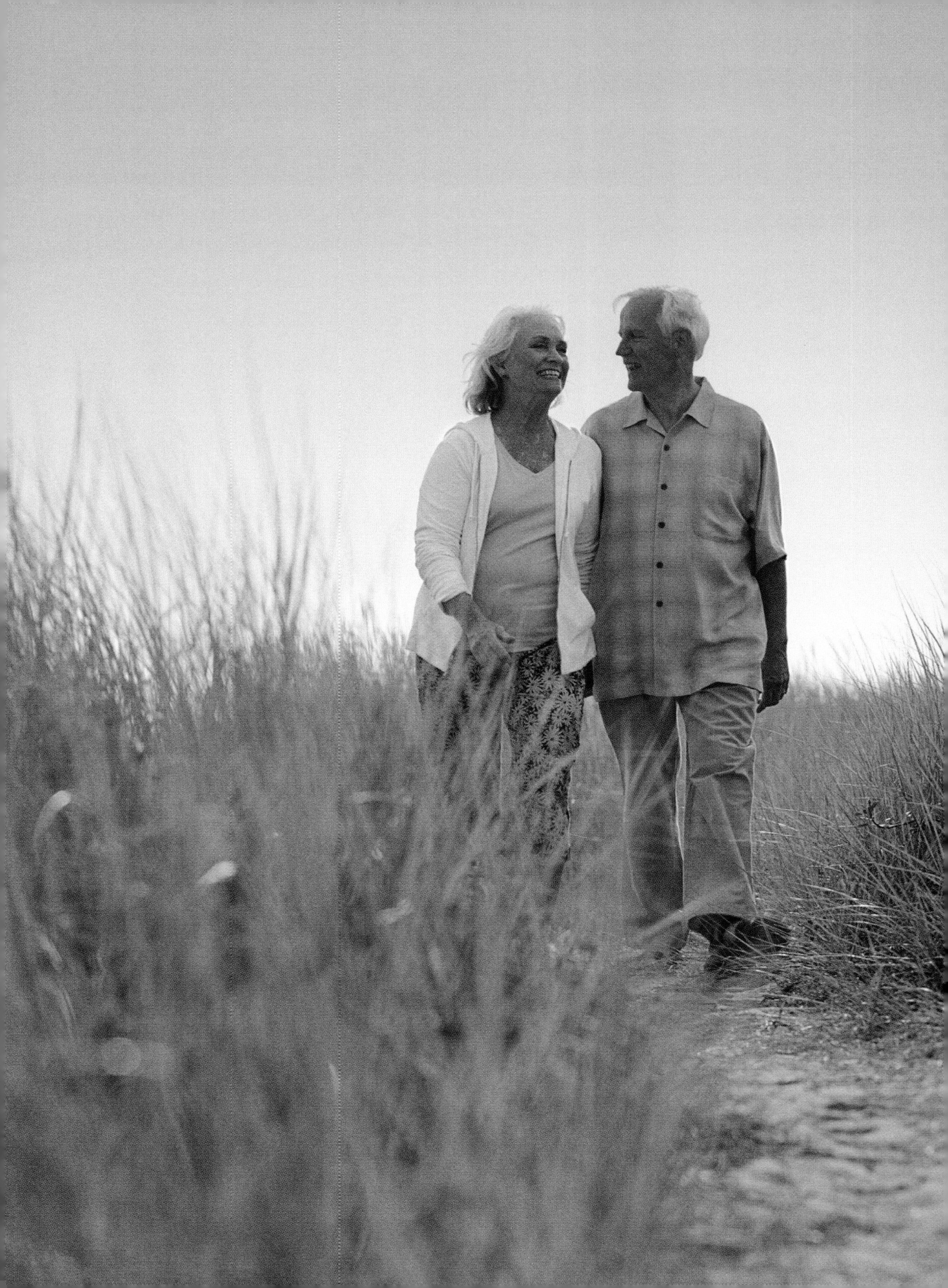

TAKING CONTROL OF LONG-TERM CONDITIONS

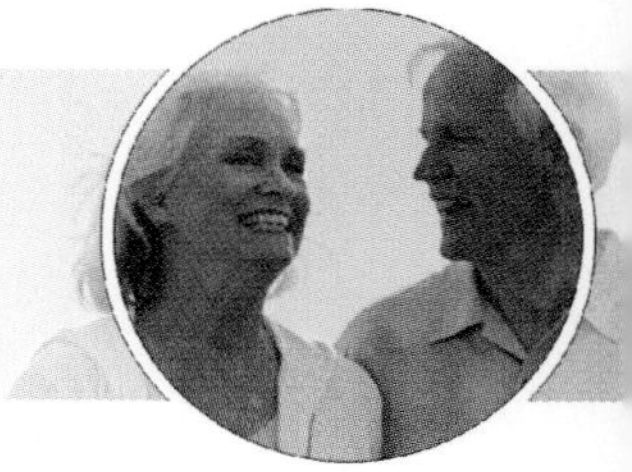

ARTHRITIS

Arthritis involves inflammation of one or more joints and the breakdown of cartilage. Cartilage normally protects the joint, allowing for smooth movement. Cartilage also absorbs shock when pressure is placed on the joint, like when you walk or otherwise bear weight. Without the usual amount of cartilage, the bones rub together, causing pain, swelling, and stiffness.

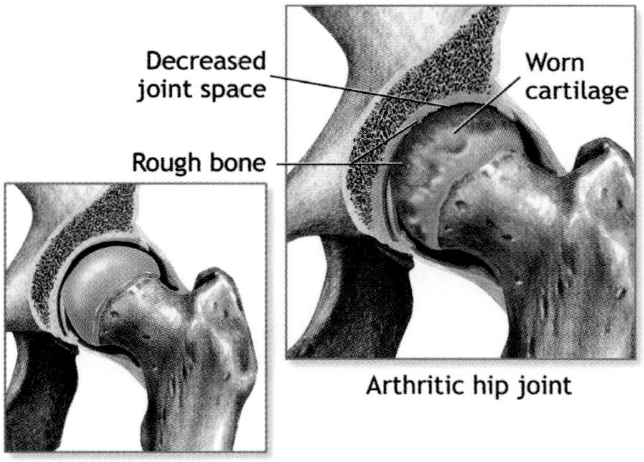

Arthritic hip joint

Normal hip joint

You may have joint inflammation for a variety of reasons, including:

- Broken bone
- Infection (usually caused by bacteria or viruses)
- An autoimmune disease (the body attacks itself because the immune system believes a body part is foreign)
- General "wear and tear" on joints

Often, the inflammation goes away after the injury has healed, the disease is treated, or the infection has been cleared.

With some injuries and diseases, the inflammation does not go away or destruction results in long-term pain and deformity. When this happens, you have chronic arthritis. **Osteoarthritis** is the most common type and is more likely to occur as you age. You may feel it in any of your joints, but most commonly in your hips, knees or fingers. Risk factors for osteoarthritis include:

- Being overweight
- Previously injuring the affected joint
- Using the affected joint in a repetitive action that puts stress on the joint (baseball players, ballet dancers, and construction workers are all at risk)

Rheumatoid arthritis is another form of arthritis. The body's own immune system attacks a joint's synovial membrane, which secretes fluid and lines the joint. The synovium becomes inflamed, produces excess fluid, and the cartilage becomes rough and pitted.

Cut-section view of knee joint

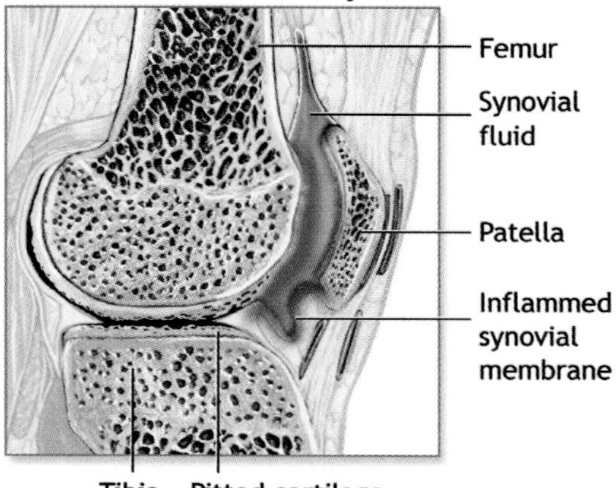

Rheumatoid arthritis in the knee.

Home care

It is possible to greatly improve your symptoms from osteoarthritis and other long-term types of arthritis without medications. In fact, making lifestyle changes without medications is *preferable* for osteoarthritis and other forms of joint inflammation. If needed, medications should be used *in addition to* lifestyle changes.

Common sites of osteoarthritis

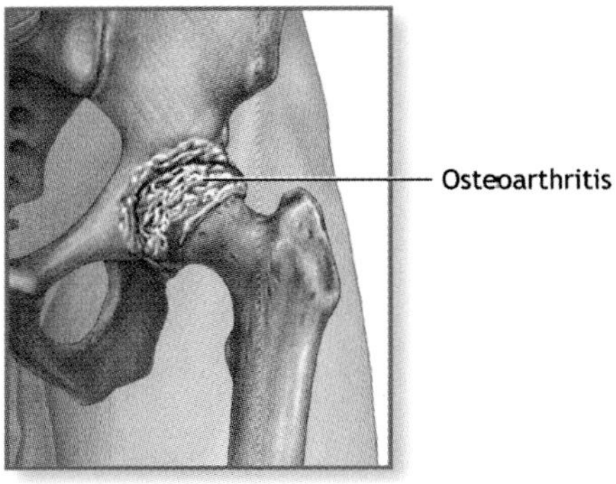

Hip joint

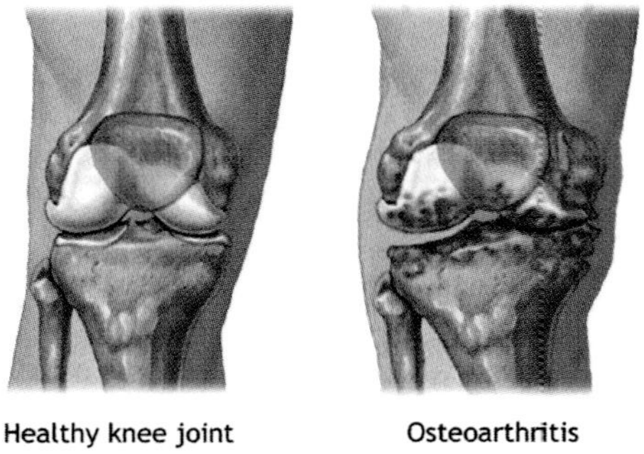

Knee joint

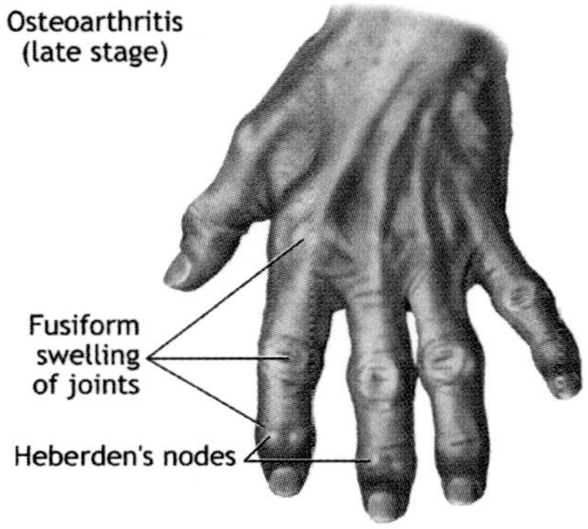

Finger joints

Exercise for arthritis is necessary to maintain healthy joints, relieve stiffness, reduce pain and fatigue, and improve muscle and bone strength. Your exercise program should be tailored to you as an individual. Work with a physical therapist to design an individualized program, which should include:

- Range of motion exercises for flexibility
- Strength training for muscle tone
- Low-impact aerobic activity (also called endurance exercise)

A physical therapist can apply heat and cold treatments as needed and fit you for splints or orthotic (straightening) devices to support and align joints. This may be particularly necessary for rheumatoid arthritis. Your physical therapist may also consider water therapy, ice massage, or transcutaneous nerve stimulation (TENS).

Rest is just as important as exercise. Sleeping 8 to 10 hours per night and taking naps during the day can help you recover from a flare-up more quickly and may even help prevent exacerbations. You should also:

- Avoid positions or movements that place extra stress on your affected joints.
- Avoid holding one position for too long.
- Reduce stress, which can aggravate your symptoms. Try meditation or guided imagery. And talk to your physical therapist about yoga or tai chi.
- Modify your home to make activities easier. For example, have grab bars in the shower, the tub, and near the toilet.

Other measures to try include:

- Taking glucosamine and chondroitin – these form the building blocks of cartilage, the substance that lines joints. These supplements are available at health food stores or supermarkets. Early studies indicate that these compounds are safe and may improve your arthritis symptoms. More research is underway.

- Eat a diet rich in vitamins and minerals, especially antioxidants like vitamin E. These are found in fruits and vegetables. Get selenium from Brewer's yeast, wheat germ, garlic, whole grains, sunflower seeds, and Brazil nuts. Get omega-3 fatty acids from cold water fish (like salmon, mackerel, and herring), flaxseed, rapeseed (canola) oil, soybeans, soybean oil, pumpkin seeds, and walnuts.
- Apply capsaicin cream (derived from hot chili peppers) to the skin over your painful joints. You may feel improvement after applying the cream for 3-7 days.

Your doctor will choose from a variety of medications as needed. Generally, the first drugs to try are available without a prescription. These include:

- **Acetaminophen (Tylenol)** – recommended by the American College of Rheumatology and the American Geriatrics Society as first-line treatment for osteoarthritis. Take up to 4 grams a day (2 extra-strength Tylenols every 6 hours). This can provide significant relief of arthritis pain without many of the side effects of prescription drugs. DO NOT exceed the recommended doses of acetaminophen or take the drug in combination with large amounts of alcohol. These actions may damage your liver.
- **Aspirin, ibuprofen, or naproxen** – these anti-inflammatory drugs are often effective in combating arthritis pain. However, they have many potential risks, especially if used for a long time. They should not be taken in any amount without consulting your doctor. The most dangerous side effects are stomach ulcers, bleeding from the digestive tract, and kidney damage. If you have kidney or liver disease, or a history of gastrointestinal bleeding, you should not take these medicines unless your doctor specifically recommends them.

It is very important to take your medications as directed by your doctor. If you are having difficulty doing so (for example, due to intolerable side effects), you should talk to your doctor.

When to Contact a Medical Professional

Call your doctor if:

- Your joint pain persists beyond 3 days.
- You have severe unexplained joint pain.
- The affected joint is significantly swollen.
- You have a hard time moving the joint.
- Your skin around the joint is red or hot to the touch.
- You have a fever or have lost weight unintentionally.

Prevention

If arthritis is diagnosed and treated early, you can prevent joint damage. Find out if you have a family history of arthritis and share this information with your doctor, even if you have no joint symptoms.

Osteoarthritis may be more likely to develop if you abuse your joints (injure them many times or over-use them while injured). Take care not to overwork a damaged or sore joint. Similarly, avoid excessive repetitive motions.

Excess weight also increases the risk for developing osteoarthritis in the knees, and possibly in the hips and hands. See the article *Body Mass Index* to learn whether your weight is healthy.

Asthma

Asthma is a chronic, inflammatory disorder of the airways. Managing asthma is easier now than in the past, thanks to new medications and a greater understanding of what causes the condition.

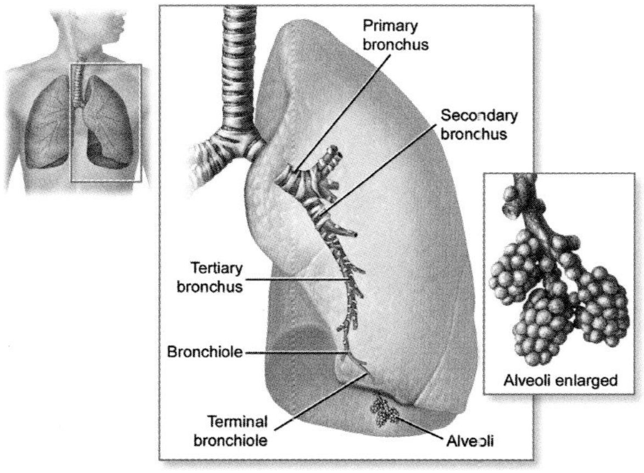

Asthma occurs throughout the lung's bronchial tubes and bronchioles.

A person with asthma may not feel symptoms all the time. But during an "asthma episode" (also called an asthma attack), it becomes hard for air to pass through the airways.

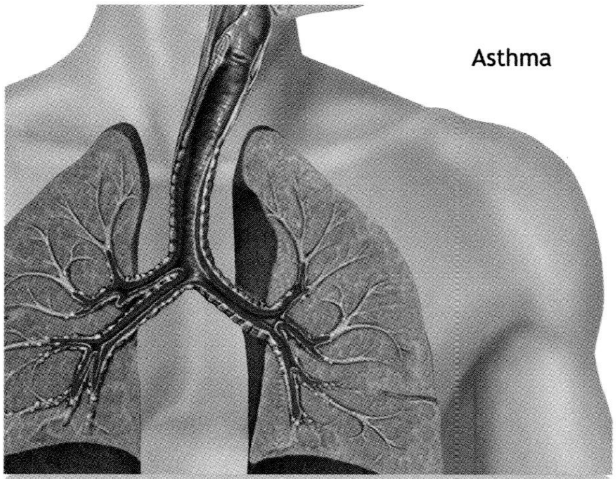

An asthma attack is indicated by the red inflammation of the airways leading into the lungs.

The most common symptoms are difficulty breathing, wheezing, chest tightness, and coughing. Even if you have only one of these signs – like chronic coughing – it may be due to asthma. Other symptoms, like sweating or rapid heart rate, may be present.

There are three things that happen during an asthma episode:

1. **Inflammation** – The lining of the airways become very inflamed, which means they swell (in response to an allergic reaction, exercise, or other trigger). Chronic inflammation is now thought to be the major cause of asthma. In fact, the purpose of steroid "control" medication is to keep inflammation as low as possible and prevent attacks.
2. **Airway muscles tighten** – The rings of muscles that wrap around the airways constrict tighter and tighter, pinching the airway closed. Drugs used to relax the muscles are called "bronchodilators."
3. **Fluid buildup** – The cells that line the airway produce excess mucus, which builds up inside the airway passage.

People with asthma have very sensitive airways that are constantly on the verge of over-reacting to asthma triggers. It doesn't take much for the airways to become inflamed, constricted, and filled with fluid.

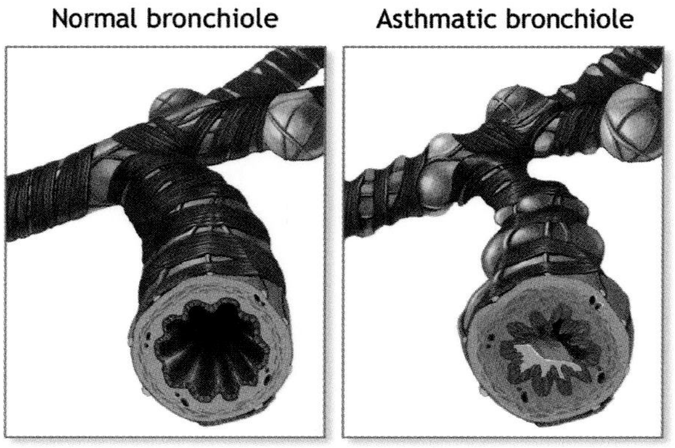

Notice in the normal airway, is there more room for air to flow when you breathe compared to an airway that is inflamed, constricted, and filled with fluid, where there is almost no room for air to flow.

What triggers asthma?

Asthma can be triggered by many of the same things that trigger allergies. It also can be triggered by cold air, exercise, and other factors. Other possible asthma triggers include:

- Pollen, dust mites, indoor and outdoor mold, pet dander, cockroaches, and other allergens
- Smoke from tobacco or a fireplace; indoor and outdoor air pollution
- Viral infections (colds, flu, acute bronchitis, pneumonia)
- Gastroesophageal Reflux (this especially affects night-time asthma)
- Strong odors, perfumes, cleaning sprays, and chemical fumes
- Sinusitis and rhinitis (hay fever)

A key step in controlling asthma is to identify which of these triggers make your asthma worse, and then work to eliminate or avoid them.

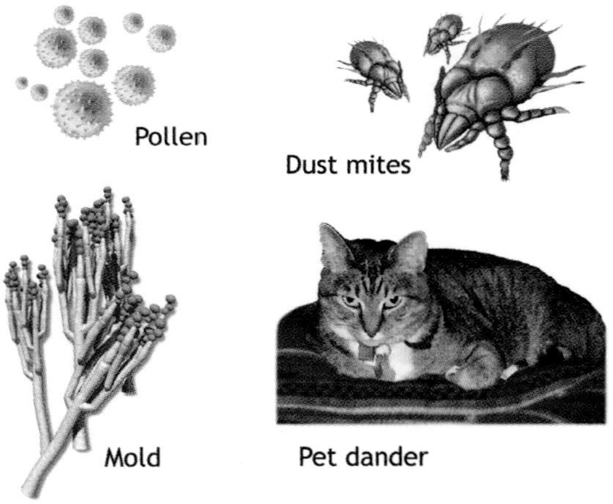

Common household asthma triggers.

Treatment

Asthma can be treated effectively with medication to keep the symptoms under control. Almost anyone with asthma should be able to prevent most asthma attacks, sleep at night without being wakened by symtoms, prevent most trips to the hospital, prevent missed work or school because of asthma symptoms, exercise normally, and find an asthma treatment plan that has minimal side effects.

Consider seeing an asthma specialist if these goals are not being met. All people with asthma should continue to visit their doctor at least twice a year to make sure that they are still achieving optimal control.

There are two major types of asthma medication. The first are called long-term control drugs, which may be used on a daily basis to PREVENT asthma attacks. Inhaled steroids, which prevent inflammation, are generally a doctor's first choice for daily control. For moderate to severe asthma, steroids are even more effective when combined with long-acting beta-agonists.

The second type are called quick-relief drugs, which are used DURING an asthma attack to bring fast relief. Short acting beta-agonists are the most effective and most widely used drugs for treating asthma attacks. They also can be used just before exercising to help prevent exercise-induced symptoms. They work by relaxing the muscles that tighten around the bronchial tubes during an attack. Albuterol is the most commonly used short-acting beta-agonist.

There are several ways to get an asthma drug into your lungs. The most common methods are metered dose inhalers (MDIs), dry powder inhalers, and nebulizers. Spacers work with your MDI to deliver medication more easily and effectively, and can reduce side effects. The appropriate method depends on personal preference, age, ability to use MDIs, and the drugs you have been prescribed.

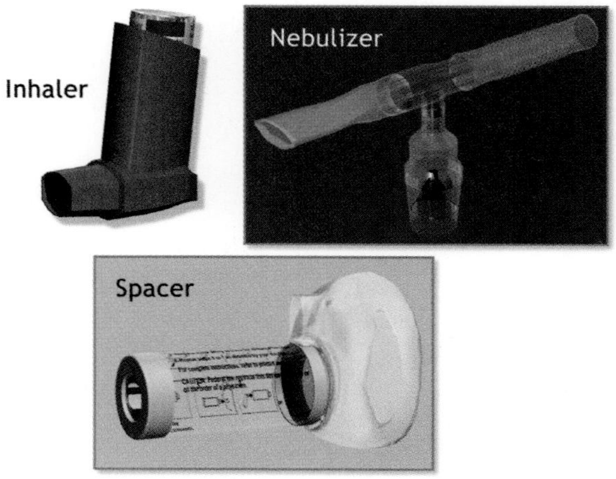

You should ask for a written action plan that explains how to take and adjust your medicines to control your asthma.

Checking your peak flow is one of the best ways to empower yourself and gain control over your asthma. It can help you make sure your asthma is not getting worse and can bring you peace of mind. Peak flow is measured at home with a small, inexpensive plastic meter.

Peak flow meter

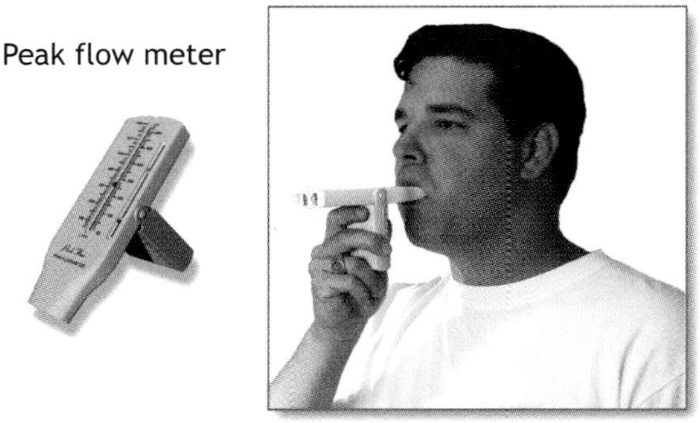

Asthma can be managed by a pediatrician, family doctor, or primary care provider. Allergists and respiratory specialists (pulmonologists) have specific training in the care of asthma and in some cases may be more familiar with current clinical guidelines, such as the 2002 National Institutes of Health asthma guidelines.

Some patients may wish to go to an allergist or other specialist for a second opinion or to get the initial treatment plan established.

> **KEY POINT**
>
> If you are having trouble breathing from an asthma attack, a visit to the emergency room will help you. However, most hospital visits are preventable through good management of your asthma. Talk to a doctor experienced in asthma care.

HEART DISEASE

Heart disease develops from the build-up of plaque (cholesterol and other material) in the coronary blood vessels. This disease process is called atherosclerosis.

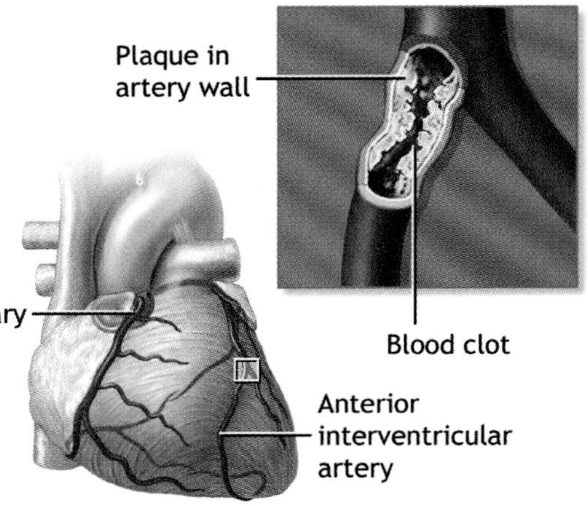

When you have plaque in your blood vessels, several things are more likely to happen. The inner lining of the blood vessel wall may not function properly, unstable plaques can rupture, and blood clots may develop. This sequence of events can lead to a heart attack or sudden, severe symptoms.

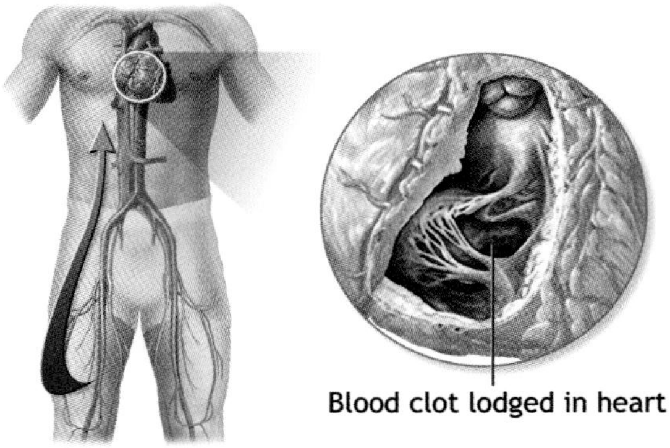

Blood clot in leg may break-off and travel through veins to the heart

If you have heart disease, you might feel:

- Chest pain
- Neck, back, jaw, abdominal, shoulder, or arm pain
- Nausea and vomiting
- Shortness of breath
- Unexplainable fatigue, especially after physical activity

The symptoms of heart disease are more likely when you are physically exerting yourself, under more stress than usual, or after eating a large, fatty meal.

You won't necessarily know if you have heart disease until it has progressed a fair amount. Nonetheless, be aware of your risk factors and try to control them. Risk factors include high cholesterol, high blood pressure, tobacco use, and diabetes. If you do have risk factors, there are many lifestyle changes that can significantly reduce your chances of getting heart disease or having problems from existing heart disease.

Lifestyle changes

Careful lifestyle choices can prevent and treat heart disease. Heart-healthy habits include:

- Control your blood pressure, cholesterol, and diabetes. Do this with diet, exercise, and medication.
- Do not smoke or use tobacco. Avoid second-hand smoke.

Smoking increases your risk of heart disease

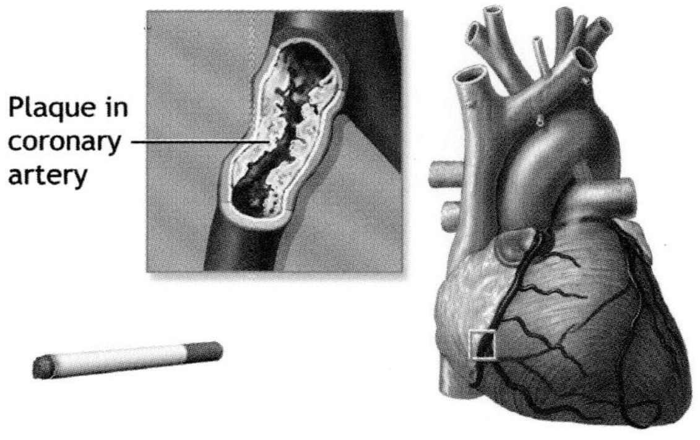

- Eat a diet low in saturated fat and rich in fiber, fruits, and vegetables.
- Exercise at least 3 hours per week (for example, 30 minutes per day, 6 days per week). If you already have any symptoms or you have several risk factors for heart disease, talk to your doctor about how to begin an exercise program safely and effectively.
- Achieve and maintain a normal weight.
- Reduce stress and learn to relax. Try yoga, tai chi, or meditation.

Here's what the American Heart Association recommends:

- Eat a variety of fruits and vegetables (5 to 9 servings / day).
- Eat a variety of grain products, especially whole grains (6 or more servings / day).
- Eat at least 2 servings of fish per week. Fish, particularly cold-water fish, have lots of omega-3 fatty acids – a good kind of fat.
- Avoid fried and hydrogenated foods, which contain saturated fats and trans-fatty acids. Instead, look for foods with monounsaturated fats (like olive oil), and polyunsaturated fats, especially omega-3 fatty acids (such as salmon and other fatty fish, walnuts, almonds, and flaxseeds).

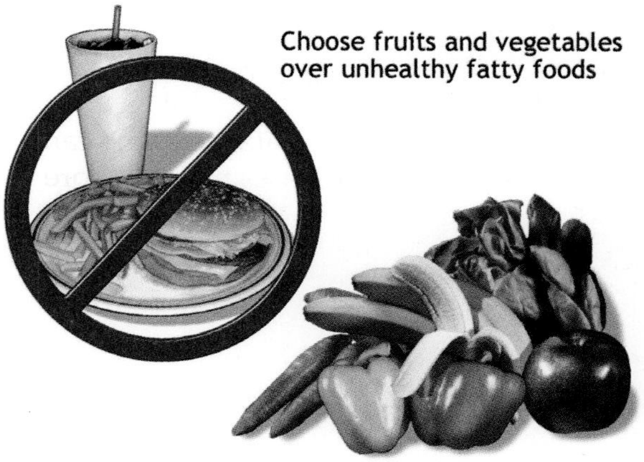

Choose fruits and vegetables over unhealthy fatty foods

- Limit dairy products to low-fat or fat-free items (2 to 4 servings / day).
- Limit sodium to 6 grams / day.
- Limit alcohol to 2 drinks / day for men and 1 drink / day for women.
- Eat soy. Avoid animal protein.

Here are other steps to consider and talk to your doctor about:

- Taking an aspirin every day or two.
- Checking your homocysteine level and, if high, taking folic acid (vitamin B9), vitamin B6, and vitamin B12. Homocysteine, similar to high cholesterol, may increase your chances of developing heart disease.

- Using prescription medications like statins to lower cholesterol, hypoglycemics or insulin to control diabetes, and beta-blockers and ACE inhibitors to lower your risk of dying if you have had a heart attack.

Recovering from a heart attack

After a heart attack, bypass surgery, or angioplasty, attending a cardiac rehabilitation program can be very helpful. Such programs offer practical advice on how to make lifestyle changes and exercise safely.

They also provide support and coping mechanisms for the feelings you will likely experience after such a scary life event. Many people feel depressed or anxious after a heart attack. This is normal, but can slow down your recovery. Getting help with such feelings, even taking medication if necessary, can make a big difference in the healing process.

When to contact a medical professional

Call 911 if:

- You have sudden crushing, squeezing, tightening, or pressure pain in your chest.
- You have shortness of breath, an irregular pulse, sweating, dizziness, or nausea.
- You know you have angina and your chest discomfort is suddenly more intense, brought on by lighter activity, occurs while you are resting, or lasts longer than usual.

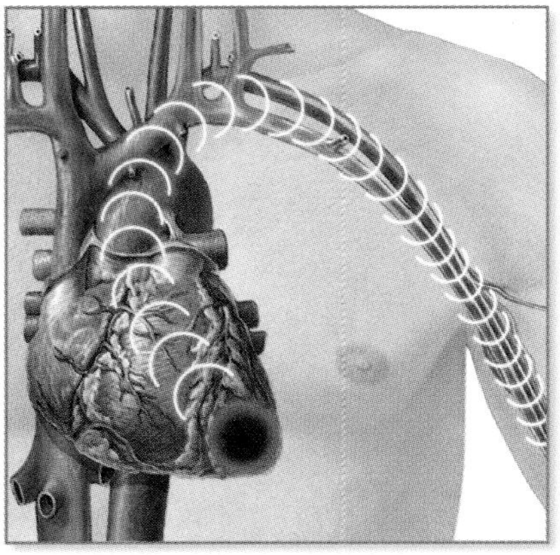

Pain radiating down arm might signal heart attack

High blood pressure

Nearly 50 million Americans have high blood pressure. That's one in every four adults. It is referred to as the "silent killer" because it often has no warning signs.

Many people are surprised to find that they have high blood pressure. But it is a serious condition – one of the leading causes of stroke and heart disease. If you've been diagnosed with high blood pressure, **take it seriously**.

It is important to realize that although high blood pressure may have no outward symptoms, it can cause problems with multiple organs. This includes stroke, heart attack, congestive heart failure, blindness, and kidney disease.

What is blood pressure?

The term **blood pressure** refers to how hard the blood is pressing against the walls of your arteries. When your heart contracts, blood is forced out of the heart, and the pressure increases. When your heart relaxes, the pressure decreases.

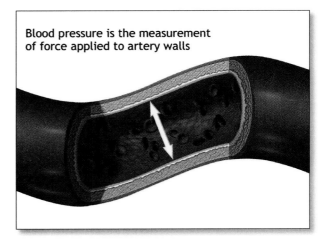

Blood pressure is the measurement of force applied to artery walls

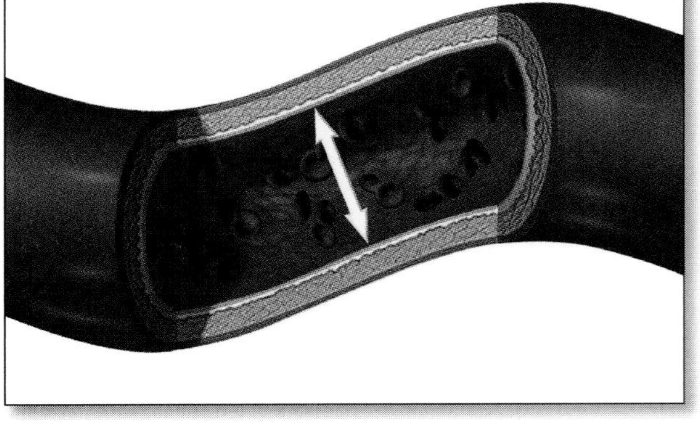

A blood pressure monitor allows you to see the pressure at both points. The higher number is called the **systolic** pressure, and the lower number is the **diastolic** pressure. For example, a normal blood pressure is "115 over 70":

115 systolic pressure (heart contracting)
70 diastolic pressure (heart relaxing)

High blood pressure, or "hypertension," often has no obvious cause, although many factors can contribute. When you have high blood pressure, your blood vessels are too narrow or they have too much blood circulating in them. High blood pressure puts a strain on blood vessels throughout your body and increases the workload on the heart. The result is that one or both of those numbers is higher than it should be.

Anyone can get high blood pressure, but some people are at greater risk than others. Some of the risk factors include:

- Age
- Excess weight
- Lack of physical activity
- Stress, anxiety, and depression
- Smoking

What should my numbers be?

The chart below shows how blood pressure is classified in adults at least 18 years old. You want your blood pressure reading to be lower than "120 over 80."

	Systolic	Diastolic
Normal	Less than 120	Less than 80
Pre-High Blood Pressure	120-139	80-89
Stage 1 High Blood Pressure	140 - 159	90 - 99
Stage 2 High Blood Pressure	160 or over	100 or over

Maintain healthy habits

There are lifestyle changes you can take to lower or prevent high blood pressure. These healthy habits are important for anyone who has been diagnosed with high blood pressure or anyone in the "pre-high blood pressure" category. Regardless of your current blood pressure or whether you are taking blood pressure medication, these steps will improve the quality of your life.

Of course, EVERYONE ELSE benefits from these healthy habits, too – by preventing high blood pressure in the future!

Keep your weight at a healthy level

If you are overweight, focus on losing those extra pounds. Reducing your weight by just 10 pounds may be enough to lower your blood pressure. Losing weight can help to enhance the effects of high blood pressure medication and may also reduce other risk factors, such as diabetes and high cholesterol.

The only way to lose weight is to eat less and burn more calories than you consume. This may not be easy, but with persistence and changing your overall eating habits, it can be done successfully. Talk with your health care provider about a diet plan appropriate for you.

Choose healthy foods

The old saying "You are what you eat" is true when it comes to maintaining a healthy weight and blood pressure. According to the National Heart, Lung, and Blood Institute, studies show that what you eat directly affects the development of high blood pressure.

One of the most effective diets is called **Dietary Approaches to Stop Hypertension (DASH).**

This diet recommends that you eat:

- Foods low in saturated fat, cholesterol, and total fat
- More fruits, vegetables, and low-fat dairy products
- More whole grain foods, fish, chicken, and nuts

- 3,500 mg of dietary potassium each day. Foods rich in potassium include green leafy vegetables, orange juice, potatoes, brown rice, avocados, and bananas
- LESS red meat, sweets, and drinks high in sugar
- No more than 3,000 mg of sodium per day. In fact, other experts from the National Institutes of Health actually recommend that sodium intake be no more than 2,400 mg per day. Some people may benefit from an additional reduction of sodium to 1500 mg daily.

Follow the DASH diet to potentially lower your blood pressure

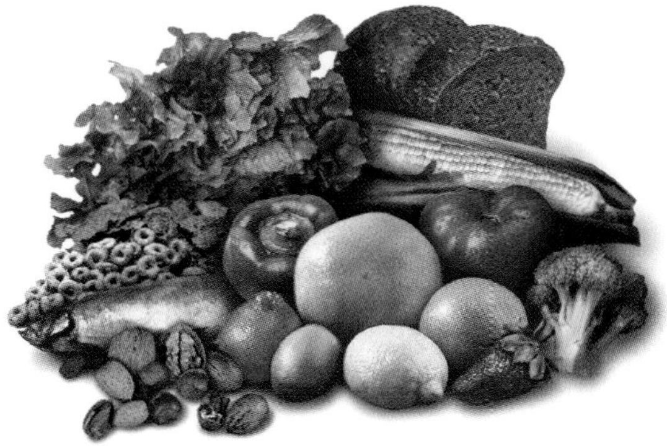

The DASH diet shows a dramatic reduction in most people's blood pressure. The reductions in blood pressure may even begin within 2 weeks of starting the diet plan.

Limit alcohol

Finally, limit the amount of alcohol you drink to no more than one ounce per day if you are a man, and no more than 1/2 ounce if you are a woman. (1 ounce of alcohol is in 24 oz of beer, 10 oz of wine, or 2 oz of 100-proof whiskey.)

Followup office visits

If your blood pressure is normal, keep up the good work! But make sure you get a checkup at least every two years. If you are in the "pre-high blood pressure" category, recheck it in a year and seriously consider making some healthy lifestyle changes.

If you DO have high blood pressure, your doctor will investigate further to see whether there is an identifiable cause. In addition, the doctor will want to determine if you have any related medical problems or risks for heart disease, such as high cholesterol and diabetes. If you do have these risks, your doctor will likely want to see you more often and start treatment sooner.

Both you and your doctor play important roles in achieving your health goals. Your doctor is responsible for providing you with complete and accurate information about your health care and treatment. Your role is important too – even though you may not feel symptoms, high blood pressure is a serious condition and it is very important that you understand and stick to your treatment plan.

If you experience problems with your medicine, **do not stop taking the drug on your own**. Talk with your doctor first. Most side effects go away over time, or your doctor

Treating high blood pressure can be safer and less expensive

A major study has concluded that good old diuretics are a better choice than commonly used ACE inhibitors and calcium channel blockers. The study, published in the *New England Journal of Medicine*, recommended that diuretics be the first-choice medication for high blood pressure.

In fact, those who took the less expensive diuretics had fewer hospitalizations, fewer strokes, and were less likely to develop heart failure than those on other popular medications. Ask your doctor for more information about diuretics.

Source: Major outcomes in high-risk hypertensive patients randomized to angiotensin-converting enzyme inhibitor or calcium channel blocker vs. diuretic: The Antihypertensive and Lipid-Lowering Treatment to Prevent Heart Attack Trial (ALLHAT). JAMA December 18, 2002;288:2981-97.

may be able to change the dosage or prescribe a different drug.

It is also very important that you **maintain your follow-up appointments** with your doctor and consider purchasing a home blood pressure monitor to keep track of your pressure between doctor visits.

High blood pressure can be controlled. By working with your doctor to follow your treatment guidelines, making healthy lifestyle changes, and staying informed about your health status, you CAN reduce your high blood pressure and decrease your risk for heart disease and stroke.

HIGH CHOLESTEROL

Have you had your cholesterol levels checked lately? High cholesterol is a major risk factor for cardiovascular disease, which kills more men and women each year than any other illness.

High blood cholesterol has no warning signs. People diagnosed with high cholesterol often feel fine and therefore may not take their condition seriously.

Excess cholesterol builds up on the inner walls of arteries throughout the body, forming scar tissue and plaque. This can lead to blood clots, heart attack, stroke, and other cardiovascular problems.

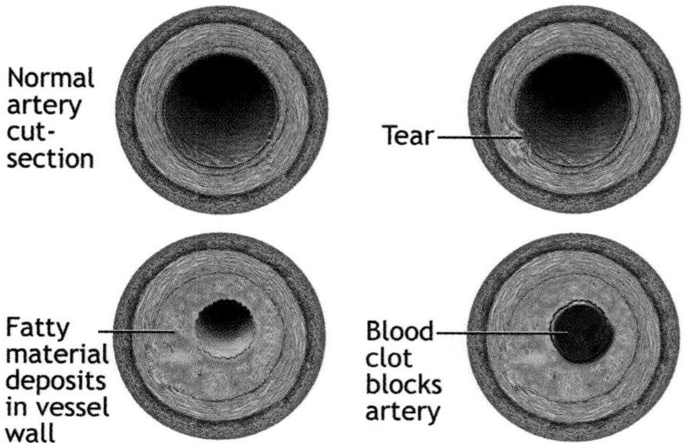

Everyone should have their blood cholesterol levels tested at least every five years.

A blood cholesterol test looks at the level of four things: total cholesterol, HDL ("good") cholesterol, LDL ("bad") cholesterol, and triglycerides

A lipoprotein profile measures the level of cholesterol in the blood

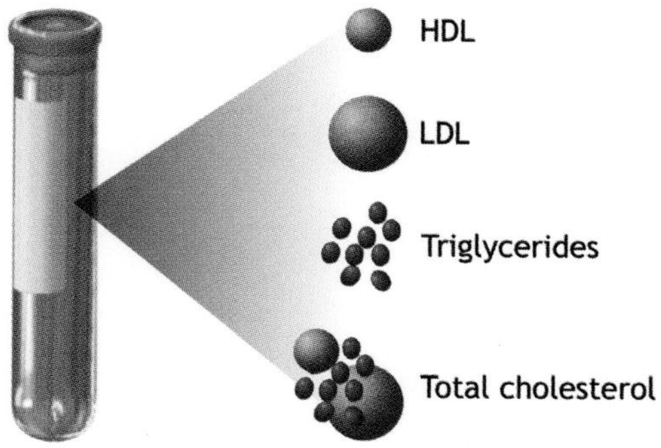

Here's a simple rule to remember: **you want HDL to be HIGH, and you want LDL to be LOW.**

Your LDL level is what doctors watch most carefully. If it gets too high, it will need to be treated. Treatment includes eating better, losing weight, and exercising more. You may also need medication.

People who do not have heart disease, or who have average cholesterol levels, still need to eat right, maintain a healthy weight, and exercise. These steps help PREVENT future heart attacks and other complications for EVERYONE.

CHOOSE FOODS LOW IN SATURATED FAT

Food labels are one of the best tools for eating healthy. In terms of lowering cholesterol, pay particular attention to these items on the label:

- total fat
- saturated fat
- cholesterol
- calories

Of these, the most important by far is saturated fat.

Here are some other considerations about food labels:

- When looking at food labels, pay very close attention to serving size.
- The % Daily Value is based on a diet of 2,000 calories a day. You may need to eat more or less than 2,000 calories a day depending on your weight.

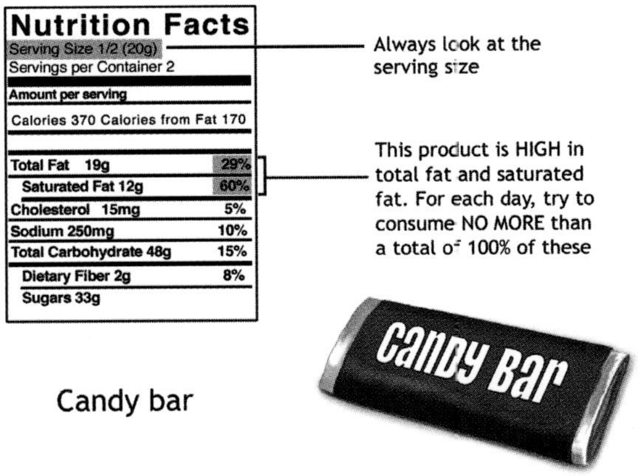
Nutrition Facts
Serving Size 1/2 (20g)
Servings per Container 2
Amount per serving
Calories 370 Calories from Fat 170
Total Fat 19g 29%
Saturated Fat 12g 60%
Cholesterol 15mg 5%
Sodium 250mg 10%
Total Carbohydrate 48g 15%
Dietary Fiber 2g 8%
Sugars 33g
Always look at the serving size
This product is HIGH in total fat and saturated fat. For each day, try to consume NO MORE than a total of 100% of these
Candy Bar

Candy bar

- Each day, your total of the "bad ingredients" (fat, cholesterol, sodium) should not go over 100%. In contrast, your total of the "good ingredients" (vitamins, fiber, protein) should be at least 100% each day.
- The % Daily Value on the food label for TOTAL fat is something to watch, especially because it usually means high calories. It is not as important as saturated fat, however, because it also may include unsaturated fats, which are healthier.

More tips for healthy eating

- Choose lean, protein-rich foods such as soy, fish, skinless chicken, very lean meat, and fat free or 1% dairy products. Substitute soy protein for animal protein in your diet, particularly if you already have high cholesterol.
- Eat foods that are naturally low in fat, like whole grains, fruits, and vegetables.

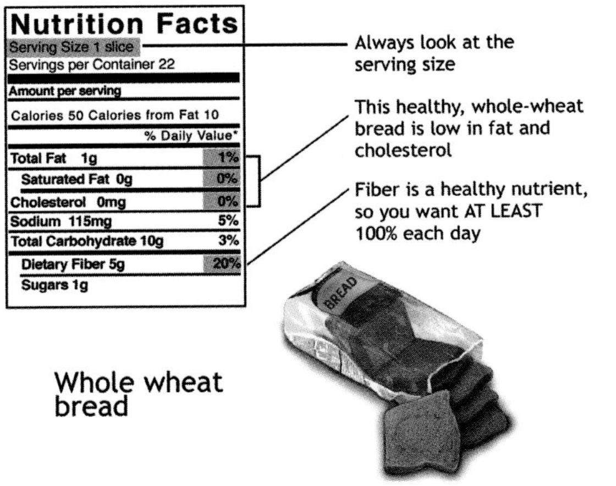
Nutrition Facts
Serving Size 1 slice
Servings per Container 22
Amount per serving
Calories 50 Calories from Fat 10
% Daily Value*
Total Fat 1g 1%
Saturated Fat 0g 0%
Cholesterol 0mg 0%
Sodium 115mg 5%
Total Carbohydrate 10g 3%
Dietary Fiber 5g 20%
Sugars 1g
Always look at the serving size
This healthy, whole-wheat bread is low in fat and cholesterol
Fiber is a healthy nutrient, so you want AT LEAST 100% each day
BREAD

Whole wheat bread

- Increase soluble fiber in your diet by selecting foods like oats, bran, dry peas, beans, cereal, and rice. Fiber may also give you a sense of fullness so that you don't eat as much, making weight loss somewhat easier.
- Choose soft margarines (liquid or tub) over stick margarine to limit trans-fatty acids.
- Foods rich in omega-3 fatty acids may reduce triglycerides, raise HDL levels, and reduce your risk of heart disease. Such food sources include cold-water fish (including wild salmon, tuna, and mackerel), fish oils, flaxseed and flaxseed oil, canola oil, soybean oil, and nuts (especially walnuts and almonds).

> **Healthy habits give you more cholesterol control**
>
> Eating right, exercising, and losing weight are essential to lower your cholesterol – whether you need to take medication or not. In fact, medication works much better when you commit to these healthy habits. Some studies even suggest that by getting enough fiber, soy, and omega-3 fatty acids – and limiting saturated fat – you may even be able to avoid medication altogether.

- Folic acid, also called vitamin B9, may help lower the risk of heart disease in those with high cholesterol.

Foods to avoid

- Limit your consumption of fried foods, processed foods, and commercially prepared baked goods (such as donuts, cookies, and crackers).
- Limit animal products like egg yolks, cheeses, whole milk, cream, ice cream, and fatty meats. These are all high in saturated fats.
- Look on food labels for words like "hydrogenated" or "partially hydrogenated" – these foods are loaded with saturated fats and trans-fatty acids and should be avoided.

Exercise regularly

You knew regular physical activity was good for you, but did you know it helped keep your cholesterol levels healthy? It actually raises HDL (good) cholesterol and lowers total and LDL (bad) cholesterol. Try to exercise at least 30 minutes on most days. Exercising also helps you to lose weight, lowers your blood pressure, strengthens your heart and blood vessels, and reduces stress.

Lose excess weight

Overweight people tend to have higher cholesterol levels than people who maintain a healthy weight. Losing weight can help to lower your LDL cholesterol. For people who have multiple risk factors for heart disease (such as high cholesterol, diabetes, and high blood pressure), losing weight is especially important.

Check with your health care provider for weight-loss recommendations. Losing 10% of your weight may improve your cholesterol levels. (For example, if you weigh 200 pounds, dropping 20 pounds can help your cholesterol.)

Congestive heart failure

Heart failure does not actually mean that your heart has failed or stopped beating. It means that your heart, a muscle that pumps blood to all parts of your body, is not working as well as it should be.

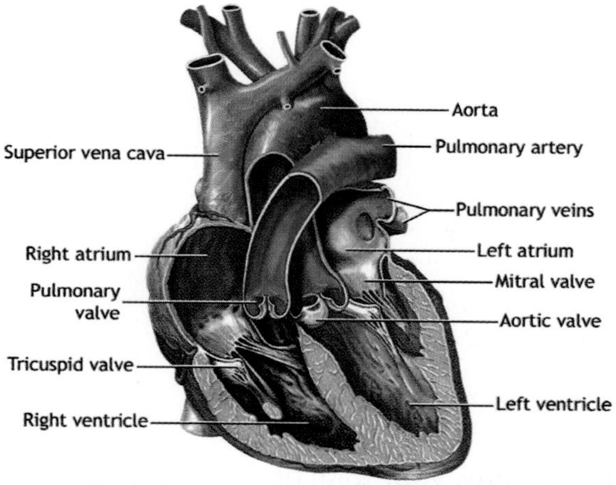

The heart is primarily made of muscle tissue that contracts to pump blood. The right ventricle pumps blood to the lungs to exchange carbon dioxide for oxygen. The oxygenated blood is then pumped by the left ventricle to your body's organs and tissues.

As your heart's pumping action lessens, blood may back up in your lungs, liver, or legs. This can cause shortness of breath, leg swelling (edema), and other problems. In addition, organs in your body may not get the oxygen and nutrients they need, reducing their ability to function properly.

You may experience one or more of the following if your heart is failing:

- Swelling of your feet, ankles, and possibly abdomen
- Weight gain
- Shortness of breath and cough
- Racing or skipping heart beat (palpitations)

- Indigestion, nausea and vomiting, and loss of appetite
- Difficulty sleeping
- Fatigue, weakness, and lightheadedness
- Diminished concentration and alertness
- Changes in urination, like needing to urinate at night. If you have decreased urine production, this is often a sign that your kidneys are failing.

The more advanced your heart failure, the more likely you are to have symptoms. Doctors use different grading or staging systems to classify your heart failure by severity.

You are at risk for developing heart failure if you:

- Have had a heart attack
- Have heart disease (see *Heart Disease*)
- Have high blood pressure or diabetes
- Are obese
- Abuse alcohol, smoke cigarettes, or use cocaine

Take control

If you have heart failure, your doctor will monitor you closely. This means having followup appointments at least every 3-6 months, figuring out any underlying cause and treating it, and periodic testing of your heart function. For example, an ultrasound of your heart, called an echocardiogram, will be done periodically to see how well your heart is pumping blood with each stroke or beat.

It is your responsibility to carefully monitor yourself and help manage your condition. Track your weight on a daily basis. Weight gain can be a sign that you are retaining fluid and that the pump function of your heart is worsening. Make sure you weigh yourself at the same time each day and on the same scale, with little to no clothes on.

Common causes of congestive heart failure

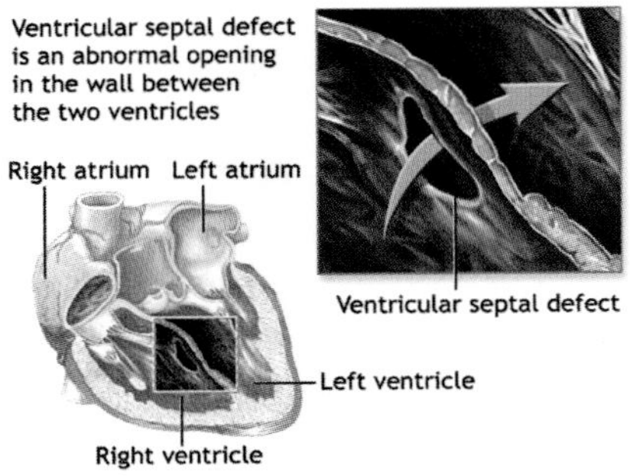

Heart defects (more common in children)

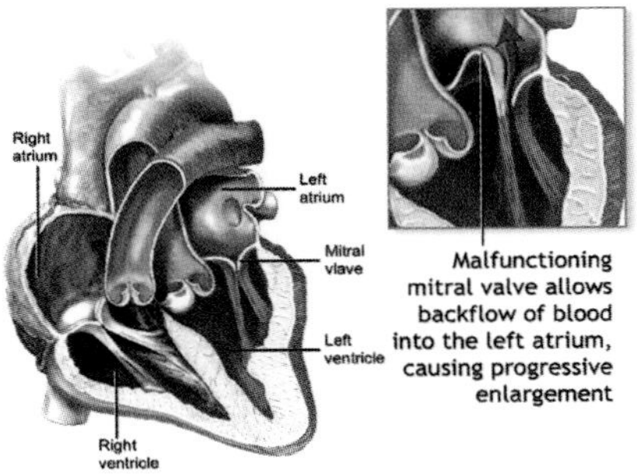

Heart valve damage

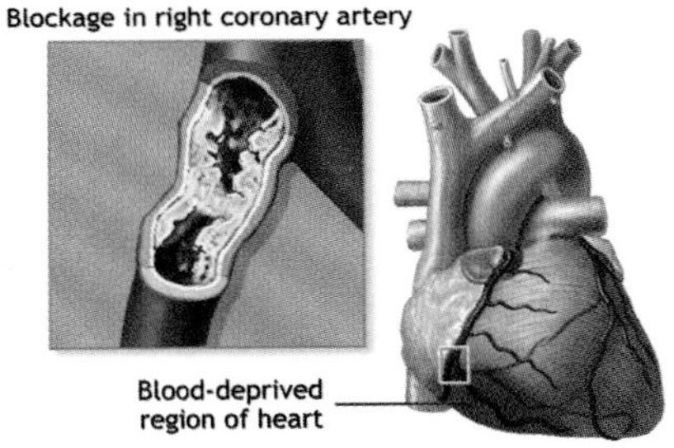

Ischemic (lack of blood flow) heart disease

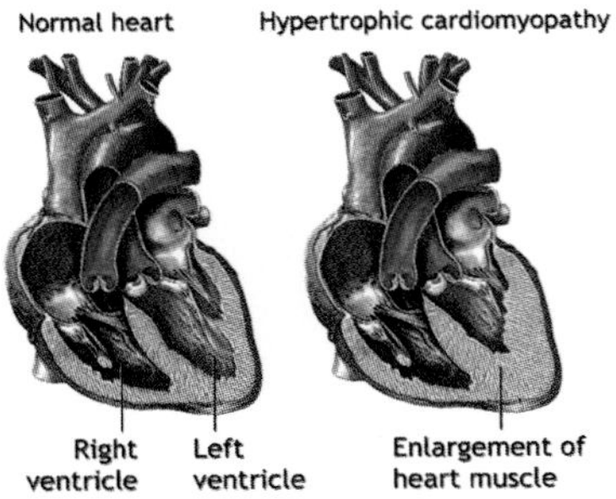

Overwork of ventricles causing heart wall thickening (hypertrophic cardiomyopathy)

Other important measures include:

- Take medications as directed. Carry a list of medications with you wherever you go.
- Limit salt and sodium.
- Don't smoke.
- Stay active. For example, walk or ride a stationary bicycle. Your doctor can provide a safe and effective exercise plan based on your degree of heart failure and how well you do on tests that check the strength and function of your heart. DO NOT exercise on days that your weight has gone up from fluid retention or you are not feeling well.
- Lose weight if you are overweight.
- Get enough rest, including after exercise, eating, or other activities. This allows your heart to rest as well. Keep your feet elevated to decrease swelling.

Tips to lower your salt and sodium

- Look for foods that are labeled "low-sodium," "sodium-free," "no salt added," or "unsalted." Check the total sodium content on food labels. Be especially careful of canned, packaged, and frozen foods. A nutritionist can teach you how to understand these labels.
- Don't cook with salt or add salt to what you are eating. Try pepper, garlic, lemon, or other spices for flavor instead. Be careful of packaged spice blends as these often contain salt or salt products (like monosodium glutamate, MSG).
- Avoid foods that are naturally high in sodium, like anchovies, meats (particularly cured meats, bacon, hot dogs, sausage, bologna, ham, and salami), nuts, olives, pickles, sauerkraut, soy and Worcestershire sauces, tomato and other vegetable juices, and cheese.

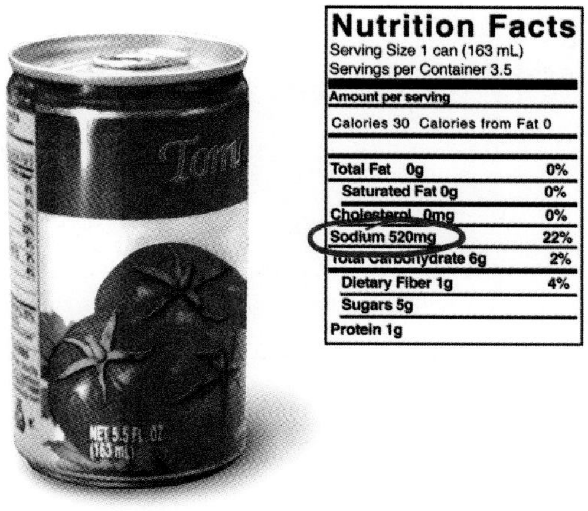

- Take care when eating out. Stick to steamed, grilled, baked, boiled, and broiled foods with no added salt, sauce, or cheese.
- Use oil and vinegar on salads rather than bottled dressings.
- Eat fresh fruit or sorbet for dessert.

When to contact a medical professional

Call 911 if:

- You have sudden pain or pressure in your chest, neck, jaw, arm, or shoulder.
- You have severe shortness of breath.
- You are dizzy or lightheaded.
- You have a rapid or irregular heartbeat.

Also call your doctor right away if:

- You have gained weight for two or more days in a row, or you gain more than 2 pounds in one day.
- You notice increased swelling in your feet, legs, or abdomen.
- You have worsened shortness of breath than usual, especially when lying down.
- You feel nauseated.
- You are more fatigued than usual.

Diabetes

Diabetes is a serious, long-term medical condition characterized by high levels of glucose in the blood. Glucose is a simple sugar that comes from the food you eat. When your stomach digests food, glucose is absorbed into the bloodstream.

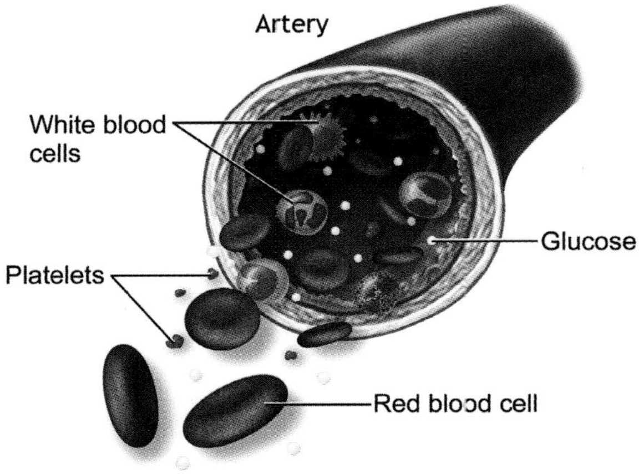

The glucose circulates in your blood and serves as the main source of fuel for all the cells in your body. The process of changing glucose into energy depends on a hormone called *insulin*.

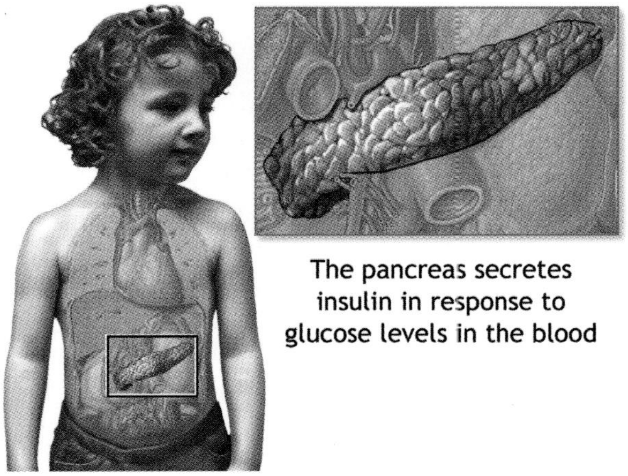

The pancreas secretes insulin in response to glucose levels in the blood

If you have diabetes, you either do not produce enough insulin or you cannot use the insulin that your body makes. As a result, glucose builds up in your blood stream.

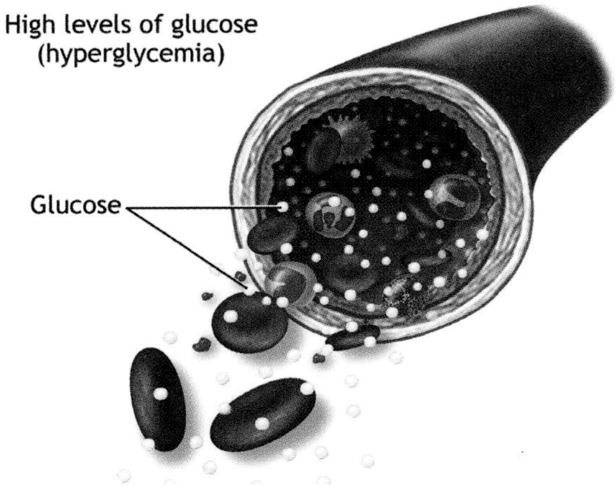

If left untreated, diabetes can lead to blindness, kidney disease, nerve damage, heart disease, and stroke.

There are two main types of diabetes:

- **Type 1** – usually starts in childhood or as a young adult. People with this type of diabetes produce little to no insulin and need to take insulin by injection.
- **Type 2** – usually starts as an adult, although the number of children with type 2 diabetes is on the rise. Accounts for more than 90% of all diabetes. Those with this type of diabetes produce some insulin, but not enough, and the body cannot properly use it. Being overweight is a significant risk factor for this type of diabetes.

While type 1 diabetes cannot be prevented, there are many things you can do to avoid type 2 diabetes. There are also many steps to control it, if you already have diabetes.

Most people with type 2 diabetes do not require insulin injections. Oral medications may be necessary. However, the key to controlling type 2 diabetes is making lifestyle changes. In fact, if you have type 2 diabetes, you may be able to avoid or eliminate medications altogether by losing weight and carefully following dietary and exercise advice.

Take control

If you have diabetes, it is important to keep tight control of your blood glucose levels.

This means maintaining levels within or near the normal range as often as possible. If you are able to do this, you are much less likely to develop complications from diabetes. To do this requires:

- A carefully calculated diet, meaning not only what types and amounts of foods you eat throughout the day but also what times of day you eat. Once this is established, try not to skip meals or snacks.
- Planned exercise times.
- Daily blood glucose testing at home, even several times per day.

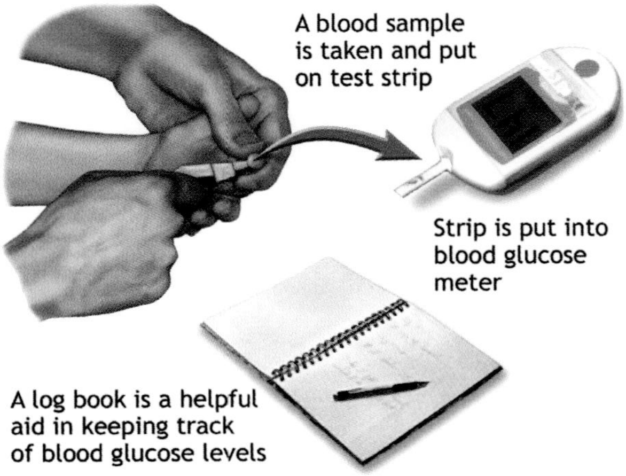
A blood sample is taken and put on test strip
Strip is put into blood glucose meter
A log book is a helpful aid in keeping track of blood glucose levels

- If on insulin, several insulin injections throughout the day. If on oral medication, take it at the same time each day.

Periodically, a blood test known as hemoglobin A1C should be performed. Check with your doctor to make sure that it is being done. The result of this test gives a sense of how close to the normal range your blood sugars have been over the previous 3 months.

Eat for Health

According to the American Diabetes Association (ADA), you should follow a healthy, low-fat diet, rich in fiber from whole grains, fruits, and vegetables. Here are some guidelines for your total daily calories:

- Eat lean protein, which you get from fish, poultry, non-fat or low-fat dairy, and certain vegetables like soy and legumes. Lean protein should be about 15-20% of your total calories. If you already have signs of kidney damage, your nutritionist or doctor may want you to have less protein than this.
- Avoid saturated fats, which are found in meats, full-fat dairy products, and many other foods. Also avoid trans-fatty acids, which come from fried foods, hydrogenated oils, and partially hydrogenated oils. Learn to read and understand food labels, including the list of ingredients on products. Your daily calories should be 30% or less from fat, with less than 7-10% coming from saturated fats.

A registered dietitian can help you best determine how to balance your diet with carbohydrates, protein, and fat. He or she can also teach you about glucose monitoring – how to use the apparatus, how often to check your blood glucose level, and how to respond to the results. It is best for any person with diabetes to receive diabetic teaching from such a trained professional, especially early on.

Exercise

Exercise not only lowers blood sugar directly, but it also helps your body use circulating insulin more efficiently. In addition, exercise improves blood flow to the heart, promotes weight loss, and lowers your blood pressure. Even with type 1 diabetes, exercise may allow you to reduce the amount of insulin you need to take. Before you begin an exercise routine, talk to your doctor about how to do so safely and effectively. If you have had diabetes for a while, your doctor may want you to undergo a stress test before starting.

Once your doctor gives you the go-ahead, follow these general guidelines:

- Include a 5 to 10 minute warm-up and cool down with each exercise session.
- Stretch before and after exercise.

- Check your glucose level before and after each exercise session. Together with your nutritionist or diabetic teacher, make appropriate adjustments to food, and insulin if you use it.
- Always carry a sugar–based food like fruit juice, soft drink, or glucose tablets, in case your blood glucose level drops from exercise. This may happen as long as 24 hours after an exercise session.
- Wear a visible ID bracelet indicating that you have diabetes.

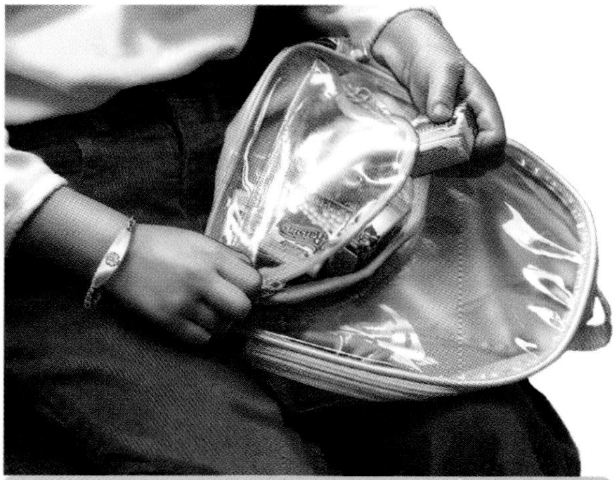

It's important to carry sugar-based food and wear a diabetes ID bracelet if you have diabetes.

Control stress

Long-term stress is likely to worsen diabetes. Tai chi, yoga, and other forms of relaxation may help you control blood sugar. Biofeedback can help motivate you to change your lifestyle habits.

See your doctor often

The ADA recommends the following:

- **Every 3 to 6 months** – a doctor's visit for weight and blood pressure. Hemoglobin (HgB) A1c is done at these visits to check your average blood sugar level over the previous 3 months. Your HgB A1c number should be below 7.
- **Every year** – urine and blood tests for signs of kidney damage; eye exam; foot

Dangers of unmanaged diabetes

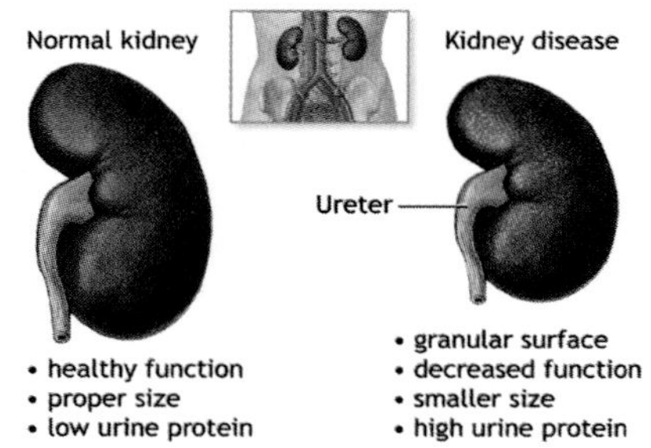

Diabetic nephropathy (kidney disease)

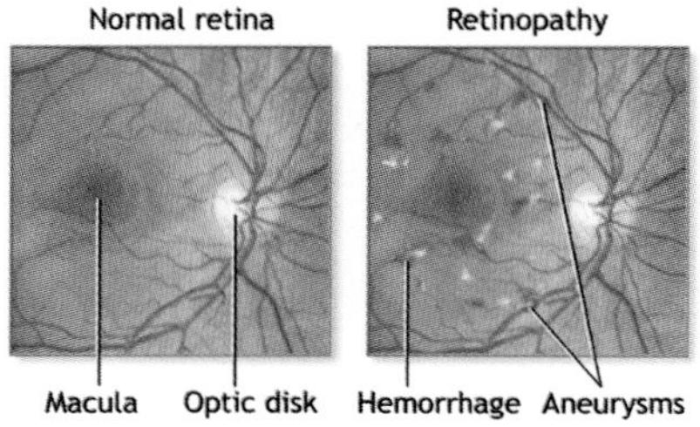

Retinopathy (hemorrhages in the retina)

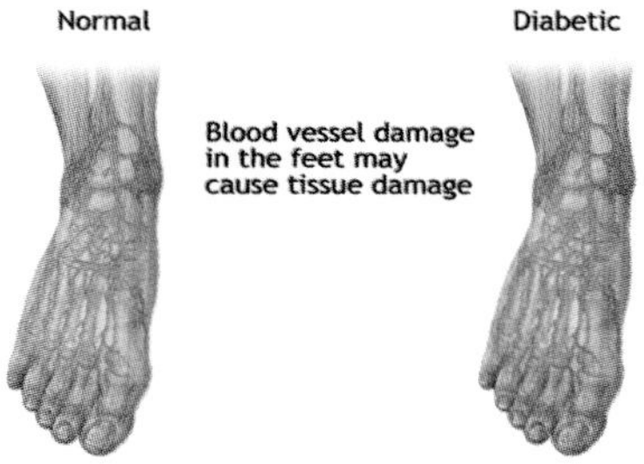

Poor foot circulation

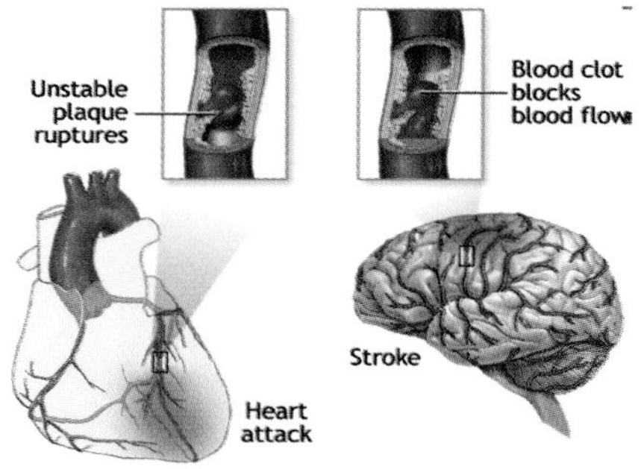

Cholesterol builds up into plaque that may rupture, causing a clot to form and block blood flow

exam focusing on circulation, nerve function, and signs of infection; cholesterol levels including HDL (the good kind of cholesterol).

For your future health

If you have diabetes, work closely with a nutritionist to gain control of your blood sugars. Doing so can greatly reduce your chances of long-term complications. Ask your doctor the value of your Hemoglobin A1C. Your number should be below 7.

Stroke

A stroke is an interruption of the blood supply to any part of the brain, resulting in damaged brain tissue.

If the flow of blood in an artery supplying the brain is interrupted for longer than a few seconds, brain cells can die, causing permanent damage. An interruption can be caused by either blood clots or bleeding in the brain.

Most strokes are due to blood clots that block blood flow. Bleeding into the brain occurs if a blood vessel ruptures or there is a significant injury.

High blood pressure is the number one reason that you might have a stroke. The risk of stroke is also increased by age, family history of stroke, smoking, diabetes, high cholesterol, and heart disease.

Cocaine use, alcohol abuse, head injury, and bleeding disorders increase the risk of bleeding into the brain.

Symptoms

The symptoms of stroke depend on what part of the brain is damaged. In some cases, a person may not even be aware that he or she has had a stroke.

How can a stroke occur?

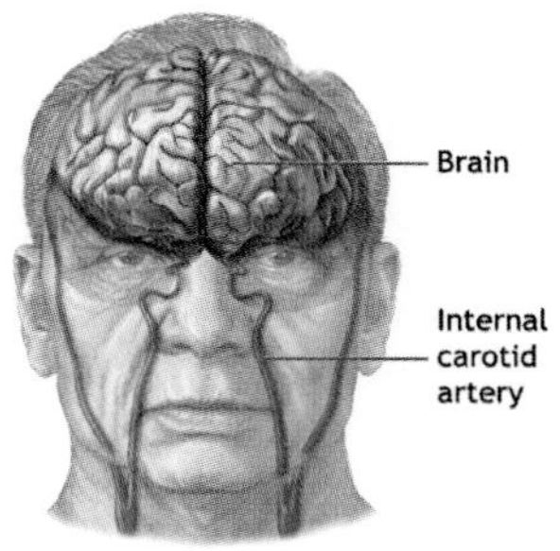

Much of the brain is supplied blood by the internal carotid arteries.

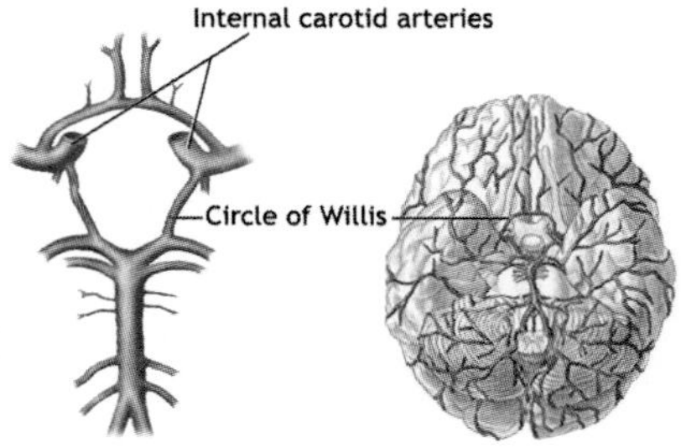

The internal carotid arteries branch at the base of the brain in an area called the circle of Willis.

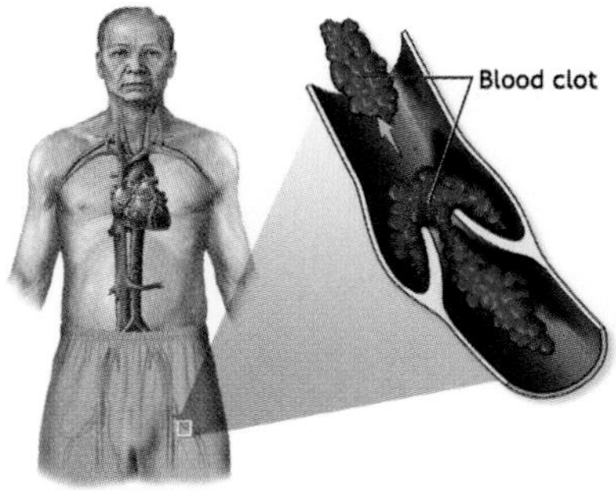

A blood clot (thrombus) may form in the body, break-off, and travel to the brain through a carotid artery and the circle of Willis.

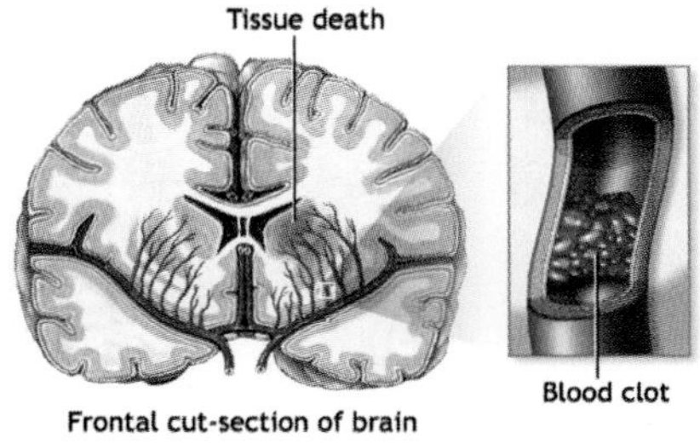

The blood clot may block the passage of blood through a brain artery, depriving nearby tissue of oxygen and nutrients. The result is a stroke.

Usually, a SUDDEN development of one or more of the following indicates a stroke:

- Weakness or paralysis of an arm, leg, side of the face, or any part of the body
- Numbness, tingling, decreased sensation
- Vision changes
- Slurred speech, inability to speak or understand speech, difficulty reading or writing
- Swallowing difficulties or drooling
- Loss of memory
- Spinning sensation
- Loss of balance or coordination
- Personality changes
- Mood changes (depression, apathy)
- Drowsiness, lethargy, or loss of consciousness
- Uncontrollable eye movements or eyelid drooping

If one or more of these symptoms is present for less than 24 hours, it may be a transient ischemic attack (TIA). A TIA is a temporary loss of brain function and a warning sign for a possible future stroke.

Tests may be performed to rule out other disorders causing stroke-like symptoms, such as poor blood flow through the carotid arteries.

Home care

A stroke is a medical emergency. Doctors have begun to call it a "brain attack" to stress that getting treatment immediately can save lives and reduce disability. Treatment varies, depending on the severity and cause of the stroke. For virtually all strokes, hospitalization is required, possibly including intensive care and life support.

The goal is to get the person to the emergency room immediately, determine if he or she is having a bleeding stroke or a stroke from a blood clot, and start therapy – *all within 3 hours of when the stroke began.*

LONG-TERM TREATMENT

The goal of long-term treatment is to recover as much function as possible and prevent future strokes. Depending on the symptoms, rehabilitation includes speech therapy, occupational therapy, and physical therapy. The recovery time differs from person to person.

Certain therapies, such as repositioning and range-of-motion exercises, are intended to prevent complications related to stroke, like infections and bed sores. People should stay active within their physical limitations. Sometimes, urinary catheterization or bladder/bowel control programs may be necessary to control incontinence.

Testing blood flow through the carotid arteries

Carotid duplex

This test assesses how well blood is flowing through the carotid arteries. Sound waves are directed from a hand-held transducer probe, which "echo" off the arterial structures to produce an image on a monitor.

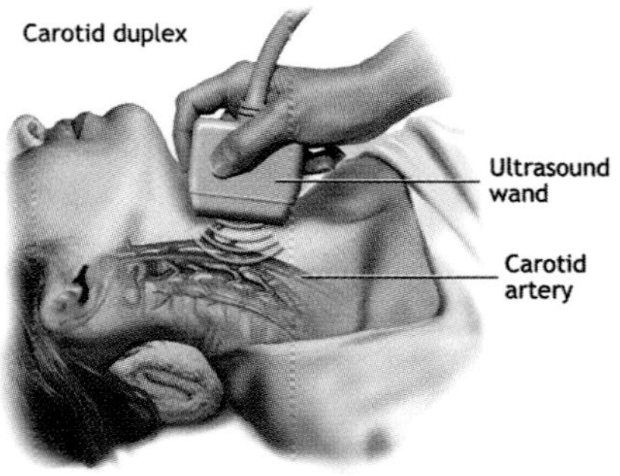

Angiogram

Contrast dye is injected into the arteries and an x-ray is taken of the carotid artery. In this example, the arrow is pointing to a location of severe narrowing (stenosis) of the right carotid artery.

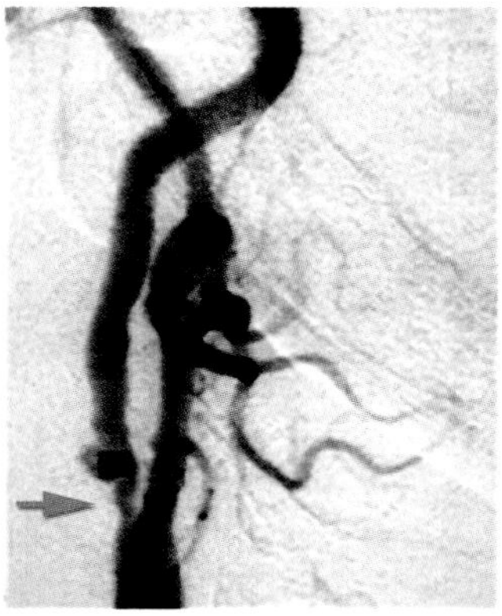

The person's safety must be considered. Some people with stroke appear to have no awareness of their surroundings on the affected side. Others show indifference or lack of judgment, which increases the need for safety precautions. For these people, friends and family members should repeatedly reinforce important information, like name, age, date, time, and where they live, to help the person stay oriented.

Caregivers may need to show the person pictures, repeatedly demonstrate how to perform tasks, or use other communication strategies, depending on the type and extent of the language problems.

In-home care, boarding homes, adult day care, or convalescent homes may be required to provide a safe environment, control aggressive or agitated behavior, and meet medical needs.

Family counseling may help in coping with the changes required for home care. Visiting nurses or aides, volunteer services, homemakers, adult protective services, and other community resources may be helpful.

Legal advice may be appropriate. Advance directives, power of attorney, and other legal actions may make it easier to make ethical decisions regarding the care of a person who has had a stroke.

When to Contact a Medical Professional

Call 911 if someone has symptoms of a stroke. Stroke requires immediate treatment!

Prevention

To help prevent a stroke:

- Get screened for high blood pressure at least every two years, especially if you have a family history of high blood pressure.
- Have your cholesterol checked.
- Treat high blood pressure, diabetes, high cholesterol, and heart disease if present.
- Follow a low-fat diet.
- Quit smoking.
- Exercise regularly.
- Lose weight if you are overweight.
- Avoid excessive alcohol use (no more than 1 to 2 drinks per day).

If you have had a TIA or stroke in the past, or you currently have a heart arrhythmia (like atrial fibrillation), mechanical heart valve, congestive heart failure, or risk factors for stroke, your doctor may have you take aspirin or other blood thinners. Make sure you follow your doctor's instructions and take the medication.

To prevent bleeding strokes, take steps to avoid falls and injuries.

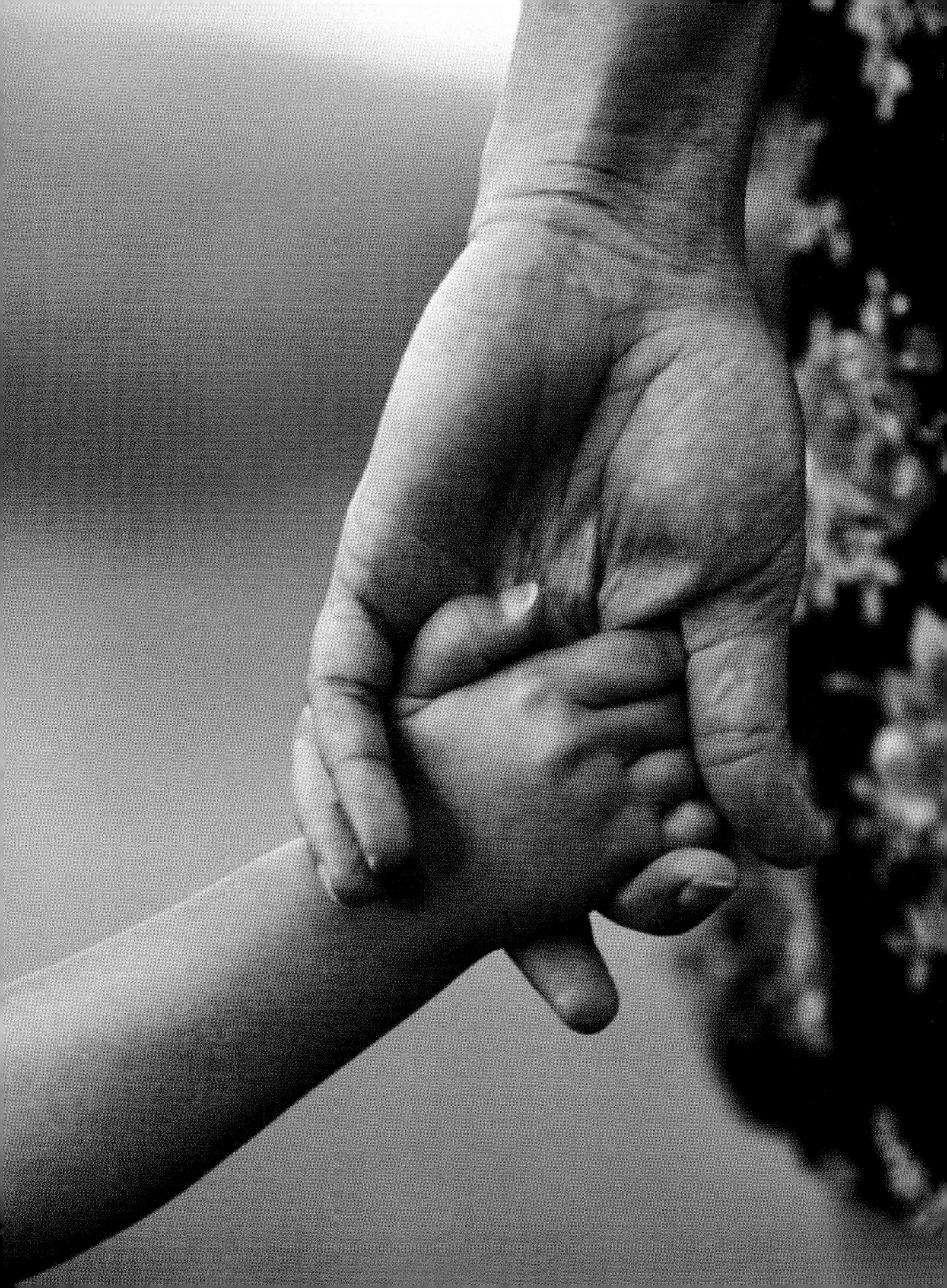

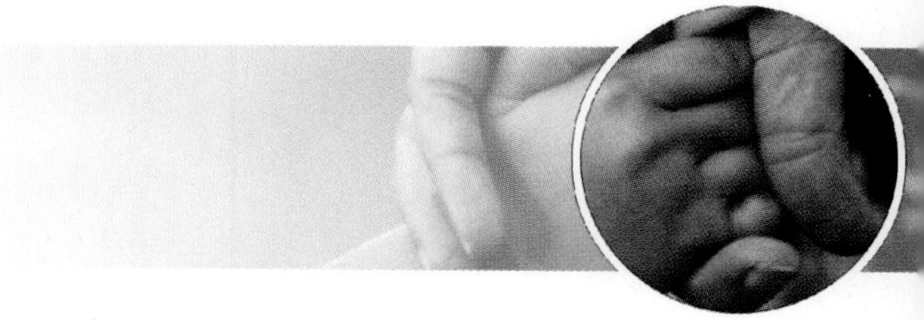

SAFETY

FAMILY SAFETY CHECKLIST

Accidents are the most common cause of death in children 14 years old and younger. In fact, accidents cause more childhood deaths than diseases, drugs, or violence. Fortunately, many accidents – for both children and adults – can be avoided if simple safety measures are taken.

FIRE SAFETY

- Install smoke detectors in hallways, sleeping areas, the kitchen, and garage. Test them once a month and change the batteries regularly.
- Do not smoke in bed.
- Keep matches and other flammable materials out of reach of children.
- Never leave a burning candle or fireplace fire unattended.
- Establish fire escape routes from every room in your house and teach family members what to do in case of a fire. Have semi-annual home fire drills to practice escaping.
- Keep fire extinguishers in handy locations. Have at least one extinguisher on each level of your home.
- Know how to use a fire extinguisher. In an emergency, you must be able to act fast.
- Teach children about fires. Explain how they are accidentally started and how to prevent them.
- Make sure household wiring is up-to-date.
- Store flammable materials away from heat sources, water heaters, and open-flame space heaters.
- Supervise children when they are using fireworks. Never assume that a child will read and follow safety instructions.

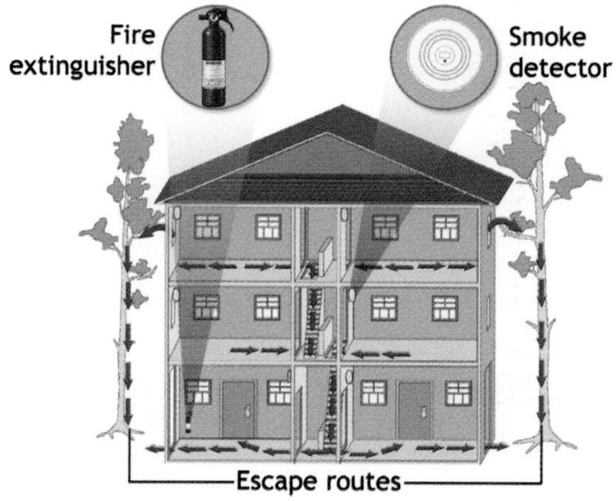

Every home needs a fire safety plan. Make sure fire extinguishers and smoke detectors are placed in key areas and that all family members know the fire escape routes from various locations in the home.

BICYCLE SAFETY

- Wear a bike helmet.
- Make sure bikes are the right size. A child should be able to straddle a bike with both feet on the ground.
- Young children should use bikes with coaster brakes – the kind that brake when you pedal backwards. With hand brakes, a child's hands should be large enough and strong enough to use the levers.
- Avoid riding at night if at all possible. Make sure your bike has reflectors.
- Stop at stop signs, check for traffic before turning, and never ride out into a street without stopping first.
- Ride on the same side of the road as the cars.

- Be predictable and ride defensively. Ride where drivers of cars can see you. Bicycles are frequently hit by cars because the driver did not even know the bike was there. Many accidents have been avoided because the biker was watching out for cars.
- Wear brightly colored clothing so that motorists can easily see you.

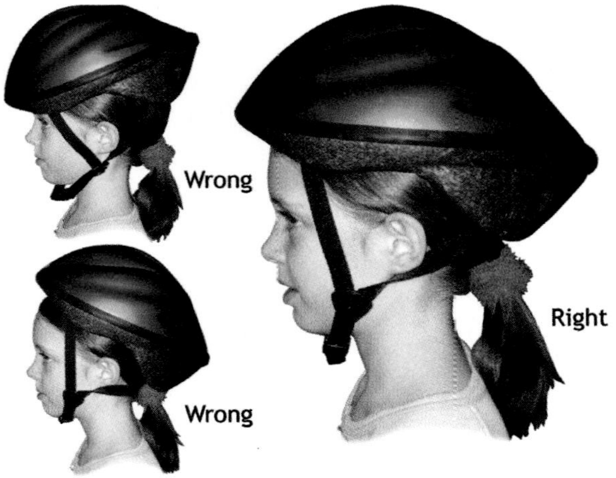

Teach children the proper way to wear a bicycle helmet. Refer to the manufacturer's instructions.

Child safety

- The space between crib bars should be no more than 2.5 inches.
- The distance from the mattress to the top of the rail should be over 2 feet.
- DO NOT put extra blankets and stuffed animals in a crib with a baby.
- DO NOT place a baby on the stomach to sleep.
- Always keep one hand on an infant who is lying on a changing table.
- Place gates at the top and bottom of each stairway.
- Cover unused electrical sockets.
- Keep cleaning fluids, bug poisons, and other chemicals well out of a child's reach. Avoid storing toxic substances in unmarked or inappropriate containers (such as food containers).
- Put safety latches on cabinets that a child should not open.
- Keep knives and matches out of reach.
- Keep plastic bags away from children.
- Buy medicines with child-resistant caps. Place all medications out of the reach of children.
- Keep children away from hot drinks and stove tops.
- When cooking on the stove, make sure that pot and pan handles are turned to the middle of the stove. Handles that hang over the edge of the stove may be reached by a curious toddler.
- Keep toys with small parts out of the reach of infants and toddlers. This includes stuffed animals with buttons.
- Avoid putting dangerous items in a waste basket where a young child might find them.
- Keep toilet lids down.
- Never leave infants and children unattended in a bathtub.
- Check water temperature in a bath before placing a child in it.
- Set the hot water heater thermostat to no more than 130°F.
- When heating a baby bottle, always test the milk temperature to prevent burning your baby's mouth.
- Inspect playground equipment for signs of deterioration, weakness, and damage.
- Teach children what to do if strangers approach them. Teach them at an early age that no one should touch private areas of the body.
- Make sure children know their address as early as possible. Teach them to call 911 when in trouble.
- Teach children to watch for cars on streets. They must stop, look both ways and listen for approaching traffic. Children must also be very aware of cars on driveways and in

parking lots. Cars backing up cannot see small children.

- Supervise young children at all times.

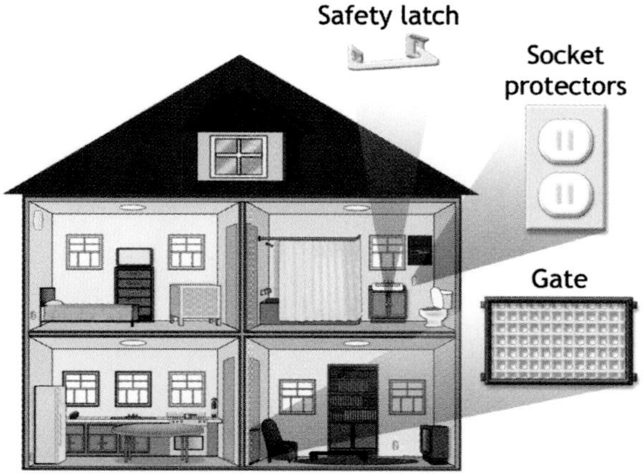

Child safety in the home includes installing safety latches on cabinets, socket protectors over electrical outlets, and gates at the entrance of stairs.

Water safety

- Learn CPR.
- Teach your children to swim.
- Never leave young children unattended, even for a minute, in a bathtub, swimming pool, lake, ocean, or stream.
- Fence all home pools and keep the gate closed and locked.
- Always wear life preservers when boating, even if you can swim.
- Avoid drinking alcohol when swimming or boating.
- Never swim alone.
- Never dive into water unless you know beforehand how deep it is.
- Know your limits. Do not over-exert yourself.
- Avoid standing on wet surfaces or being in water during a lightening storm.
- Stay out of strong currents.
- Do not overload your boat. If your boat turns over, stay with the boat until help arrives.

Infant and Child Car Seats

As many of us know, accidents are one of the major causes of injury and death in children. To keep children safer while driving, it is important to use child car seats properly. Car seats are required by law for children under 40 pounds. Unfortunately, studies show that **most people do NOT have their car seats installed properly**. The confusion is understandable – there are different car seats for different heights, weights, and ages of children.

Follow the manufacturer's instructions carefully. In addition, police inspection services can help you identify installation problems.

Here are the most critical points:

- The safest position for an infant seat is rear facing in the car's back seat.

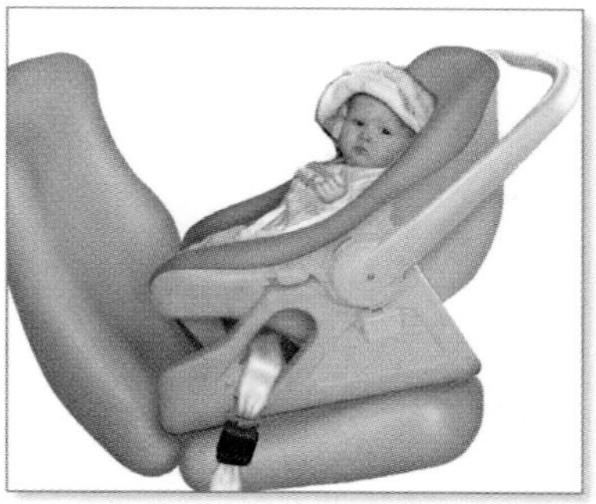

Place children under one year old and weighing under twenty pounds in the back seat of the car in a rear-facing seat

- In most models, the infant seat is used AT LEAST until the child reaches 20 pounds and 1 year of age. At that point, a forward-facing seat can be used. This may require a new car seat – it depends on the model.
- As children get older and bigger (usually 40 pounds and over), they should use a booster seat. With a booster seat, the child is restrained by the car's seat belt, but the booster raises the child high enough to make sure the car's seat belt is positioned properly over the shoulder.

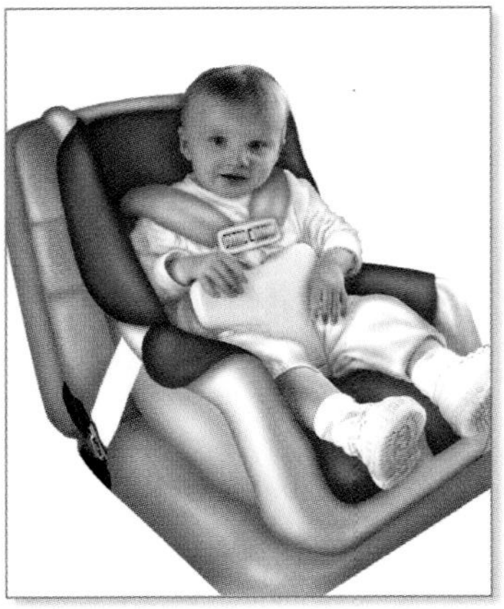

Place children over one year old and weighing between 20 to 40 pounds in the back seat of the car in a forward-facing seat

- The final stage is moving to a regular adult car seat once the child reaches about 80 pounds.

Some models are convertible seats that can be used at different stages. However, as your child grows up, you will need to buy at least two car seats, since no model covers the range from newborn all the way up to 80 lbs.

There are flat car seats for preterm babies to help them get enough oxygen. The American Academy of Pediatrics recommends that all preterm babies be observed in a car seat for fit and breathing stability before discharge from the hospital.

Additional guidelines

- Many people install a car seat far too loosely, even though they think the seat is tight. While the seat does not have to be completely immobile, re-read the instructions to see how much "give" is safe.
- Many seats are also installed at an improper angle. If the instructions are unclear, call the seat manufacturer.
- 5-point harnesses are generally considered safer than 3-point harnesses. With 5-point harnesses, make sure the upper retainer clip is armpit level – not too close to the child's neck.
- Read your car owner's manual to determine the safest place to install a car seat in YOUR car. Beware of airbag locations. Avoid placing child car seats in the front passenger location of a car, especially if it has an airbag.
- Follow the exact instructions for the installation and use of your specific car seat. Recommendations change somewhat depending on the model and type of seat.
- Some states have passed laws requiring that children up to 8 years old or 80 pounds be put in booster seats.
- It is best to use a new car seat. Avoid used car seats – these may lack instructions, be out-of-date, or have cracks or other problems.
- For more information call your car seat manufacturer, car manufacturer, or the State Highway Safety Office. A more extensive car safety seat guide can be found at www.app.org.
- Finally, remember to wear a seat belt when you are pregnant, before the baby is even born. Position the lap belt as low as possible under your abdomen and unborn child.

Tip

If your baby's head slumps at an awkward angle while in the car seat, she may not be getting enough oxygen. Be sure your car seat is the right one for your baby. And that it is installed correctly.

Teens and safe driving

Learning to drive is a major rite of passage for teens (and their parents). It's a time of exciting possibilities and achievements. It's also a time of grave risk.

Driving is fatal for almost 50,000 Americans every year. People between 15 and 24 years old (especially males) have the highest rate of auto-related deaths, even though people in this age group may be smart, skilled, and have great reflexes. A collision is the most likely tragedy to kill or cripple a teenager.

All new drivers should take a driver's education course. These courses have been proven to reduce accidents, but they are not enough. Teens often feel like serious accidents will not happen to them. Thankfully, smart teens can take steps to tilt the odds in their favor.

Teen driving deaths frequently occur...

- **After dark.** Automatic reflexes and driving skills are just developing during the first months of driving. Darkness is an extra variable to cope with.
- **When driving with friends.** Teens are safer driving by themselves or with family. They should drive as much as possible with an experienced driver, who can help develop good driving habits. As tempting as it may be, new drivers should wait until they have a consistent, safe driving record before taking friends as passengers. Friends, to the new driver, are a big distraction and a significant liability. (This liability may extend to the parent.)
- **With recreational driving.** For the first 3 to 6 months after obtaining a license, new drivers should try to gain their experience driving for school and work, not for fun.
- **When not buckled-up**. Use safety gear like a pro.
- **When drowsy**. Anyone who is sleepy should stop driving until fully alert. Sleepiness may cause even more accidents than alcohol!
- **After drinking alcohol.** Drinking slows reflexes and impairs judgment. These effects happen to anyone who drinks. So, NEVER drink and drive: ALWAYS find someone to drive who has not been drinking – even if this means an uncomfortable phone call!

Reducing accidents

Parents should discuss "household driving rules" with their teens and help their new drivers stick to them. For example, parents may want to encourage their teens to call without consequence rather than to get in a car with a driver who has been drinking. However, should the parents discover that their teenager has been driving and drinking, the parent might ask the state to suspend the license until the teenager is 18. (In many states the parent must sign for a teenager under 18 to obtain a driver's license. At any time before the 18th birthday a parent can refuse responsibility and the state will take the license.)

Remember...

Teaching good driving habits is one of the most important things you can do to save your teen's life.

A message to teens

These suggestions are not intended to be a punishment, but to prevent accidents, lifelong disability, and death. You are worth far more than the inconvenience and hassle.

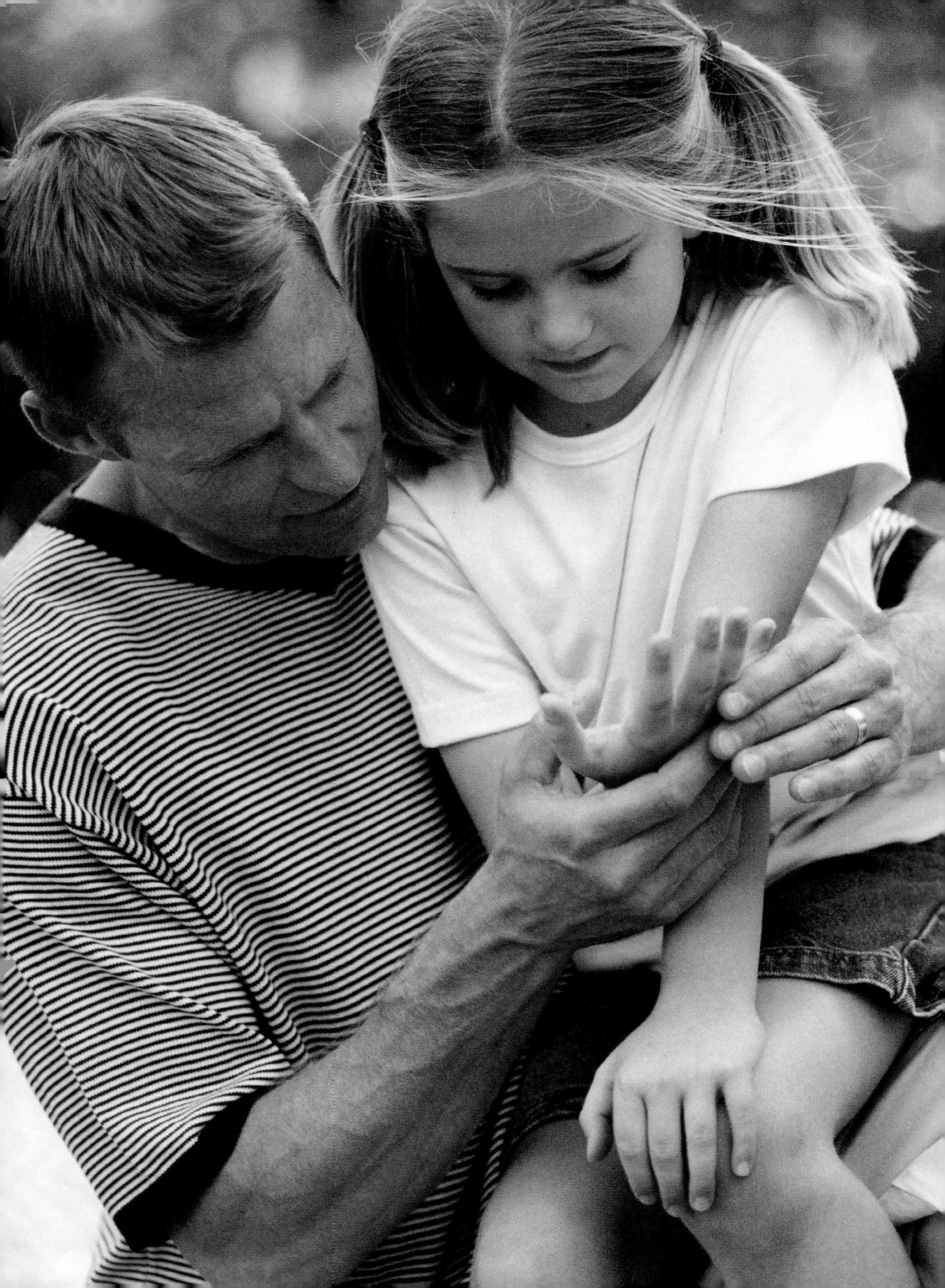

STOCKING YOUR MEDICAL SUPPLY CABINET

FIRST AID KIT

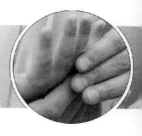

You should make sure that you and your family are prepared to treat common symptoms, injuries, and emergencies. By planning ahead, you can create a well-stocked home first aid kit. Keep all of your supplies in one location so you know exactly where they are when you need them.

The following items are basic supplies. You can get most of them at a pharmacy or supermarket.

Bandages and dressings:

- Adhesive bandages (Band-Aid or similar brand); assorted sizes
- Sterile gauze pads and adhesive tape
- Elastic (ACE) bandage for wrapping wrist, ankle, knee, and elbow injuries
- Triangular bandage for wrapping injuries and making an arm sling
- Aluminum finger splints
- Eye shield, pads, and bandages

Home health equipment:

- Thermometer
- Syringe, medicine cup, or medicine spoon for giving specific doses of medicine
- Disposable, instant ice bags
- Tweezers, to remove ticks and small splinters
- Sterile cotton balls
- Sterile cotton-tipped swabs
- Blue "baby bulb" or "turkey baster" suction device
- Save-A-Tooth storage device in case a tooth is broken or knocked out; contains a travel case and salt solution
- First-aid manual

Medicine for cuts and injuries:

- Antiseptic solution, such as hydrogen peroxide or wipes
- Antibiotic ointment, such as bacitracin, polysporin, or mupirocin
- Sterile eyewash, such as contact lens saline solution
- Calamine lotion for stings or poison ivy
- Hydrocortisone cream, ointment, or lotion for itching

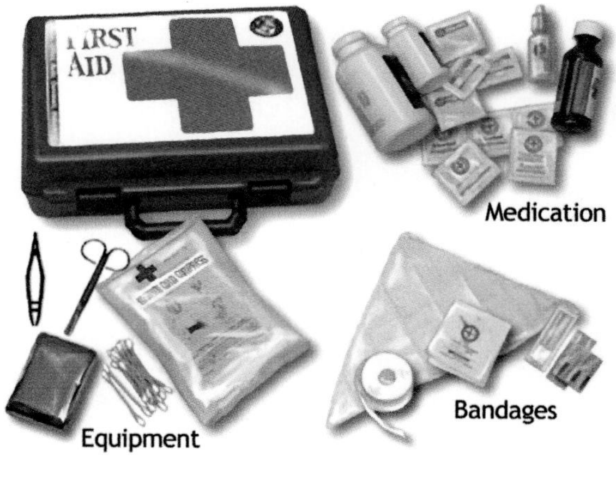

Be sure to check your kit regularly, and replace any supplies that are getting low or which have expired.

Home pharmacy

For common minor symptoms and illnesses, over-the-counter medicines are available. Always follow the manufacturer's directions and warnings when using these products. If you have any questions, consult with your doctor before starting a new over-the-counter drug. All medications lose their effectiveness (expire) over time and eventually should be replaced. Check the expiration date before using any product.

DO NOT give aspirin to children under 12. Consult your health care provider before giving aspirin, ibuprofen, or similar medicines to children. Pepto-Bismol contains aspirin-like salicylates, so talk with your doctor before using it in children.

Women should consult their doctor before taking over-the-counter medicines while pregnant or breastfeeding.

The chart on the next page includes some examples of over-the-counter medicines for common symptoms. This list is not comprehensive, nor does it imply an endorsement of some brands over others. Many of these have less expensive "store brand" equivalents. Always look at the ingredients. There are many "multi-symptom" combination versions – you should select products with the fewest ingredients needed to address your actual symptoms.

Storing medicines safely

Many people store their medications in the bathroom. But this popular spot is actually one of the worst places to keep medicine. Bathroom cabinets tend to be warm and humid, an environment that accelerates a drug's decomposition. Instead, keep medicines in a cool, dry place away from the bathroom and out of a child's reach.

If medicines are to be stored in a kitchen, store them away from the stove, sink, and any heat-releasing appliances.

In rare cases, an improperly stored medication can actually become toxic. To prevent danger, follow these tips:

- Store drugs out of harm's way. Always keep them out of the reach of children.
- Don't leave the cotton plug in a medication vial. Doing so can draw moisture into the container.
- Check the expiration date each time you take a drug. Discard and replace any medications that are out of date.
- Never use a medication that has changed color, consistency, or odor, regardless of the expiration date. Throw away capsules or tablets that stick together, are harder or softer than normal, or cracked or chipped.
- Ask your pharmacist about any specific storage instructions.

Travel tips

Travelers need to follow additional tips for safe storage of their medications:

- Before leaving home, list all your medications, as well as the name and number of your pharmacist and doctor.
- To prevent your medicine from making a detour while on vacation, keep your medicine in a carry-on bag rather than a checked suitcase.
- Bring an extra supply with you in case your return is delayed.
- Never leave medicines in an automobile, where heat can rapidly destroy the drug.
- Watch time changes. Set a separate watch to your usual time so you can remember when to take any medication.

Symptom	Over-the-counter medicines
Aches and pain **Fever** **Headache**	■ Acetaminophen (Tylenol) ■ Acetaminophen/Aspirin/Caffeine (Excedrin) ■ Aspirin (Bayer, Bufferin, Echotrin) ■ Ibuprofen (Advil, Motrin), naproxen (Aleve)
Stuffy nose **Congestion**	■ Oral decongestants: pseudoephedrine (Contact non-drowsy, Simply Stuffy, Sudafed) ■ Decongestant nasal sprays: oxymetazoline (Afrin, Neo-Synephrine, Sinex) and phenylephrine (Neo-Synephrine, Sinex) NOTE: Decongestant nasal sprays may work more quickly but have a rebound effect if you use them more than 3-5 days. They are best for short-lived colds and not for persistent allergies.
Cough with sputum, phlegm	■ Expectorant: guaifenesin (Robitussin)
Dry cough	■ Menthol throat lozenges: Halls, Robitussin, Vicks ■ Liquid cough suppressant: dextromethorphan (Benylin, Delsym, Robitussin DM, Simply Cough, Vicks 44).
Sore throat	■ Sore throat lozenges: Chloraseptic, Luden's, Sucrets ■ Anesthetic spray: dyclonine (Cepacol), phenol (Chloraseptic) ■ General pain-killers: acetaminophen (Tylenol), ibuprofen (Advil, Motrin)
Allergies	■ Non-sedating antihistamines: loratadine (Alavert, Claritin, Dimetapp ND) ■ Sedating antihistamines: brompheniramine (Dimetapp), diphenhydramine (Benadryl), chlorpheniramine (Chlor-Trimeton) or clemastine (Tavist) ■ Preventative nasal spray: Cromolyn sodium (NasalCrom)
Skin rashes **Itching**	■ Hydrocortisone cream (Cortaid, Cortizone 10), Domeboro
Cuts and scrapes	■ Antibiotic creams: bacitracin, Neosporin, Polysporin ■ Antiseptics: Bactine, Betadine, hydrogen peroxide solution, Lanacane First Aid Spray
Diarrhea	■ Anti-diarrheal: loperamide (Imodium), bismuth (Kaopectate, Pepto-Bismol) ■ Rehydration fluids: Enfalyte, Pedialyte
Nausea **Vomiting**	■ Emetrol, Pepto-Bismol ■ Rehydration fluids: Enfalyte, Pedialyte ■ Motion sickness: dimenhydrinate (Dramamine)

Herbs and supplements

More Americans than ever are taking herbs and supplements to enhance their standard health care. In many countries throughout the world, herbs are considered part of mainstream medicine. German doctors, for example, can prescribe herbs that have been established as safe and appropriate by a body called the Commission E. In the United States, however, herbs and dietary supplements are not controlled or regulated. Therefore, if you are seeking an alternative to prescription medicine or using these substances in addition to medicine, you need to understand certain safety issues.

Unlike prescription and non-prescription drugs, herbs and supplements are not regulated by the FDA (Food and Drug Administration). The availability of these products in stores does NOT mean that they are safe, and labeling of ingredients does NOT guarantee exactly what (or how much) is in each pill.

The United States Pharmacopeia (USP) has set up a voluntary, self-regulating system for companies that make and sell herbs and supplements. To date, very few companies have participated in this process. But, for your own protection, you should look for the USP seal.

The study of herbs

Herbs have been used for thousands of years. Their recommendation by an herbal specialist (herbalist) is often based mainly on the wisdom and experience over time of many clinicians, rather than formal research studies.

Whole herbs are difficult to study because climate, soil quality, and exposure to insects can affect the ingredients within the plant. Thus, scientists try to isolate one or two active ingredients from herbs for greater control. But this approach has limitations – whole herbs may contain a variety of active ingredients that work together, not just one or two. And whole herbs may cause fewer side effects.

Despite these and other limitations, researchers are beginning to successfully evaluate herbs. But remember that for most herbs on the market, a scientific understanding of the effectiveness and risks is not yet known.

Side effects and interactions

Contrary to the popular belief that *natural* means *safe*, herbs and supplements do have side effects. They can also interact with medications or deplete important vitamins and minerals in your body. This makes sense – if they were completely inert, how would they have any beneficial effect? Here are two highly publicized and concerning interactions:

- St. John's wort (for mild to moderate depression) causes sensitivity to the sun's ultraviolet rays, and may cause an allergic reaction, stomach upset, fatigue, and restlessness. Studies show that St. John's wort also interferes with the effectiveness of many drugs. These include warfarin (a blood thinner), protease inhibitors for HIV, possibly birth control pills, and many others. St. John's wort must not be taken with anti-depressant medication. The Food and Drug Administration (FDA) has issued a public health advisory concerning many of these interactions.

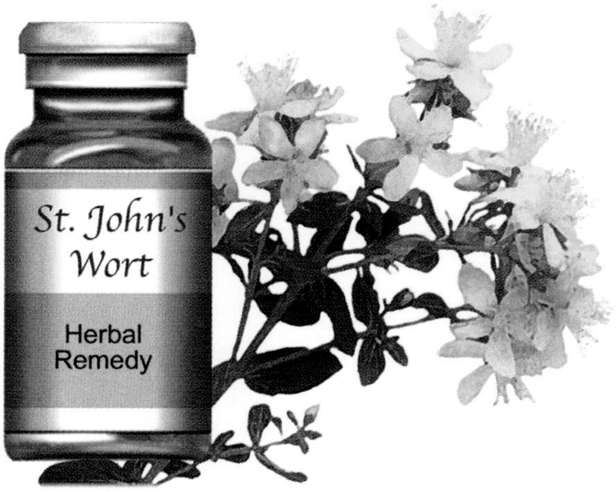

- Garlic, ginkgo, ginger, and ginseng affect bleeding time. Use of these herbs with the blood thinner warfarin, therefore, should be avoided.

If you are going to have surgery, it is very important to tell your doctor and anesthesiologist about any herbs or supplements you are taking. They will advise you on which ones need to be stopped, and when. Some may need to be stopped as long as two weeks prior to surgery.

Tips for using herbs and supplements

Herbs and supplements can be a wonderful addition to your usual medical care. However, keep in mind a few basic principles:

- Try to work with a qualified, well-trained herbalist, rather than self-treating with store-bought products. Make sure that the practitioner is licensed. Find out if he or she carries malpractice insurance.
- Tell your doctor about *any* herbs or supplements that you are taking or thinking about taking.
- Take care selecting a product if you are choosing one in the store. Look for reputable companies that, preferably, participate in the USP self-regulating system.
- Know the safety issues regarding the specific herb or supplement you are considering. Talk to your doctor or herbalist. Find a reliable source of information that explains about interactions, potential depletions of vitamins and minerals, and side effects.
- Take extra precaution if you are considering herbs for infants, children, and even teens. Herbs that are fairly harmless in adults may cause dehydration in infants and young children, who are more susceptible to fluid loss. In addition, since the central nervous and immune systems are just developing in young children, they are more sensitive to side effects from many herbs. Teens are especially vulnerable to advertising that promises things like weight-loss, body-building, and other factors to enhance one's appearance.
- Like medications, herbs can cause allergic reactions. Take special care if you or your child has a history of allergies or asthma. For example, you may be more likely to have an allergy to Echinacea, a popular herb used for colds and flu.

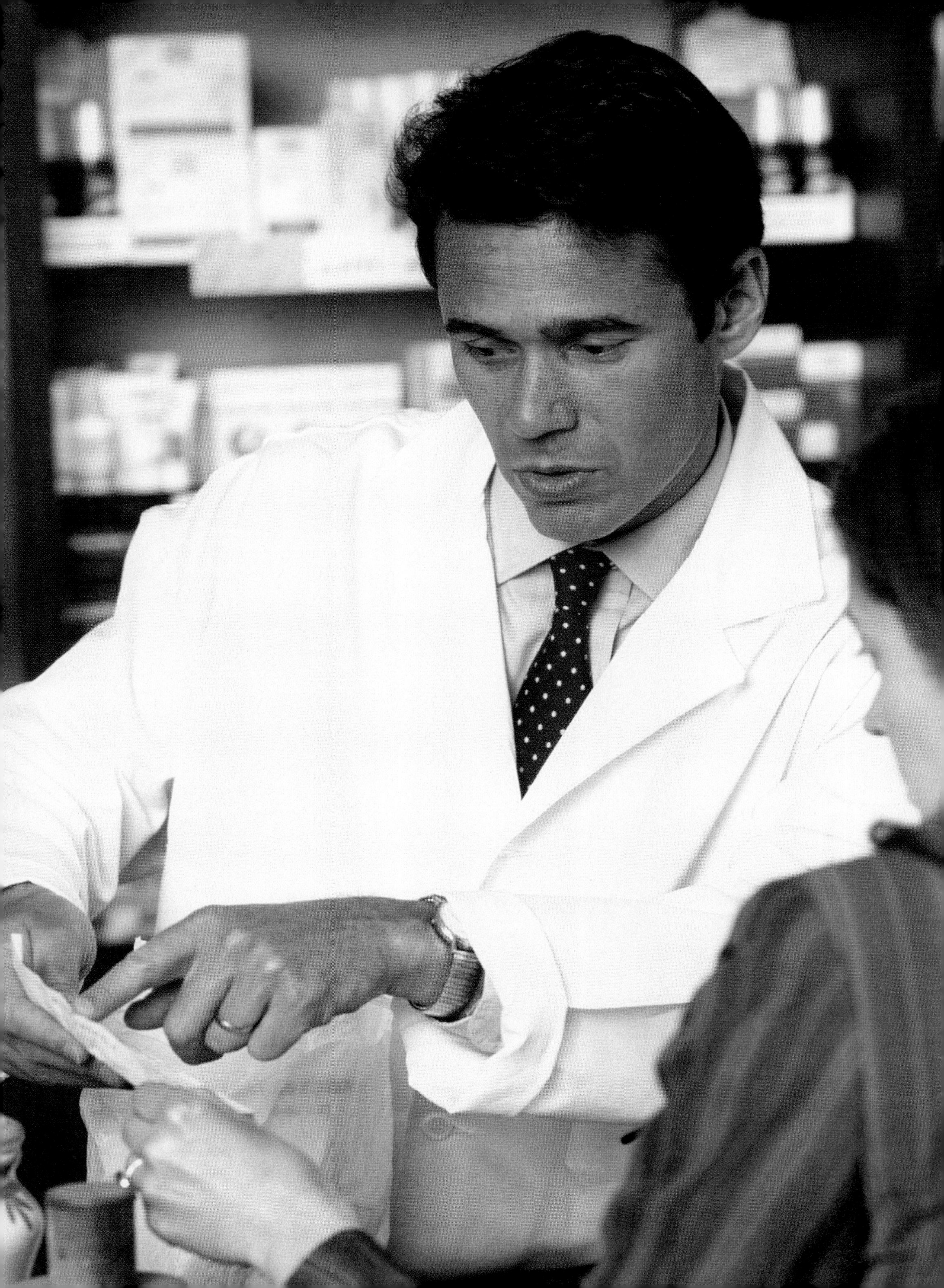

USING PRESCRIPTION DRUGS WISELY

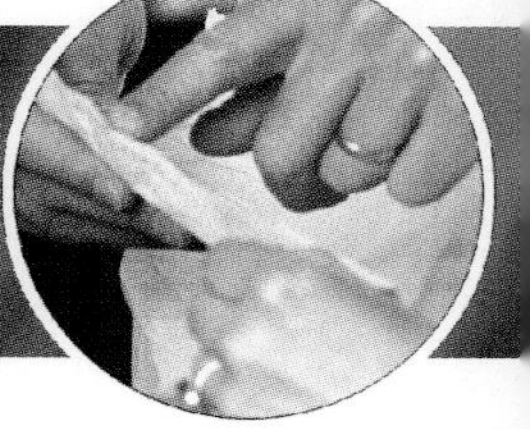

We live in an era where it's difficult to watch a television show or read a magazine without seeing advertisements trying to sell you the wonders of prescription drugs.

These advertisements work. They influence consumers, who ask their doctors about these drugs, or dangerously obtain them from other sources. But the best interests of advertisers aren't always the same as yours.

The same drugs that are advertised to consumers are also heavily advertised to doctors. Again these advertisements work. And because manufacturers fund research studies, these same drugs are often prominently featured in medical journals.

All other things being equal, choose an older medicine over a newer one. New medicines are important, and they are often the wisest choice for specific situations. However, important side effects may not be discovered until after a medicine has been on the market for awhile. Where two drugs have similar profiles, we usually have a longer safety track record on the older medicine – and it probably costs less, helping to keep healthcare more affordable for all of us.

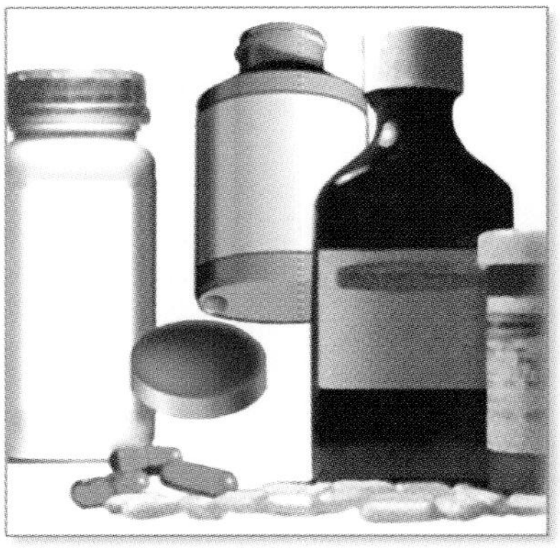

Choose established medicines over newer ones if profiles are similar

Instead of asking your doctor about the latest marketer's miracle, ask your doctor, "What are the gentlest, most effective ways to treat my condition?" Also ask, "Is there anything I can do besides medication that can make a real difference?"

Once you've decided on a medication, you might want to ask if a generic form is available (to keep costs down) and whether a smaller dose would be effective (to keep side effects down).

For whatever drug you take, find out what results and side effects to expect. Your doctor and pharmacist are both good resources. If the results or side effects are different than expected, be sure to report back to your doctor.

Remember to take the medication as directed. Taking partial prescriptions often leads to poor results. Ask your pharmacist about medication and refill reminder systems.

All of this becomes even more important if you are taking more than one medicine.

TAKING MULTIPLE DRUGS

Medicines can interact with each other in powerful and sometimes dangerous ways. All of your health care providers should be aware of all of the prescription and over-the-counter medicines you are taking.

Whenever someone prescribes you something new, make sure he or she has a list of everything you are taking, including over-the-counter products and any herbal or natural remedies.

Try to fill all of your prescriptions at the same pharmacy, so its computers can alert the pharmacist of possible drug interactions. If you purchase over-the-counter products at the same pharmacy, you can check with the pharmacist to see if they interact with any of your prescriptions they have on record.

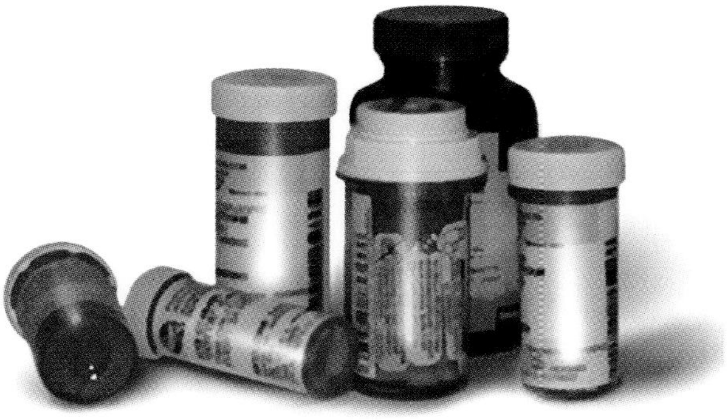

Write down all prescription, over-the-counter, and herbal medications you are taking. Bring a current list with you when you have an appointment with a health care provider.

Antibiotic overuse

Antibiotics can be wonderful, life-saving tools, but their overuse is dangerous. Over the past few decades, antibiotics have become overused for minor illnesses, because many people think there can be no harm in taking them "just to be on the safe side."

Now we know that overuse of antibiotics IS harmful. The practice selectively breeds more resistant bacteria. People become sick more often – with longer, more stubborn infections.

Many people do not realize that antibiotics have NO effect on viruses – the cause of colds and flu. Furthermore, antibiotics can cause side effects and allergic reactions.

Nevertheless, up to 60% of people with common colds are treated with antibiotics. For children, who average 3-8 colds each year, this translates into many rounds of unnecessary (and therefore harmful) antibiotics.

Why does this happen? One major reason is that people want or expect a prescription. They are looking for something, anything, to cure their cold (or a child's cold.) The doctor wants to help you and your child get through this faster. Prescribing an antibiotic seems like a fairly harmless thing to try.

Work together with your doctor to avoid antibiotics

When you see a doctor and explain the symptoms, add the sentence, "If there is any way to safely feel better without antibiotics, that is what I prefer." This tells your doctor up front that you aren't pushing for antibiotics. It takes the pressure off of him or her to write a prescription. It also shows the doctor that you want to be partners in your care or your child's care.

To be on the safe side, antibiotics should not be given unless they are clearly needed.

When NOT to use antibiotics!

The Centers for Disease Control and the Academy of Pediatrics are very concerned about the overuse of antibiotics. They have made addressing this problem a top priority. The following are some guidelines for when to use (and not to use) antibiotics for common infections. These guidelines should not be *rigidly* followed, but they do give a good idea of when to avoid antibiotics. Use them as excellent discussion points with your doctor.

Sore Throats

1. Antibiotics should NOT be given for a sore throat unless you have a positive throat swab for Strep or another bacterial infection.
2. Penicillin has been traditionally recommended. However, resistance to penicillin is increasing, and cephalosporins may be more effective in some situations.

Bronchitis and Cough

1. Regardless of how long it lasts, bronchitis or a nonspecific cough illness rarely warrants antibiotics.
2. If the cough has lasted for more than 10 days and specific bacteria are suspected, one round of antibiotics may be worthwhile.
3. If you have an underlying lung disease (except asthma), antibiotics might be beneficial if your disease flares up.

Colds

1. Antibiotics should not be given for the common cold.
2. Thick, discolored nasal discharge is normal for a cold and is not a reason for antibiotics unless it lasts longer than 10-14 days.

Sinus Infections

1. Most people should not be given antibiotics for a sinus infection unless there are both nasal discharge and cough without any improvement after more than 10-14 days. If there is some improvement by day 10, antibiotics are probably not helpful.
2. People with severe symptoms (facial swelling, facial pain, a fever over 102.2°F) may benefit from earlier treatment.
3. Use the most narrow-spectrum antibiotic practical (to kill the suspected bacteria and as few others as possible).

Ear Infections

1. Some ear infections require antibiotics to clear the infection and to prevent them from becoming worse. This is especially likely if the child is under age 2, has a fever, is acting sick (beyond just the ear), or is not improving over 24-48 hours. Most ear infections, however, would heal well without antibiotics. Talk with your doctor about whether your child can be safely treated in other ways. Many times, a pain reliever is enough. Antibiotics can cause unpleasant side effects and may even make it more difficult to treat future ear infections for your child.
2. You can also ask your doctor for a **SNAP**. This stands for "Safety Net Antibiotic Prescription." This simply means you are given a prescription, but don't fill it unless the pain is getting worse or your child still has symptoms in 48 hours. In the meantime, use a pain reliever.
3. Short courses of antibiotics (as little as **5 days**) are often sufficient for ear infections in healthy children beyond the second birthday.
4. The presence of fluid still in the ear at an ear recheck is to be expected. This does not require another round of antibiotics, except in the less common situation where signs of acute infection are still present.

Note to Parents

Children fight off most childhood illnesses better without antibiotics. The doctor's job is to gently treat children so they can get the rest and fluids they need. Occasionally, antibiotics are a vital part of the healing process.

You are in an excellent position to remove the "pressure to prescribe" and to work with your doctor to offer your child the very best care.

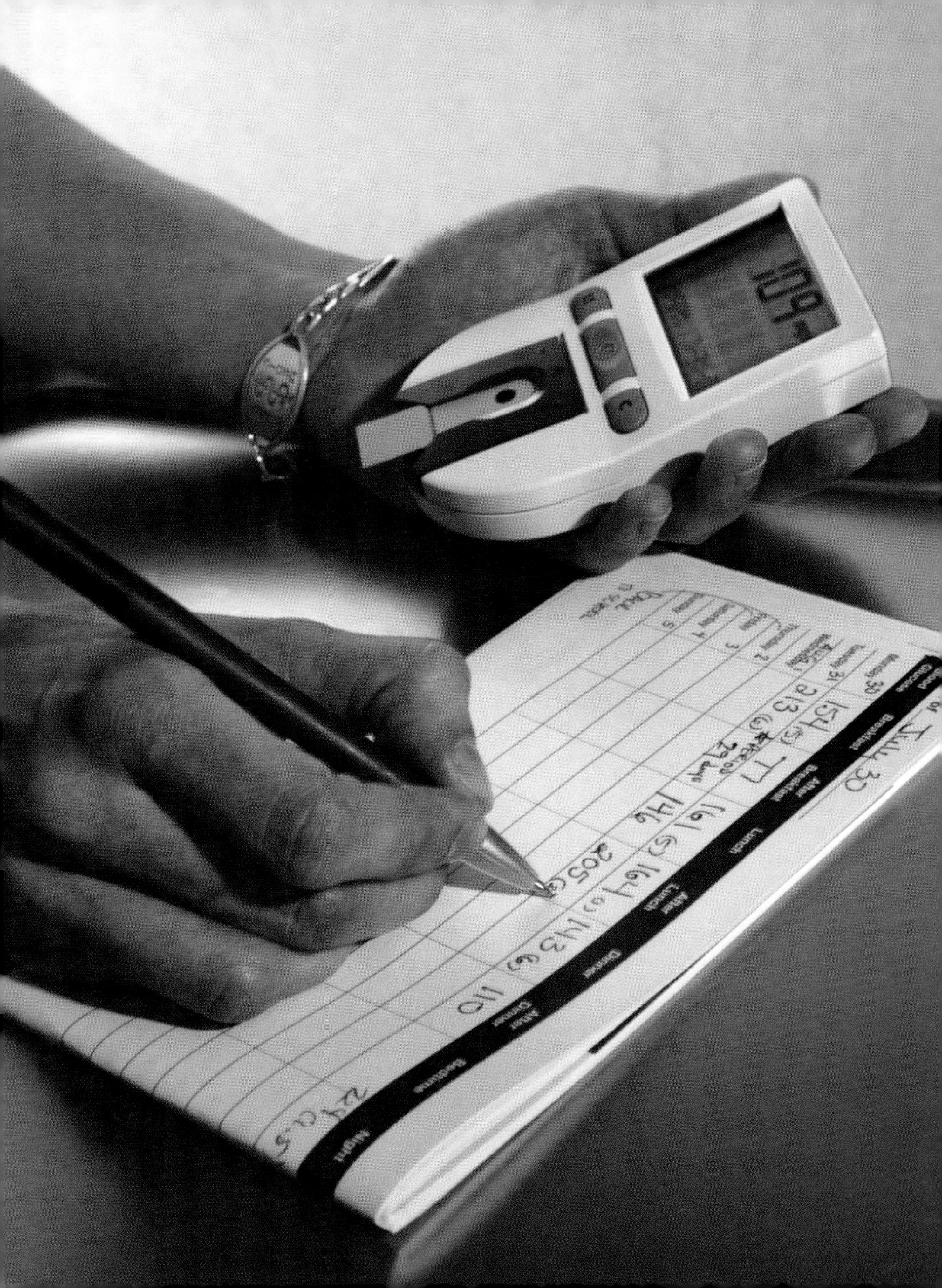
Glucose
Breakfast
After Breakfast
Lunch
After Lunch
Dinner
After Dinner
Bedtime
Night
Monday 30
Tuesday 31

TAKING CHARGE OF YOUR HEALTHCARE

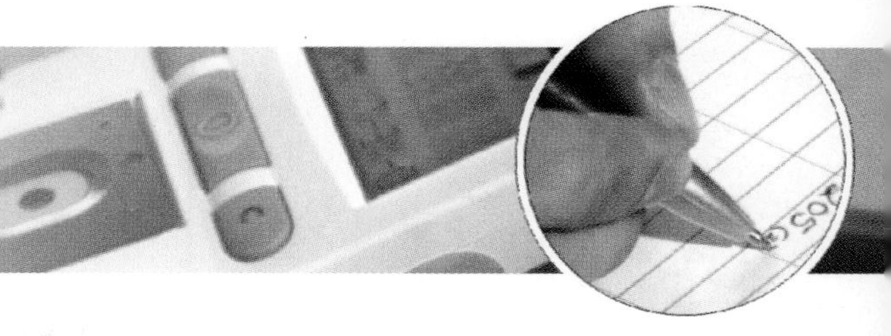

KEEP MEDICAL RECORDS

> **"During home renovation I cut myself on an old rusty nail. I couldn't remember when I'd had a tetanus shot. My doctor didn't have any record of it because I got the shot before I started seeing her."**
>
> **– Lisa, age 30**

Many of us see a lot of doctors in the course of our lives, and our medical information becomes scattered throughout multiple offices. By keeping your own paperwork and notes, you can give current and future health care providers detailed information about your medical history and that of your family.

For example, knowing when your cholesterol was last checked, as well as the results of this test, may save you from unnecessary blood work. Or it may let your doctor know that your numbers were better in the past than they are currently.

Since many conditions tend to run in families, ask parents, siblings, and other relatives what they know about their medical histories. This information may provide you and your doctor with valuable insight to possible health risks, allowing you to work together to come up with a plan for prevention.

MAKING AND ACQUIRING RECORDS

Before an office visit for a specific problem, fill out a copy of the symptom worksheet provided in this book. The worksheet can become part of your files, and you'll be glad that you took the time to keep track of the information.

During the visit, jot down notes. Record your weight, blood pressure, and anything your doctor tells you about preventing or treating a problem. It is easy to leave the office and forget important details and instructions.

Ask for the following pieces of information at the end of a doctor's appointment:

- Clinical notes
- Lab results
- Letters to and from specialists
- Results of important procedures
- Any other records your doctor keeps

After the visit, it is helpful to flesh out your notes, because you may have difficulty writing down everything you and your doctor discuss during the actual visit. Also, keep copies of prescriptions, written instructions, referrals, notes from telephone conversations, consent forms you have signed, insurance forms, patient education brochures, and anything else related to your health. Organize these papers in a logical way that makes sense to you.

Try not to be shy about requesting this information from your doctor or the office. Many doctors are glad (and impressed) that you want to actively participate in your care. Therefore, they are generally happy to give you copies of such documents. And, if not, remember that it is your right. Not to mention your health.

Family Medical History

Use this space to record significant health conditions of your near relatives. Try to have a complete picture of your family's history of chronic disease, heart conditions, stroke, eye problems, cancers, and other health problems. This information can help you and your doctor focus on key prevention steps for you to take.

Mother	
Father	
Sisters and Brothers	
Children	
Grandparents	
Aunts and Uncles	

Home Medical Record

Use this space to track key health indicators and diagnoses from each office visit.

Date	Blood Pressure	Cholesterol	Weight	Diagnosis/Vaccinations/Notes

Describe your symptoms

Before going to the doctor to discuss any symptoms you may have, think about the following questions so that you can give as detailed a picture as possible.

You might want to photocopy this worksheet, fill it out, and bring it with you to your office visit. Jot down things your provider tells you, like probable diagnosis and steps to take at home to get better. Then, you could save this sheet in your permanent home medical record, as it might be useful for future reference.

Date the symptom started	____/_____/______ or rough guess: ____________
Have you had it before?	☐ Yes ☐ No
How did it start?	☐ Suddenly ☐ Came on gradually
List things that make it better	
List things that make it worse	
Is it worse at a particular time of day?	
Does it get worse during certain activities?	
How have you tried to treat it at home? Which home care measures helped?	
List other symptoms you have	
Diagnosis	
Provider's recommendations	

NOTE: If you have ongoing or recurring symptoms, such as headaches or abdominal discomfort, you may want to keep a daily **symptom diary**. Create a chart that allows you to fill in where you were each day, what you were doing, what you had eaten, what you were thinking about or feeling, and what medications you had taken when the symptoms got better or worse. Such a diary can be one of the most effective tools for discovering important associations.

Personal Medications

If your doctor prescribes you medication, use the following chart to keep track of important information about it. You may want to photocopy this chart and fill it in for each medication that you or any family member is prescribed. This helps you keep a permanent record of all medicines that your family has ever taken. Ask your doctor or pharmacist if you don't know the answers to any of this information.

Name of drug	
Color and shape	
Date prescribed	
How much to take each time	
How many times a day (And at what times of day)	
Other instructions (For example: take with food)	
How long to take this drug (For example: two weeks)	
Reason for taking this drug (Symptoms or condition)	
Possible side effects	
Possible interactions (Interactions with other drugs, foods, herbs, or supplements)	
Other comments	

Let the prescribing doctor know

- Any other prescription medications, over-the-counter remedies, herbs, or supplements you are taking. This includes vitamins, antacids, eye drops, and non-prescription pain relievers like aspirin or ibuprofen.
- If you are pregnant or breastfeeding.
- If you have any allergies.
- If you have diabetes or heart, liver, or kidney disease.
- If you follow a special diet or drink alcohol regularly.
- If you experience any side effects.

Questions to ask your doctor

- Are there any non-medication alternatives?
- Are there less expensive medications that would work as well? For example, is the generic version just as good?
- When will I begin to see the beneficial effects from the medication?
- Should I call you about any specific problems from the medications?
- If I am going to be taking this long-term to manage a chronic condition, will you be able to consider a lower dose in the future?

Choosing a primary care provider

A primary care provider (PCP) is a general practitioner who sees people of all ages for common medical problems. This person is usually a doctor, but may be a physician's assistant or a nurse practitioner. Your PCP is often involved in your care for a long time, so it is important to select someone with whom you will work well.

A PCP is your main health care provider in non-emergency situations. Your PCP's role is to:

- Provide preventive care and teach healthy lifestyle choices.
- Identify and treat common medical conditions.
- Make referrals to medical specialists when necessary.

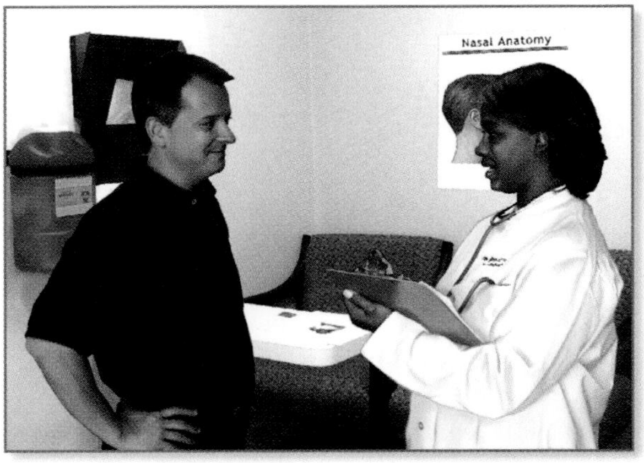

Primary care is usually provided in an outpatient setting. However, if you are admitted to the hospital, your PCP may assist in or direct your care, depending on the circumstances.

Having a primary care provider can give you a trusting, ongoing relationship with one medical professional over time. You can choose from several different types of PCPs:

- **General practitioners** – doctors who have completed an internship but not a residency.
- **Family practitioners** – doctors who have completed a family practice residency and are board certified, or board eligible, for this specialty. The scope of their practice includes children and adults of all ages and may include obstetrics and minor surgery.
- **Pediatricians** – doctors who have completed a pediatric residency and are board certified, or board eligible, in this specialty. The scope of their practice includes the care of newborns, infants, children, and adolescents.

- **Internists** – doctors who have completed a residency in internal medicine and are board certified, or board eligible, in this specialty. The scope of their practice includes the care of adults of all ages for many different medical problems.
- **Obstetricians/gynecologists** – doctors who have completed a residency and are board certified, or board eligible, in this specialty. They often serve as a PCP for women, particularly those of childbearing age.
- **Nurse practitioners and physician's assistants** – practitioners who go through a different training and certification process than doctors. They are often referred to as "physician extenders." They may be your key contact in some practices. All PAs or NPs consult with doctors.

When choosing a PCP, also consider the following:

- Is the office staff friendly and helpful? Is the office good about returning calls?
- How easy is it to reach the provider? Does the provider use email?
- Do you prefer a provider whose communication style is friendly and warm, or more formal?
- Do you prefer a provider focused on disease treatment, or wellness and prevention?
- Does the provider have a conservative or aggressive approach to treatment?
- Does the provider order a lot of tests?
- Does he or she refer to other specialists frequently or infrequently?
- What do colleagues and patients think about the provider?
- Does the provider invite you to be involved in your care? Does he or she view your patient-doctor relationship as a true partnership?

You can get referrals from:

- Friends, neighbors, or relatives
- State-level medical associations, nursing associations, and associations for physician assistants
- Your dentist, pharmacist, optometrist, previous provider, or other health professional
- Advocacy groups – especially to help you find the best provider for a specific chronic condition or disability

Another option is to request an appointment to "interview" a potential provider. There may be no cost to do this, or you may be charged a co-payment or other small fee. Some practices, particularly pediatric practice groups, may have an open house where you have an opportunity to meet several of the providers in that particular group.

ACKNOWLEDGEMENTS

About A.D.A.M.

A.D.A.M. is a leading provider of consumer health information. Our content is used by hospitals, health care organizations, government agencies, web sites, and academic institutions. Our knowledge base includes thousands of diseases, symptoms, tests, surgeries, and other medical topics.

A.D.A.M. is dedicated to helping people better understand their health and the way their bodies work. Drawing from one of the largest medical image and animation libraries in the world, our goal is to create visually rich explanations that help illuminate medical concepts. We believe that if we can connect you and your loved ones to accurate and engaging health information, we can help improve the overall quality of your health and healthcare delivery. Our mission is to deliver the most trusted, accurate, and engaging information possible.

Medical review

A.D.A.M.'s health information is physician-written, physician-reviewed, and physician-updated under the guidance of skilled consumer medical editors. All of the articles in this book have been reviewed by at least two physicians. The key reviewers and editors are listed below.

Alan Greene, M.D., F.A.A.P., Chief Medical Officer, A.D.A.M. Inc.
Dr. Greene is one of the nation's leading pediatricians. He is an attending physician at Stanford University's Packard Children's Hospital and Assistant Clinical Professor at Stanford University School of Medicine. Dr. Greene earned his Bachelor's degree from Princeton University, graduated from medical school at UC San Francisco, and passed the pediatric boards in the top 5% of the nation. He is the President of Hi-Ethics, Inc. (Health Internet Ethics), the non-profit organization formed to address privacy, advertising, and content quality issues for Internet health consumers. Dr. Greene has been recognized by Advance for Health Information Executives as one of the top 25 most influential forces in health care IT. He is a respected author and appears frequently on television and radio shows as a medical expert. He has appeared in numerous publications, including the *Wall Street Journal, Parenting, Child, Baby Talk, Woman's World, Better Home's & Gardens,* and *Reader's Digest*. Dr. Greene is also the Founder of DrGreene.com, cited by the AMA as the first physician Web site on the Internet.

Jacqueline A. Hart, M.D., Senior Medical Editor, A.D.A.M., Inc.
Dr. Hart is board certified in internal medicine. She holds an MD from the George Washington and an AB in psychology from Harvard-Radcliffe University. Dr. Hart completed her residency at Brown University in primary care internal medicine. As A.D.A.M.'s Senior Medical Editor, she performs extensive writing and editorial review in areas related to internal medicine and adult primary health care. Dr. Hart also serves as co-medical director of the Cardiovascular Lifestyle Modification (C.A.L.M.) program at Newton-Wellesley Hospital, Boston, MA. She writes extensively on preventive and integrative medicine, including a chapter for *Clinical Trials in Cardiovascular Disease: A Companion to Braunwald's Heart Disease.*

Greg Juhn, M.T.P.W., Editorial Director, A.D.A.M., Inc.
Greg Juhn has a bachelor's degree in molecular biology and a master's degree in professional writing. He has ten years of experience in medical education, public health program development, adult learning theory, and instructional design. He authored *Understanding the Pill, A Consumer's Guide to Oral Contraceptives* and co-authored numerous articles in peer-reviewed publications. As A.D.A.M.'s Editorial Director, he oversees all writing and editing, defines editorial objectives and processes, and ensures the editorial quality of the entire product line.

Additional article review

The majority of articles are part of A.D.A.M.'s extensive medical encyclopedia, which has been reviewed by over 100 physicians from many of the country's top medical schools and academic departments. Physicians review articles only in clinical areas in which they have been formally trained and actively practice. A.D.A.M. works with VeriMed Healthcare Network to identify appropriate physician reviewers around the country. A.D.A.M.'s goal is to reflect well-established, centrist medical opinion and knowledge. Our physicians rely on primary sources such as recognized textbooks, consensus guidelines, peer-reviewed journals, and professional society reports.

Medical illustrations and design

Meredith A. Nienkamp, M.S.M.I., Director of Visual Production, A.D.A.M., Inc.
Meredith joined A.D.A.M. in 1992 as a medical illustrator, completing hundreds of original medical illustrations and animations for the company's products. As the Director of Visual Production, she is responsible for the art direction and visual content development. Meredith earned her Masters of Science degree in Medical Illustration from the Medical College of Georgia and a Bachelor's of Science in Medical Illustration from Doane College in Crete, Nebraska.

Medical illustrations created by:

Lisa Higginbotham, M.S.M.I., Senior Medical Illustrator, A.D.A.M., Inc.
Dan Johnson, M.S.M.I., Senior Medical Illustrator, A.D.A.M., Inc.
Michael B. Gleason, M.S.M.I., Senior Medical Illustrator, A.D.A.M., Inc.
Kyle A. McNeir, M.A.M.S., Vice President of Production, A.D.A.M., Inc.

Cover design by: Wallace Beeson, Graphic Designer, A.D.A.M., Inc.

Index by: Carolyn Weaver, Weaver Indexing Service

We want your feedback!

Please let us know whether or not this book has helped you. Which information was most useful? How can the book be even more helpful to you and your family? While we cannot respond individually, all comments will be logged and tracked. We will take this feedback into consideration for the next edition of the book.

Send your comments to **guidecomments@adamcorp.com**

INDEX

M

N

O

R

S

Notes

Notes

Notes

Notes

Notes

Notes

Notes

NOTES

Notes